T0200294

SECOND EDITION

Handbook of
Nephrology

SECOND EDITION

Handbook of
Nephrology

Irfan K. Moinuddin, MD, FASN

General Nephrologist and Transplant Nephrologist
Kidney Care Center
Schaumburg, Illinois
Health System Clinician
Northwestern University
Chicago, Illinois
Assistant Professor of Medicine
Rosalind Franklin University School of Medicine
North Chicago, Illinois

David J. Leehey, MD, FASN

Professor of Medicine
Loyola University of Chicago Medical Center
Maywood, Illinois
Associate Chief of Staff for Clinical Affairs and Education
Hines Veterans Affairs Hospital
Hines, Illinois

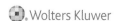. Wolters Kluwer

Philadelphia • Baltimore • New York • London
Buenos Aires • Hong Kong • Sydney • Tokyo

Acquisitions Editor: Kate Heaney
Development Editor: Ariel S. Winter
Editorial Coordinator: Shruti Bhartiya
Editorial Assistant: Latrice Jamison
Production Project Manager: Sadie Buckallew
Design Coordinator: Steve Druding
Manufacturing Coordinator: Beth Welsh
Prepress Vendor: S4Carlisle Publishing Services

Second edition

9 8 7 6 5 4 3 2 1

Printed in China

Library of Congress Cataloging-in-Publication Data
Names: Moinuddin, Irfan K., author. | Leehey, David J., author.
Title: Handbook of nephrology / Irfan Moinuddin, David J. Leehey.
Other titles: Nephrology
Description: 2nd edition. | Philadelphia, PA: Wolters Kluwer, [2020] |
    Includes bibliographical references and index.
Identifiers: LCCN 2019008151 | ISBN 9781975109400
Subjects: | MESH: Kidney Diseases | Outline
Classification: LCC RC918.D53 | NLM WJ 18.2 | DDC 616.6/1—dc23 LC record
    available at https://lccn.loc.gov/2019008151

To Abulfaiz, Momin, Sana, Ihsan,
and Iman Moinuddin,
and Patrick, Dorothy,
and Roslyn Leehey

Because of its inherent logic, focus on pathophysiology, and clinical relevance to a broad group of patients, nephrology has always appealed to some of the sharpest minds and most profound thinkers in medicine. The teaching of this discipline has always been challenging, and many learners find nephrology to be a difficult subspecialty of medicine.

The idea of writing the *Handbook of Nephrology*, first edition, was not ours. Over many years, our students have told us that our teaching provided them with learning strategies and learning content not always found in current books. Indeed, the first edition of the *Handbook of Nephrology* has been well appreciated by medical students, interns, and residents. Nephrology fellows and faculty have also found the first edition to be a helpful teaching aid. Many people assisted us in bringing the first edition to fruition. We would like to especially acknowledge two of them: Dr. John Daugirdas, Clinical Professor of Medicine at the University of Illinois Medical Center, Chicago, Illinois, and Dr. Todd Ing, Professor Emeritus of Nephrology at Loyola University Medical Center, Maywood, Illinois.

The second edition of the *Handbook of Nephrology* takes education one step further by attempting to make the subject of nephrology come to life! Albert Einstein once said that "education is what remains after one has forgotten everything he has learned in school"! Indeed, in the everyday process of education, the learner may learn the material needed to do well in the final exam and then forget everything as time passes. However, one tends to remember one's clinical experience, and the best way to learn is through such experience, coupled with reading and study. The second best way is to learn vicariously through vivid descriptions of clinical experience. The authors believe that trainees learn and retain concepts best when the concepts are described through patient cases. Storytelling, that is, case-based learning, is a powerful way of inculcating concepts into one's comprehension and one's memory, whether it is about humanities, science, or medicine. Indeed, Janice McDrury, an educator and health researcher at Otago Polytechnic, Dunedin, New Zealand, says that "when storytelling is formalized in meaningful ways, it can capture everyday examples of practice and turn them into an opportunity to learn—encouraging both reflection, a deeper understanding of a topic and stimulating critical thinking skills."

This edition of the *Handbook of Nephrology* is not only more detailed and expansive but also told primarily from a case-based approach. Patient cases are used to illustrate key concepts in nephrology, from history, physical examination, differential diagnosis, laboratory findings, and medical management. Standard textbooks can sometimes read as a collection of facts. The *Handbook of Nephrology* has facts and concepts nestled in interesting case studies that promote understanding and retention. Essentially, this book employs teaching strategies that the authors use in their rounds, lectures, morning reports, and in their own self-improvement and practice.

The *Handbook of Nephrology* is a concise introduction to the field of nephrology; it is not intended to be a comprehensive textbook of nephrology. Medical students, interns, and residents stand to benefit greatly from it. We believe primary care physicians, internists, surgeons, nurse practitioners, pharmacists, and physician assistants will also find the book very useful. Nephrology fellows and board-certified nephrologists should find the case-based storytelling approach fun, interesting, helpful, and enlightening.

CONTENTS

Urinalysis

INTRODUCTION

The urinalysis (UA) is critically important in the diagnosis of renal and urologic diseases (Akin et al., 1987; Kroenke et al., 1986). Indeed, it is generally the first test that the nephrologist looks at in evaluating acute kidney injury or chronic kidney disease (CKD). It would not be inaccurate to state that the UA is to nephrology what the electrocardiogram (EKG) is to cardiology (Sheets & Lyman, 1986). It is usually abnormal in patients with kidney disease and may reveal abnormalities in patients without proteinuria. If proteinuria is detected, it should be quantitated by a random urine albumin to creatinine ratio (UACR) and/or urine protein to creatinine ratio (UPCR) (see below and Chapter 3).

There are three portions of a complete UA: the **appearance** of the urine, the **dipstick** evaluation, and the **microscopic** examination. With a few exceptions (i.e., urine samples positive for glucose or ketones give a larger proportion of false negatives for leukocytes, and patients with clinically significant crystalluria will typically have negative dipsticks), a negative dipstick obviates the need to examine the sediment (Bonnardeaux et al., 1994; Schumann & Greenberg, 1979). However, with current automated UA techniques, both are often done in tandem.

APPEARANCE

The color of the urine should be assessed. The color of normal urine varies from clear (dilute) to yellow (concentrated). Macroscopic (gross) hematuria will make the urine appear red. Smoky red or cola-colored urine suggests glomerulonephritis. Dark yellow to orange urine is typical of bilirubinuria. Cloudy urine suggests pyuria or crystalluria (usually phosphates). Milky urine suggests chyluria (lymphatic/urinary fistula).

- Red urine
  - Dipstick positive for blood indicates heme is present
    - Red blood cells (RBCs) in urine sediment—hematuria
    - No RBCs in urine sediment—hemoglobinuria (hemolysis), myoglobinuria (rhabdomyolysis), lysis of RBCs in dilute and/ or alkaline urine (suspect if specific gravity <1.010 and/or pH >8)

- Dipstick negative
  - Porphyria
  - Beet ingestion in susceptible patients (beeturia)
  - Food dyes
- Other colors
  - Orange—rifampin, phenazopyridine (pyridium), carotene
  - Yellow—bilirubin
  - White—pyuria, chyluria, amorphous phosphate crystals
  - Green—methylene blue, amitriptyline, propofol, asparagus, *Pseudomonas* infection
  - Black—ochronosis (alkaptonuria) and melanoma

DIPSTICK

- Blood
  Dipstick positive for blood indicates heme is present (see above).
  - Microscopic hematuria, by definition, is hematuria in the absence of a visual change in color of the urine. As few as 2 to 3 RBC per high-power field (RBC/hpf) may make the dipstick positive.
  - Heme pigments will make the dipstick positive in the absence of hematuria (see above).
  - Ascorbic acid may mask true hematuria (i.e., false-negative dipstick).
- pH
  Normal pH range is 4.5 to 8 (usually 5–7).
  - Low urine pH (<5.3)
    - High-protein diet (increased endogenous acid production from sulfur-containing amino acids)
    - Metabolic acidosis (e.g., chronic diarrhea)
  - High urine pH (usually >7)
    - Metabolic alkalosis (e.g., vomiting)
    - Distal renal tubular acidosis (RTA) (urine pH is >5.3 in face of acidosis)
    - Urea-splitting organisms (e.g., *Proteus*) (urine pH often ~9)
    - Urine that is infected will become alkaline over time because of the formation of ammonia (NH_3) from bacterial urease
    - Urine that is exposed to air for a long time can also have elevated pH because of the loss of CO_2 from the urine
- Specific gravity
  Specific gravity is the weight of urine relative to distilled water and reflects the number and size (weight) of particles in urine. Osmolality is dependent only on the number of particles (solute concentration) in urine. Specific gravity is usually directly proportional to osmolality. However, iodinated contrast and, to a lesser extent, protein will increase specific gravity but have little effect on osmolality. The normal range of urine specific gravity is 1.001 (very dilute) to 1.030 (very concentrated). Urine specific gravity of 1.010 is the same as plasma (isosthenuria). If specific gravity is not >1.022 after a 12-hour overnight fast (food and water), renal concentrating ability is impaired.

- In an oliguric patient, a specific gravity >1.020 suggests normal ability to concentrate urine and prerenal failure (decreased renal blood flow), whereas ~1.010 suggests loss of tubular function (acute tubular necrosis [ATN]/acute kidney injury).
- In a hyponatremic patient, an inappropriately high specific gravity (>1.010) suggests antidiuretic hormone secretion (see Chapter 5).
- In a hypernatremic patient, an inappropriately low specific gravity (<1.010) suggests diabetes insipidus (central or nephrogenic) (see Chapter 5).

- Protein

  The dipstick detects primarily albumin. Normal urine has no protein by dipstick, but occasionally very concentrated urine will be trace positive for protein in healthy individuals. A positive dipstick should lead to a quantitative measurement. Classically, this is done by a 24-hour collection, but as creatinine is excreted at a constant rate, a UACR or UPCR is sufficient in most patients.

  - *Albumin versus total protein* (Shihabi et al., 1991). Healthy subjects excrete up to 30 mg of albumin and 150 to 200 mg of total protein per day (and on average 1,000 mg of creatinine per day). Thus, the normal UACR is <30 mg/g and the normal UPCR is <150 to 200 mg/g. UACR of 30 to 300 mg/g is considered to be microalbuminuria and >300 mg/g overt albuminuria. UPCR >500 mg/g indicates overt proteinuria.
  - Classically, sulfosalicylic acid (SSA) is added to the urine to detect total protein. A discrepancy between the dipstick and the SSA test (e.g., 1+ protein in dipstick and 4+ by SSA) suggests the presence of a paraprotein (e.g., myeloma protein) in the urine. A marked discrepancy between UACR and UPCR gives the same information.

- Glucose

  Normal urine does not contain glucose because filtered glucose is reabsorbed by the proximal tubule.

  - Glycosuria with elevated blood glucose—diabetes mellitus (Singer et al., 1989)
  - Glycosuria with normal blood glucose—renal glycosuria
    - Isolated
    - Associated with other proximal tubular dysfunction (phosphaturia, aminoaciduria, bicarbonaturia) (Fanconi syndrome). One should exclude multiple myeloma.

- Ketones

  Normally, there are no ketones in the urine.

  - Ketonuria without ketoacidosis—starvation, low-carbohydrate (Atkins) diet, isopropyl alcohol ingestion
  - Ketonuria with ketoacidosis—diabetic or alcoholic ketoacidosis. Note that in some patients with ketoacidosis, the dipstick may be negative because of reduction of acetoacetate to beta-hydroxybutyrate.

- Bilirubin

  Normally, there is no bilirubin in the urine. If present, this suggests hepatobiliary disease (failure to conjugate and/or excrete bilirubin into the gut).

- Urobilinogen
  Bilirubin is secreted in bile into the gut, where it is metabolized by microorganisms into urobilinogen. Urobilinogen is then absorbed and partially excreted into the urine. In the presence of liver disease, urobilinogen can accumulate in plasma and appear in the urine. Bilirubin without urobilinogen in the urine suggests biliary obstruction.
- Leukocyte esterase
  This is an enzyme found in white blood cells (WBCs) and indicates the presence of pyuria.
  - Urinary tract infection (UTI)
  - Sterile pyuria (see below)
  - Nitrite
    Enterobacteria convert urinary nitrate to *nitrite*, and therefore a positive test suggests UTI. Note that not all organisms make nitrite, so UTI may be present with a negative nitrite too.

MICROSCOPIC EXAMINATION

- RBCs
  Hematuria (see Chapter 4) (Fig. 1.1)
- WBCs
  Infection (Ditchburn & Ditchburn, 1990) or sterile pyuria. With sterile pyuria, one should exclude interstitial nephritis; other causes include nonbacterial infection, prostatitis, nephrolithiasis, and glomerulonephritis. Eosinophiluria suggests interstitial nephritis (Fig. 1.2).
- Squamous epithelial cells
  Squamous epithelial cells from the skin surface or the outer urethra can appear in urine. Their significance is that they represent possible contamination of the specimen.

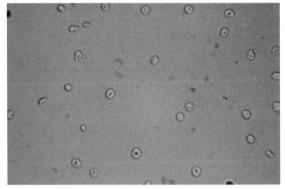

FIGURE 1.1. Red blood cells. (Image courtesy of Medcom, Inc.)

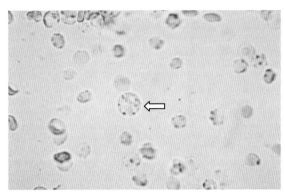

FIGURE 1.2. White blood cell (*arrow*). (Image courtesy of Medcom, Inc.)

- Bacteria
  Indicate possible infection (Fig. 1.3)
- Yeast
  Could be infection versus contamination. Presence of pseudomy-celia suggests infection. Risk factors include indwelling catheters, recent antibiotics, immunosuppression, and diabetes.
- Crystals
  - Calcium oxalate—dihydrate: tetragonal (envelopes); mono-hydrate: dumbbells—can be seen in normal urine; if present in large amounts, it suggests calcium oxalate kidney stones or

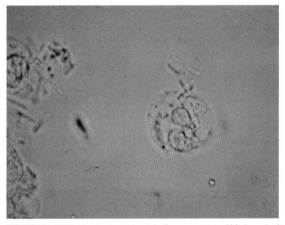

FIGURE 1.3. White blood cells and bacteria. (Image courtesy of Medcom, Inc.)

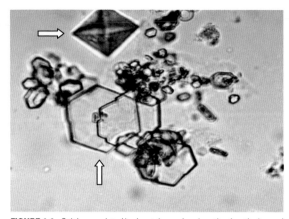

FIGURE 1.4. Calcium oxalate (*horizontal arrow*) and cystine (*vertical arrow*) crystals. (Image courtesy of Jessie Hano, M.D.)

ethylene glycol poisoning (which is metabolized to oxalate) (Fig. 1.4)
- Calcium phosphate—form in alkaline urine—amorphous; in large amounts, it suggests calcium phosphate kidney stones (seen in RTA)
- Uric acid—form in acid urine—pleomorphic, yellow/brown; when in large amounts, it suggests uric acid kidney stones or nephropathy (Fig. 1.5)
- Cystine—hexagonal—indicates cystinuria (Fig. 1.4)
- Magnesium ammonium phosphate (triple phosphate)—coffin lids—suggests struvite stones (a urea-splitting organism must be present to produce NH_3 and elevate urine pH) (Fig. 1.6)

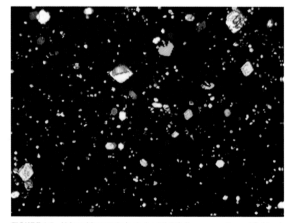

FIGURE 1.5. Uric acid crystals (polarized light). (Image courtesy of Subhash Popli, M.D.)

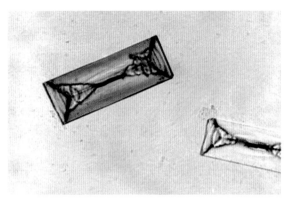

FIGURE 1.6. Triple phosphate crystals. (Image courtesy of Jessie Hano, M.D.)

- Casts
  Urinary casts are formed in the distal convoluted tubule (DCT) or the collecting duct (distal nephron).
  - Hyaline casts are composed primarily of a mucoprotein (Tamm-Horsfall protein) secreted by tubule cells. They are formed in concentrated urine and can be seen in small numbers in healthy patients; large amounts suggest low urinary flow (prerenal or postrenal state) (Fig. 1.7).
  - RBC casts are indicative of glomerulonephritis, with leakage of RBCs from glomeruli, or severe tubular damage (rare) (Fig. 1.8).
  - WBC casts indicate acute pyelonephritis or kidney inflammation (usually tubulointerstitial) (Fig. 1.9).
  - Granular casts are nonspecific but indicate kidney disease (Fig. 1.10). Acute kidney injury (ATN) is characterized by pigmented granular ("muddy brown") casts.

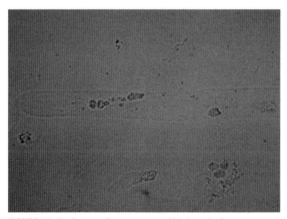

FIGURE 1.7. Hyaline cast. (Image courtesy of Medcom, Inc.)

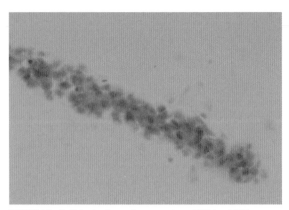

FIGURE 1.8. Red blood cell cast. (Image courtesy of T.S. Ing, M.D.)

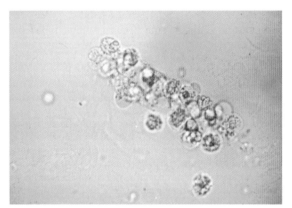

FIGURE 1.9. White blood cell cast. (Image courtesy of Jessie Hano, M.D.)

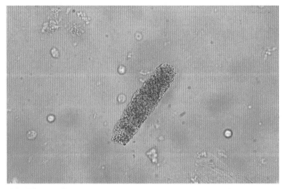

FIGURE 1.10. Granular cast. (Image courtesy of Medcom, Inc.)

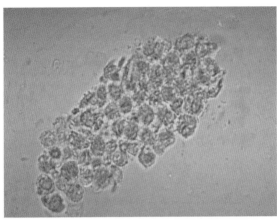

FIGURE 1.11. Renal tubular epithelial cell cast. (Image courtesy of Medcom, Inc.)

- Renal tubular epithelial cell casts are seen in acute kidney injury and CKD (Fig. 1.11).
- Broad waxy casts are seen in CKD (Fig. 1.12).
- Fatty casts and oval fat bodies (lipid-laden macrophages) can be seen in nephrotic syndrome. Under polarizing light, characteristic "Maltese crosses" can be seen (Fig. 1.13).

CLINICAL SYNDROMES SUGGESTED BY THE UA

- Normal UA with elevated creatinine:
  - Prerenal
  - Obstruction (postrenal)
  - Hypercalcemia

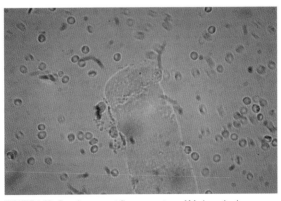

FIGURE 1.12. Broad waxy cast. (Image courtesy of Medcom, Inc.)

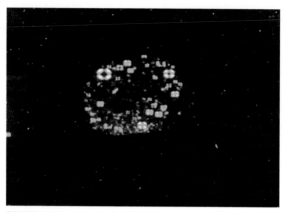

FIGURE 1.13. Oval fat body (polarized light). (Image courtesy of Jessie Hano, M.D.)

- Multiple myeloma
- Nephrosclerosis
- Vasculopathies of medium-sized vessels
  - Scleroderma
  - Cholesterol emboli
  - Polyarteritis nodosa
  - Ischemic nephropathy
- Hematuria/proteinuria
  - Glomerulonephritis
  - Small-vessel vasculitis
- Massive proteinuria
  - Diabetes
  - Amyloid
  - Membranous nephropathy
  - Minimal-change disease
  - Focal segmental glomerulosclerosis (FSGS)

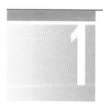

VIGNETTE **1**

A 40-year-old male with a history of intermittent abdominal pain, seizures, and psychosis complains of abdominal pain and cramping. He also complains of light sensitivity. He was out in the sun yesterday and developed blistering, redness, and swelling of the skin. He has been vomiting and complains of constipation. He has noted that his urine turned red. He also has muscle pain, muscle weakness, and pain in the arms, legs, and back. He has not eaten well for several days. Physical examination reveals blisters, erythema on the forehead and upper extremities, and diffuse guarding and tenderness in the abdomen.

Blood chemistry:
Sodium: 141 mmol/L
Potassium: 4.6 mmol/L
Chloride: 106 mmol/L
Total CO_2: 25 mmol/L
Urea nitrogen: 40 mg/dL (urea 14.3 mmol/L)
Creatinine: 2.0 mg/dL (177 mcmol/L)
Glucose: 80 mg/dL (4.4 mmol/L)

Complete blood count:
WBCs: 12,000/mm^3
Hemoglobin: 11.0 g/dL (110 g/L)
Hematocrit: 35%
Platelets: 410,000/mm^3

Urinalysis:
Color: red
pH: 6.0
Specific gravity: 1.025
Protein: negative
Blood: negative
Glucose: negative
Ketones: 1+
Bilirubin: negative
Urobilinogen: negative
Leukocyte esterase: negative
Nitrite: negative
WBC: 3/hpf
RBC: 0/hpf
Bacteria: negative

Q: Which of the following best explains this patient's presentation?

1. Volume depletion
2. UTI
3. Porphyria
4. Hemolysis
5. Rhabdomyolysis
6. Starvation

A: The most prominent finding is that the color of the urine is red. However, the sediment is negative for RBCs and the dipstick is negative for blood, thus excluding hemoglobinuria or myoglobinuria. The urine specific gravity is high, suggesting volume depletion from vomiting. The renal failure is likely to be prerenal failure with an elevated plasma urea nitrogen to creatinine ratio, mild hypernatremia, lack of proteinuria, and absence of symptoms of renal obstruction. Ketonuria is suggestive of recent lack of food intake. The absence of pyuria or bacteriuria and negative leukocyte esterase and nitrite rules out urinary infection. Red urine in combination with the recurrent abdominal pain/cramps, sunburned rash, history of seizures, and history of psychosis suggests acute intermittent porphyria.

VIGNETTE 2

1

An 82-year-old male with a history of calcium oxalate kidney stones and cold agglutinin disease presents for evaluation after a fall in the bathroom. He has chronic bilateral knee and hip pain and could not get back up by himself. He stayed down on the floor for 6 hours and was found by the home health nurse who called an ambulance and brought him to the emergency room. He denies syncope or head trauma. He does complain of chronic abdominal pain, which his primary care physician attributes to irritable bowel syndrome and/or kidney stones. Medications include hydrochlorothiazide, potassium citrate, and acetaminophen. On examination, he has limited range of motion of the hips and knees with pain with extremes of range of motion. There is mild right upper quadrant tenderness. He has 3/5 strength of the lower extremities with intact sensation and generalized hyporeflexia.

Blood chemistry:
Sodium: 138 mmol/L
Potassium: 5.6 mmol/L
Chloride: 102 mmol/L
Total CO_2: 22 mmol/L
Urea nitrogen: 30 mg/dL
    (urea 10.7 mmol/L)
Creatinine: 2.5 mg/dL
    (221 mcmol/L)
Glucose: 135 mg/dL
    (7.5 mmol/L)
Total calcium: 8.0 mg/dL
    (2 mmol/L)
Inorganic phosphorus: 5.5 mg/
    dL (1.8 mmol/L)

Complete blood count:
WBCs: 10,000/mm^3
Hemoglobin, 9.0 g/dL (90 g/L)

Hematocrit: 30%
Platelets: 300,000/mm^3
Antinuclear antibodies (ANAs):
    1:40
Plasma haptoglobin: 200 mg/dL
    (2 g/L) (normal)
Creatine kinase (CK): 10,000 U/L
    (normal < 200)
Chest X-ray: broken
R eleventh rib
Renal ultrasound: 2 mm stone
    in the right kidney, no
    hydronephrosis
Review of the medical record indicates that the plasma urea nitrogen and creatinine were 10 mg/dL (3.6 mmol/L) and 0.8 mg/dL (71 mcmol/L), respectively, 1 month ago.

Q: Which of the following urinalyses is most consistent with the above patient?

1. Color: yellow
pH: 5.5
Specific gravity: 1.025
Protein: 2+
Blood: 1+
Glucose: negative
Ketones: 1+
Bilirubin: negative
Urobilinogen: negative
Leukocyte esterase: negative
Nitrite: negative
WBC: 2/hpf
RBC: 10/hpf
Bacteria: negative
2. Color: yellow
pH: 5.0

Specific gravity: 1.025
Protein: negative
Blood: 1+
Glucose: negative
Ketones: 1+
Bilirubin: negative
Urobilinogen: negative
Leukocyte esterase: negative
Nitrite: negative
WBC: 3/hpf
RBC: 6/hpf
Bacteria: negative
Calcium oxalate crystals present
3. Color: yellow
pH: 5.5
Specific gravity: 1.025

Protein: 1+
Blood: 4+
Glucose: negative
Ketones: 1+
Bilirubin: 2+
Urobilinogen: 2+
Leukocyte esterase: negative
Nitrite: negative
WBC: 2/hpf
RBC: 2/hpf
Bacteria: negative
4. Color: yellow
pH: 5.0

Specific gravity: 1.025
Protein: 1+
Blood: 4+
Glucose: negative
Ketones: 1+
Bilirubin: negative
Urobilinogen: negative
Leukocyte esterase: negative
Nitrite: negative
WBC: 2/hpf
RBC: 0/hpf
Bacteria: negative

A: The patient has acute renal failure. It is thus possible that he has glomerulonephritis. Option 1 is consistent with glomerulonephritis because the prominent finding in this UA is the combination of proteinuria and hematuria. The ANA is positive, which seems consistent with nephritis associated with systemic lupus erythematosus or another collagen vascular disease. However, a weakly positive ANA is frequently seen in the elderly and is unlikely to be meaningful.

Because of the history of nephrolithiasis and right upper quadrant pain, kidney stones are also a possibility. Option 2 is consistent with kidney stones; here, the UA lacks proteinuria and has hematuria in combination with calcium oxalate crystals. However, there is only a 2-mm parenchymal kidney stone without hydronephrosis, which is unlikely to explain this patient's abdominal pain. The pain is more likely caused by a fractured rib detected on the chest X-ray. He has chronic abdominal pain as well.

Hemolysis is another possibility. The patient has a history of cold agglutinin disease that can render RBCs susceptible to lysis mediated by complement. Option 3 is consistent with hemolysis because there is bilirubinuria, urobilinogenuria, and heme-positive urine consistent with hemoglobinuria. With hemolysis, the released hemoglobin binds haptoglobin; hence, plasma haptoglobin is reduced. However, in this patient, it is not low.

This case is most consistent with rhabdomyolysis. The patient had a fall and was unable to get up for 6 hours. This trauma and immobility is sufficient for significant muscle breakdown to occur. The plasma CK is high, which is consistent with rhabdomyolysis. There is also diffuse weakness in the lower extremities resulting from muscle breakdown. Rhabdomyolysis is also characterized by hyperkalemia and hyperphosphatemia because these substances are released from damaged muscle cells, both of which are present in this patient. The UA has large blood without hematuria (consistent with the presence of myoglobin, which is a heme pigment).

References

Akin BV, Hubbell FA, Frye EB, et al. Efficacy of the routine admission urinalysis. *Am J Med*. 1987;82:719–722.

Bonnardeaux A, Somerville P, Kaye M. A study on the reliability of dipstick urinalysis. *Clin Nephrol*. 1994;41:167–172.

Ditchburn RK, Ditchburn JS. A study of microscopical and chemical tests for the rapid diagnosis of urinary tract infections in general practice. *Br J Gen Pract*. 1990;40:406–408.

Kroenke K, Hanley JF, Copley JB, et al. The admission urinalysis: impact on patient care. *J Gen Intern Med*. 1986;1:238–242.

Schumann GB, Greenberg NF. Usefulness of macroscopic urinalysis as a screening procedure. *Am J Clin Pathol*. 1979;71:452–456.

Sheets C, Lyman JL. Urinalysis. *Emerg Med Clin North Am*. 1986;4:263–280.

Shihabi ZK, Konen JC, O'Connor ML. Albuminuria vs urinary total protein for detecting chronic renal disorders. *Clin Chem*. 1991;37:621–624.

Singer DE, Coley CM, Samet JH, et al. Tests of glycemia in diabetes mellitus: their use in establishing a diagnosis and in treatment. *Ann Intern Med*. 1989;110:125–137.

Measurement of Renal Function

MEASUREMENT OF GLOMERULAR FUNCTION

Renal function is best determined by measuring the glomerular filtration rate (GFR) (Bröchner-Mortensen & Rödbro, 1976). The most common methods use the endogenous substance creatinine, which is formed by metabolism of creatine in skeletal muscle (Fuller & Elia, 1988) and excreted by glomerular filtration (although it is not a perfect marker of GFR, because there is also some tubular secretion) (Shemesh et al., 1985). Other methods of measuring GFR include (1) measurement of levels of the serum protease cystatin, which is produced at a constant rate by nucleated cells (Kyhse-Andersen et al., 1994) and (2) clearance of an exogenous substance that is excreted by glomerular filtration and neither reabsorbed nor secreted by renal tubules, such as inulin, iohexol, iothalamate, and diethylenetriaminepentaacetic acid (DTPA). These methods can be used if a more exact measurement of GFR is required.

CREATININE-BASED MEASUREMENTS

- *Plasma creatinine* (PCr) (Doolan et al., 1962): This is the most commonly used indirect measure of GFR. The PCr concentration will reflect both the production rate of creatinine (which is proportional to muscle mass) and the excretion rate of creatinine (which depends on renal function). In the steady state, that is, when PCr is stable, production equals excretion; this equality is also true when there is chronic kidney disease (CKD), although there will be a higher level of PCr, which will be inversely proportional to GFR (see Vignette 1).
- *Measured creatinine clearance* (CCr) (DeSanto et al., 1991; Sawyer et al., 1982): When a substance is cleared from the blood by glomerular filtration, the excretion rate of the substance (urine concentration $\times$ urinary flow rate) will equal the volume of plasma that is totally cleared of the substance. Therefore,

  Plasma concentration $\times$ Clearance = Urine concentration $\times$ Urinary flow rate

  or

  Clearance = (Urine concentration $\times$ Urinary flow rate)/Plasma concentration

  For example, if a patient excretes 1,440 mg of creatinine in 24 hours (1 mg/min) and the plasma concentration is 1.0 mg/dL (0.01 mg/mL), then the CCr = 1 mg/min/0.01 mg/mL = 100 mL/min. Using SI units, if a patient excretes 12.7 mmol of creatinine in 24 hours (8.84 mcmol/min) and the plasma concentration is 88.4 mcmol/L, then the CCr = (8.84 mcmol/min)/(0.0884 mcmol/mL) = 100 mL/min.

- *Creatinine-based formulae* (note that all these formulae require a steady-state [stable] level of PCr and cannot be used in patients whose renal function is rapidly changing) (Levey et al., 1989):
  - Inverse creatinine: CCr being inversely proportional to plasma creatinine (Cr), symbolically, CCr ~ 1/Cr, a rough approximation of renal function can be obtained in this manner. For example, if CCr is 100 mL/min when Cr is 1.0 mg/dL (88.4 mcmol/L), then CCr would be 50 mL/min when Cr is 2 mg/dL (177 mcmol/L) and 25 mL/min when Cr is 4 mg/dL (354 mcmol/L) (assuming stable but elevated creatinine levels).
  - Cockroft–Gault equation. This formula was developed empirically during the 1970s by Cockroft and Gault (1976).

    CCr (mL/min) = [(140 − age) × body wt (kg)/(72 × serum Cr)] × 0.85 (females), where serum Cr is in mg/dL.

    Other modifications of this formula have been made (e.g., using correction factors of 0.8 for paraplegia and 0.6 for quadriplegia). It has now essentially been replaced by formulae for estimated GFR (eGFR) in laboratory medicine, although it still has value, because it is easy to calculate at the bedside and can be useful for estimating GFR in special populations (e.g., spinal cord–injured patients).
  - Estimated GFR
    - These formulae were initially developed from data obtained in the Modification of Diet in Renal Disease (MDRD) Study (Levey et al., 1989). Because this study did not include many non-Caucasian or diabetic patients and was based on subjects with fairly advanced renal failure, the Chronic Kidney Disease Epidemiology Collaboration (CKD-EPI) equation was subsequently developed on the basis of data from several clinical trials, including a much broader range of patients, which is more applicable to patients with normal or near-normal renal function (Levey et al., 2009).

      MDRD: eGFR(mL/min/1.73m^2) = 186 × SCr$^{-1.154}$ × Age$^{-0.203}$ × [0.742 if female] × [1.21 if black], where SCr is in mg/dL.

      CKD-EPI: eGFR (mL/min/1.73 m^2) = 141 × min(SCr/k,1)^a × max(SCr/k,1)$^{-1.209}$ × 0.993^{Age} × [1.018 if female] × [1.159 if black], where SCr is serum creatinine (mg/dL), k is 0.7 for females and 0.9 for males, a is −0.329 for females and −0.411 for males, min indicates the minimum of SCr/k or 1, and max indicates the maximum of SCr/k or 1.
    - The MDRD and CKD-EPI formulae are available as web-based and downloadable calculators at various websites, including www.hdcn.com, www.nephron.com, and www.renal.org. Note that these formulae use SCr, although this can be substituted by PCr.
- *Mean of creatinine and urea clearance*: Because creatinine is secreted and urea is reabsorbed by tubules, the mean of the creatinine and urea clearance has been used to estimate GFR (Lubowitz

et al., 1967). However, one should keep in mind that this formula was validated in a population of patients with severe CKD (GFR measured by inulin clearance of <20 mL/min) and is not applicable to other populations, especially when urea reabsorption is markedly enhanced, as in congestive heart failure (CHF) and cirrhosis.

OTHER METHODS OF MEASURING RENAL FUNCTION

■ *Serum cystatin C*: Cystatin C is a serine protease inhibitor produced by all nucleated cells. It has a constant production rate, and it is filtered and completely reabsorbed by renal tubules. Therefore, clearance measurements cannot be used. An advantage over PCr is that its concentration is less influenced by gender, age, or muscle mass. However, certain conditions such as thyroid disease, inflammation, diabetes, and fat mass can affect cystatin C. Its plasma concentration increases before the increase in PCr when renal function is rapidly declining, that is, in acute renal failure. It is not currently in widespread clinical use.

■ *Isotopic GFR*: Several radiopharmaceuticals are freely filtered by the glomerulus and not reabsorbed or secreted and can be used to measure GFR. The most commonly used is ^{99}Tc-DTPA. After an intravenous injection, timed plasma samples allow the determination of disappearance rate from plasma and thus renal clearance. These techniques are expensive and somewhat labor intensive and, in the clinical setting, are best reserved for cases in which an accurate measurement of GFR is required for clinical decision making. For example, they may be useful in deciding whether to start dialysis in patients in whom formulae may not apply (e.g., marked obesity or malnutrition/muscle wasting) and standard clearance measurements are not possible.

MEASUREMENT OF TUBULAR FUNCTION

With CKD, loss of nephrons leads to defects in tubular as well as glomerular function. However, it is possible to have isolated defects in tubular function in the presence of normal or near-normal GFR.

■ Physiology
  ■ The proximal tubule (PT) reabsorbs the bulk of solutes and water filtered by the glomeruli.
  ■ The loop of Henle actively reabsorbs electrolytes (sodium, potassium, and chloride). The thick ascending limb (TAL) is impermeable to water, allowing formation of dilute urine.
  ■ The distal convoluted tubule (DCT) and collecting duct (CD) fine-tune sodium excretion and regulate potassium and acid–base balance. In the absence of antidiuretic hormone (ADH), the CD is also impermeable to water, allowing excretion of dilute urine. ADH increases water permeability in the CD, allowing urine concentration.

■ Pathophysiology
  ■ Proximal tubular dysfunction leads to a characteristic disorder called Fanconi syndrome. Failure to reabsorb glucose,

phosphate, bicarbonate, potassium, amino acids, and low–molecular-weight proteins such as β_2-microglobulin filtered by the glomeruli leads to renal glycosuria (normal plasma glucose), phosphaturia with hypophosphatemia, metabolic acidosis (proximal renal tubular acidosis [RTA]), hypokalemia, aminoaciduria, and tubular proteinuria. Isolated proximal RTA can also occur (see below).

- Loop of Henle dysfunction leads to Bartter syndrome, characterized by salt wasting, hypokalemia, and metabolic alkalosis. Hypomagnesemia is mild, and hypercalciuria is present. Loop diuretics such as furosemide (Lasix) can cause identical metabolic disturbances.
- DCT dysfunction results in Gitelman syndrome, characterized primarily by hypokalemia, hypomagnesemia, and hypocalciuria. Thiazide-type diuretics cause similar disturbances, although, for reasons not well understood, hypomagnesemia is much more severe in Gitelman syndrome than in patients taking thiazides.

- Renal tubular acidosis
  - Renal acidification mechanisms (also see Chapter 7):
    • Bicarbonate is freely filtered and then almost completely reabsorbed (reclaimed) by the PT.
    • Bicarbonate that has been titrated by endogenously produced acid is then regenerated by the distal nephron via renal acid excretion by one of the following three mechanisms:
      • Excretion of H^+ (lowering urine pH) (minor mechanism)
      • Excretion of acid phosphate $HPO_4^{2-} + H^+ \rightarrow H_2PO_4^-$
      • Excretion of ammonium $NH_3 + H^+ \rightarrow NH_4^+$
  - Thus, metabolic acidosis can result from failure to reclaim bicarbonate in the PT or failure to secrete acid in the distal tubule.
  - Hypokalemic distal RTA (type 1) is due to impaired secretion of H^+ from the alpha-intercalated cells in the CD. Increased secretion of K^+ also occurs, resulting in hypokalemic hyperchloremic acidosis. The most common causes are hereditary, autoimmune disease, tubulointerstitial disease, and dysproteinemias. Urine pH is increased (>5.3) despite systemic acidosis. There is decreased NH_4^+ excretion, resulting in decreased excretion of the accompanying Cl^- anion; thus, urinary $Na^+ + K^+ > Cl^-$ (this is referred to as positive urine "net charge" or urine anion gap [defined as $UNa^+ + UK^+ - UCl^-$]).
  - Proximal RTA (type 2) results from failure to reabsorb filtered bicarbonate. It is often accompanied by other features of Fanconi syndrome. The most common causes are dysproteinemias and drugs (carbonic anhydrase inhibitors). Urine pH is <5.3. Calculation of urine net charge or anion gap is not useful because it has been shown to be variable in different studies.
  - Hyperkalemic distal RTA (type 4) is usually due to hypoaldosteronism or aldosterone resistance in the setting of CKD. The resultant hyperkalemia leads to decreased NH_4^+ excretion (because of inhibition of ammonia formation). Most common causes are diabetes (hyporeninemic hypoaldosteronism, thought to be primarily due to glycation of prorenin with impaired activation to

renin), drugs (renin–angiotensin–aldosterone [RAAS] axis inhibitors, aldosterone synthesis inhibitors such as heparin, and inhibitors of tubular K^+ secretion such as trimethoprim and calcineurin inhibitors). Nonsteroidal anti-inflammatory drugs (NSAIDs) inhibit the RAAS as well as tubular K^+ secretion. Urine pH is <5.3. Urinary $Na^+ + K^+ > Cl^-$ (positive urine "net charge").

Summary of Major Laboratory Findings in RTA

RTA	Type 1	Type 2	Type 4
Plasma K^+	Low	Low	High
Urine pH	>5.3	<5.3	<5.3
Urine net charge	Positive	Variable	Positive
Aldosterone to K^+ ratio	Normal	Normal	Usually low (unless aldosterone resistance)

2

Q1: A 22-year-old male medical student weighing 72 kg undergoes blood chemistry measurements as part of a class project to study renal physiology. His PCr is 1.0 mg/dL (88.4 mcmol/L). Although his PCr is in the normal range, he is concerned that he may have kidney disease, and so he does a urinalysis, which is normal, and collects a 24-hour urine for measurement of CCr. His 24-hour urine creatinine excretion is 1,440 mg (12.7 mmol) in a volume of 1,440 mL. What is his CCr?

A1: The first consideration is whether the 24-hour urine was completely collected. The student relates that he voided all the urine in his bladder at 7:00 AM into the toilet and then collected all his urine until 7:00 AM the following day, which is the correct procedure. The amount of creatinine in the urine is 20 mg/kg (177 mcmol/kg). Creatinine excretion depends on muscle mass, and normal ranges are 14 to 26 mg/kg (124–230 mcmol/kg) for men and 11 to 20 mg/kg (97–177 mcmol/kg) for women. Thus, this appears to be a complete collection.

Now we wish to determine the CCr. As CCr = [(urine creatinine concentration) × (urine flow rate)]/plasma creatinine concentration, and creatinine excretion rate = urine creatinine concentration × urine flow rate, CCr = creatinine excretion rate/plasma creatinine. The only problem is that creatinine excretion rate is in mg (or mmol)/24 hours, and plasma creatinine is in mg/dL (or mmol/L), so we need a correction factor to arrive at a CCr in mL/min. In the above example, this can be determined as follows:

$$CCr = \text{creatinine excretion rate } (1{,}440 \text{ mg/24 h}) / \text{plasma creatinine } (1.0 \text{ mg/dL}) = 1{,}440 \text{ dL/24 h}.$$

In order to convert to mL/min, one needs to do the following:

$1{,}440$ dL/24 h $\times$ 100 mL/dL $\times$ 24 h/1,440 min $= 100$ mL/min. Since $100/1{,}440 = 0.07$, a quick way to calculate this is as follows:

$$CCr \text{ (mL/min)} = [\text{creatinine excretion rate (mg/24 h)} / \text{plasma creatinine (mg/dL)}] \times 0.07$$

Another option is to convert mg/24 h to mg/min and plasma creatinine to mg/mL (as we did in the example at the beginning of the chapter), which will give you $(1.0 \text{ mg/min})/(0.01 \text{ mg/mL}) = 100$ mL/min. However, this method, although good for illustration with nice numbers, as in this case, does not work out as well in practice as the "0.07 correction factor" method.

Why not calculate CCr the more "usual" way taught in medical school? That is,

$$CCr = (\text{urine creatinine concentration} \times \text{urine flow rate}) / (\text{plasma creatinine concentration} \times 1{,}440)$$

In the above example, since the 24-hr urine volume is (conveniently) 1,440 mL, and the urine creatinine concentration can be calculated to be 100 mg/dL (1 mg/mL), then

$$CCr = (100 \text{ mg/dL}) (1{,}440 \text{ mL})/(1.0 \text{ mg/dL}) (1{,}440 \text{ min}) = 100 \text{ mL/min}$$

The problem with the "usual way" is that one may lose track of the creatinine excretion rate, which allows for assessment of whether the collection was complete. Also, the alternate way ("0.07 correction factor" method) is faster. Note that for those that use international units for recording creatinine, the correction factor will be 0.7 (actually 0.69), not 0.07.

Q2: The same student becomes an attending nephrologist and 10 years later repeats his blood chemistries and is dismayed to find that his PCr is now 2.0 mg/dL (177 mcmol/L). He does not believe it, so he repeats it 3 days later and finds that it is again 2.0 mg/dL (177 mcmol/L). He repeats his CCr. Recall the 24-hour creatinine excretion was 1,440 mg (12.7 mmol) 10 years ago. What is the 24-hour creatinine excretion rate now?

A2: Most trainees (and many experienced physicians, including some nephrologists!) will answer 50% of the original value, but this is incorrect. Remember that in the steady state (i.e., with a stable PCr concentration), creatinine excretion rate depends on the rate of creatinine generation by skeletal muscle, not by renal function. Therefore, the creatinine excretion rate is still 1,440 mg/24 hours (12.7 mmol/24 hours) (it could be a little less if the attending nephrologist is not as muscular as he was when he was a student, but for the purpose of this discussion, we will assume that his muscle mass and thus creatinine generation rate by muscle remained unchanged over the 10-year interval).

Since CCr = creatinine excretion rate/plasma creatinine, if creatinine excretion rate remains the same and plasma creatinine doubles, then CCr halves. Assuming our former medical student now attending nephrologist has progressive renal dysfunction (CKD), the following table will be true:

Plasma Creatinine (mg/dL)	Creatinine Excretion Rate (mg/24 h)	Creatinine Clearance (mL/min)
1.0	1,440	100
2.0	1,440	50
4.0	1,440	25
8.0	1,440	12.5

Using SI units:

Plasma Creatinine (mcmol/L)	Creatinine Excretion Rate (mmol/24 h)	Creatinine Clearance (mL/min)
88.4	12.7	100
177	12.7	50
265	12.7	25
354	12.7	12.5

Thus, renal function (CCr or GFR) and plasma creatinine are inversely proportional, with the plasma creatinine doubling for every halving of CCr. This same relationship can be seen in the Cockroft–Gault formula, where plasma creatinine is in the denominator, as well as in all the eGFR formulae, because of the negative exponents on the plasma creatinine term.

VIGNETTE **2**

A 22-year-old female medical student complains of weakness. Her friends tell her that she is just anxious about her upcoming exams, but she seeks medical attention and goes to the student health department. Her medical history is unremarkable. She denies vomiting or diarrhea and denies use of any drugs, either prescribed or illicit. Vital signs include the following pulse: 90/min (supine), 110/min (standing); blood pressure: 110/70 mm Hg (supine), 90/60 mm Hg (standing). Her neck veins are flat while supine. Otherwise, the physical examination is unremarkable. The following labs are obtained:

Blood chemistry:
Sodium: 135 mmol/L
Potassium: 2.4 mmol/L
Chloride: 94 mmol/L
Total CO_2: 29 mmol/L
Urea nitrogen: 20 mg/dL (urea: 7.1 mmol/L)
Creatinine: 1.2 mg/dL (106 mcmol/L)
Glucose: 100 mg/dL (5.5 mmol/L)
Total calcium: 9.0 mg/dL (2.25 mmol/L)
Inorganic phosphorus: 3.5 mg/dL (1.1 mmol/L)
Magnesium: 0.9 mg/dL (normal 1.8–2.4) (0.37 mmol/L, normal 0.75–1)

Complete blood count:
WBC: 7,000/mm³
Hemoglobin: 13.0 g/dL (130 g/L)
Hematocrit: 39%
Platelets: 300,000/mm³
ANA: negative
Urinalysis: normal
Urine chemistries:
Sodium: 84 mmol/L
Potassium: 65 mmol/L
Chloride: 138 mmol/L
Calcium: 3 mg/dL (0.75 mmol/L)
Magnesium: 5 mg/dL (2 mmol/L)
Creatinine: 67 mg/dL (5,923 mcmol/L)

Q: What is the most likely cause of her electrolyte abnormalities?

1. Anxiety
2. Poor dietary intake
3. Diuretic abuse
4. Bartter syndrome
5. Gitelman syndrome

A: This patient has a combination of hypokalemia, hypomagnesemia, and metabolic alkalosis and appears volume depleted on examination. Although these plasma electrolyte disorders could be seen with poor dietary intake, the inappropriately elevated urine sodium and chloride concentrations in the face of volume depletion and the elevated urinary potassium and magnesium concentrations in the face of profound hypokalemia and hypomagnesemia suggest a renal tubular disorder, which could be either genetic or acquired. Calculation of the fractional excretions of these electrolytes will allow a more quantitative assessment.

The fractional excretion of a substance is the ratio of the amount of the substance excreted in the urine (urine concentration × urine flow rate) relative to the amount of the substance filtered (plasma concentration × GFR). For sodium, fractional excretion of sodium (FENa) would be as follows:

$$\text{FENa} = \text{(urine sodium concentration} \times \text{urine flow rate)}/\text{(plasma sodium concentration} \times \text{GFR).}$$

Substituting CCr for GFR, we have

$$\text{FENa} = \text{(urine sodium concentration} \times \text{urine flow rate)}/\text{(plasma sodium concentration} \times \text{CCr), or}$$

$$(\text{UNa} \times \text{V})/(\text{PNa} \times [(\text{UCr} \times \text{V})/\text{PCr}]).$$

The V term cancels out, leaving

$$UNa/(PNa \times [UCr/PCr]) = (UNa/PNa)/(UCr/PCr) = (UNa/PNa) \times (PCr/UCr).$$

To express as a percentage rather than a fraction, it must be multiplied by 100, so the most useful final formula is

$$(UNa/PNa) \times (PCr/UCr) \times 100 \, (\%)$$

Normally, the FENa will be ~1%, depending on the dietary sodium intake. This means that with a usual diet in a healthy person, about 1% of the filtered sodium is excreted into the urine. In the presence of volume depletion, the kidneys reabsorb sodium, leading to a FENa <1, unless the kidneys are causing the problem, in which case FENa is >1.

In this case, FENa = $84/135 \times 1.2/67 \, (106/5,923) \times 100 = 1.1\%$, suggesting inappropriate natriuresis, as the kidneys should be conserving sodium in the face of volume depletion.

The fractional excretion of potassium (FEK) is

$$(UK/PK) \times (PCr/UCr) \times 100 \, (\%) = 65/2.4 \times 1.2/67$$
$$(106/5,923) \times 100 = 48.5\%,$$

indicating inappropriate kaliuresis, because the kidneys should be conserving potassium, that is, FEK $<10\%$ or transtubular potassium gradient of <2.5 (see Chapter 6), in the face of hypokalemia.

The fractional excretion of magnesium (FEMg) is

$$(UMg/[PMg \times 0.7]) \times (PCr/UCr) \times 100 = 5/(0.9 \times 0.7)$$
$$\times 1.2/67 \times 100 = 14\%, \text{ or, using SI units, } 2/$$
$$(0.37 \times 0.7) \times 106/5,923 \times 100 = 14\%,$$

indicating magnesium wasting, because the kidneys should be conserving magnesium in the face of hypomagnesemia (FEMg is expected to be $<2\%$ in hypomagnesemic patients, if the kidneys are not the cause). Note that we multiply PMg by 0.7, because only 70% of the plasma magnesium is filterable by the glomeruli (30% is bound to plasma proteins and does not cross the glomerular filtration barrier).

Thus, our student has a renal tubular defect characterized by inappropriate loss of salt, potassium, and magnesium into the urine. Diuretic abuse can cause these abnormalities, but she was not taking diuretics. It is concluded that she has Gitelman syndrome. Gitelman syndrome is a defect in the distal sodium chloride cotransporter and is also characterized by renal magnesium wasting. Gitelman syndrome is similar to being on a thiazide diuretic and is associated with hypomagnesemia and elevated urine magnesium and decreased calcium excretion. She was not just anxious!

References

Bröchner-Mortensen J, Rödbro P. Selection of routine method for determination of glomerular filtration rate in adult patients. *Scand J Clin Lab Invest.* 36:35–43, 1976.

Cockroft DW, Gault MH. Prediction of creatinine clearance from plasma creatinine. *Nephron.* 16:31–41, 1976.

DeSanto NG, Coppola S, Anastasia P, et al. Predicted creatinine clearance to assess glomerular filtration rate in chronic renal disease in humans. *Am J Nephrol.* 11:181–185, 1991.

Doolan PD, Alpen EL, Theil GB. A clinical appraisal of the plasma concentration and endogenous clearance of creatinine. *Am J Med*. 32:65–79, 1962.

Fuller NJ, Elia M. Factors influencing the production of creatinine: implications for the determination and interpretation of urinary creatinine and creatine in man. *Clin Chim Acta*. 175:199–210, 1988.

Kyhse-Andersen J, Schmidtl C, Nordin G, et al. Serum cystatin C, determined by a rapid, automated particle-enhanced turbidimetric method, is a better marker than serum creatinine for glomerular filtration rate. *Clin Chem*. 40:1921–1926, 1994.

Levey AS, Berg RL, Gassman JJ, et al. Creatinine filtration, secretion, and excretion during progressive renal disease. *Kidney Int*. 36(suppl 27):S73–S80, 1989.

Levey AS, Stevens LA, Schmid CH, et al; CKD-EPI (Chronic Kidney Disease Epidemiology Collaboration). A new equation to estimate glomerular filtration rate. *Ann Intern Med*. 150(9):604–612, 2009.

Lubowitz H, Slatopolsky E, Shankel S, et al. Glomerular filtration rate. Determination in patients with chronic renal disease. *JAMA*. 199(4):252–256, 1967.

Sawyer WT, Canaday BR, Poe TE, et al. A multicenter evaluation of variables affecting the predictability of creatinine clearance. *Am J Clin Pathol*. 78:832–838, 1982.

Shemesh O, Golbetz H, Kriss JP, et al. Limitations of creatinine as a filtration marker in glomerulopathic patients. *Kidney Int*. 28:830–838, 1985.

3 | Proteinuria

CASE STUDY 3.1 A 26-year-old male with a past medical history of hyperlipidemia and asthma presents for evaluation of proteinuria that was detected on a urinalysis done as part of a preinsurance examination. He subsequently underwent a 24-hour urine collection, which revealed 600 mg of protein. He has no other complaints. He takes simvastatin and fish oil capsules and uses an albuterol inhaler as needed. He does not use other over-the-counter (OTC) medications, including nonsteroidal anti-inflammatory drugs (NSAIDs). His vital signs are normal. Physical examination is unremarkable. His body mass index (BMI) is 22 kg/m^2.

Question 3.1.1: What is proteinuria and how can it be classified?

DEFINITION AND TYPES

Proteinuria is a condition in which urine contains an abnormal amount of protein and can be divided into three types:

- *Glomerular proteinuria:* Most proteins are too big to pass through the normal glomerular filtration barrier, and thus proteinuria is usually a sign that the glomeruli are damaged. Glomerular proteinuria can be transient if it results from increased hydrostatic pressure (such as in congestive heart failure) or variables such as exercise (Poortmans et al., 1988) or fever, where the mechanism may be due to increased glomerular permeability by substances such as angiotensin II and norepinephrine. Postexercise proteinuria is due to both increased glomerular permeability and partial tubular reabsorption inhibition (Poortmans et al., 1988). Glomerular proteinuria is pathologic if the proteinuria is persistent. Albuminuria ("selective proteinuria") or, more frequently, excretion of abnormally large amounts of albumin and globulin ("nonselective proteinuria") results.

- *Tubular proteinuria:* This is due to damaged tubules resulting from one or more of the following mechanisms:
  - Impaired tubular reabsorption of filtered proteins (e.g., light chains, α_1-microglobulin, β_2-microglobulin). Excretion of high amounts of polyclonal light chains indicates tubular damage; however, excretion of large amounts of monoclonal light chains indicates paraproteinuria resulting from plasma cell dyscrasia and can damage tubules (see below)

- Excretion of tubular enzymes from damaged cells (e.g., *N*-ace-tyl-D-glucosaminidase, NAG; neutrophil gelatinase-associated lipocalin, NGAL)
■ *Overflow proteinuria:* This occurs in situations in which large concentrations of small proteins (such as light chains, hemoglobin, or myoglobin) are produced and are freely filtered by the glomerulus. These filtered proteins overwhelm the capacity of the renal tubules to completely reabsorb and catabolize these proteins, so they appear in the urine.

Question 3.1.2: How is proteinuria measured? How is albuminuria different from proteinuria?

MEASUREMENT OF PROTEINURIA

■ *Albumin versus total protein:* Urine albumin and/or urine total protein can be measured. The urine dipstick for protein is a screening test, as it is semiquantitative, reacts primarily to albumin and is affected by urine concentration. Classically, urine total protein was assessed by addition of sulfosalicylic acid to the specimen, which precipitated protein and increased turbidity of the urine. Urine total protein is now more commonly measured by dye-based assays, which react predominantly to albumin but also, to a lesser extent, to globulins, including monoclonal paraproteins. Thus, a disproportionate increase in urine total protein relative to urine albumin suggests possible paraproteinuria (see below).
■ *Urine albumin to creatinine ratio (UACR) and urine protein to creatinine ratio (UPCR):* Because albumin, protein, and creatinine are usually excreted at a constant rate, measurement of ratios in a random urine specimen can generally be substituted for 24-hour urine measurements.
  ■ Creatinine excretion reflects generation of creatinine by muscle. Thus, it can vary greatly depending on muscle mass (with a median of about 1 g/day) (8.84 mmol/day). If excretion of 1 g/day is assumed, then an UACR or UPCR of 1.0 (g/g) would indicate 1.0 g of daily albumin or protein excretion. Note that some labs measure UACR and UPCR as mg/g, so this ratio would then be 1,000 (mg/g). The corresponding ratio in SI units would be 113 mg/mmol.
  ■ UACR is commonly used to assess low amounts of albumin excretion that cannot be detected by standard urine dipsticks for protein. This is referred to as "microalbumin"; however, what is being measured is albumin. The upper limit of albumin excretion is 30 mg/day. Excretion of between 30 and 300 mg of albumin in the urine per day is referred to as microalbuminuria. Macroalbuminuria (overt albuminuria) is the excretion of >300 mg of albumin in the urine per day (this amount is detectable by dipstick, i.e., "dipstick proteinuria").
  ■ In most laboratories, the upper limits for albumin and protein excretion are 30 and 150 mg/day, respectively, although, depending

on the method, up to 300 mg/day of protein excretion may be normal in healthy kidney donors (Leischner et al., 2006).
- A disproportionately elevated UPCR versus UACR suggests either tubular proteinuria or overflow proteinuria. For instance, if the UACR is 15 mg/g (1.7 mg/mmol) but the UPCR is 500 mg/g (56.5 mg/mmol), tubular or overflow proteinuria should be suspected and should raise the suspicion for paraproteinuria.

Question 3.1.3: What is the clinical significance of proteinuria?

CLINICAL SIGNIFICANCE OF PROTEINURIA (ALBUMINURIA)

- Progression of kidney disease and cardiovascular risk
  - Albuminuria is one of the first signs of kidney disease. Urinalysis is done routinely as an initial test to detect albuminuria. If detected, UACR is used for quantitation (see section on Measurement of Proteinuria). If two consecutive urine samples show high levels of albumin, persistent albuminuria is present.
  - Albuminuria has no signs or symptoms in the early stages. Large amounts of albumin in the urine may cause it to look foamy in the toilet. Nephrotic syndrome is characterized by the daily excretion of >3.5 g of protein in the urine per day, that is, UPCR > 3.5 g/g or 3,500 mg/g (396 mg/mmol). It is also characterized by edema (due to low oncotic pressure and renal sodium retention), hypoalbuminemia (due to loss of protein in the urine), hyperlipidemia (due to increased hepatic synthesis of proteins, including lipoproteins), and lipiduria (due to loss of lipoproteins into the urine). Hypercoagulability is also common (in part, due to loss of antithrombin III in the urine).
  - The degree of albuminuria is correlated with severity of kidney disease and likelihood of decline in kidney function (Leehey et al., 2005) and/or end-stage kidney failure (Klag et al., 1997). It is also an important cardiovascular risk factor (Bigazzi et al., 1998).

Question 3.1.4: How should proteinuria be evaluated?

- Most diseases that cause albuminuria can present with or develop nephrotic syndrome (see Chapter 11). When proteinuria is detected by the laboratory in the absence of clinical manifestations, this is termed "asymptomatic" or "isolated" proteinuria.
- In the United States, nephrotic syndrome is most commonly caused by diabetes. Other causes include primary glomerular disease (i.e., in the absence of systemic disease) and other systemic diseases (such as lupus and amyloidosis). The most common primary glomerular diseases are focal segmental glomerulosclerosis (most common in blacks), membranous nephropathy (most common in whites), and minimal-change disease (most common in children). Biopsy is usually required to establish the diagnosis, unless diabetes is thought to be the cause (see Chapter 13). Serum creatinine may or may not be elevated, glomerular filtration rate (GFR) may or may not be reduced, and hypertension may or may not be present.

Question 3.1.5: What is the likely cause of proteinuria in this patient?

CASE STUDY 3.1 CONTINUED

The following laboratory results are obtained:

Blood chemistry:
Urea nitrogen: 11 mg/dL (urea: 3.6 mmol/L)
Creatinine: 1.0 mg/dL (88.4 mcmol/L)
Albumin: 4.4 g/dL (44 g/L)

Complete blood count:
WBC: 6,200/mm^3
Hemoglobin: 14.9 g/dL (149 g/L)
Hematocrit: 44%
Platelets: 258,000/mm^3
Serum and urine protein electrophoresis—no abnormal protein bands
Serum kappa:lambda light chain ratio: 0.51 (normal 0.26–1.65)
Complement C3: 135 mg/dL (normal)
Complement C4: 25 mg/dL (normal)
Antinuclear antibodies (ANA): negative
HIV: negative
Hepatitis panel: nonreactive
Renal ultrasound—normal-sized kidneys, normal echogenicity, no hydronephrosis
Glycated hemoglobin (HbA$_{1c}$): 5.4% (normal)
Urine protein: 60 mg/dL
Urine albumin: 450 mg/L
Urine creatinine: 100 mg/dL
UPCR: 600 mg/g
UACR: 450 mg/g

Question 3.1.6: Is this glomerular, tubular, or overflow proteinuria?

Because proteinuria is predominantly albuminuria, this is likely glomerular proteinuria.

Question 3.1.7: Should this patient undergo a renal biopsy?

Biopsy is generally reserved for patients in whom 24-hour protein is >1 g (or UPCR is >1,000 mg/g). However, in view of the patient's age and his desire for life insurance, a biopsy should be contemplated in this case for diagnosis and prognosis.

Question 3.1.8: A renal biopsy is done, revealing mild membranous nephropathy. Is there any treatment indicated?

- Treatment of albuminuria (glomerular disease)
  - If possible, treatment should be directed at the cause(s) of the kidney disease. Primary glomerular disease is discussed in

Chapters 10 and 11. Treatment of secondary glomerular disease is directed at the underlying disease.

- Control of blood pressure (BP) is a very important intervention in any type of glomerular disease (Peterson et al., 1995). In diabetic patients, glucose control (Adler et al., 2003; UKPDS, 1998) is also important, although BP remains of paramount importance (Mogensen, 1998). Strict BP control (<130 systolic) has been shown to prevent progression of glomerular disease. This may require a combination of two or more antihypertensive medications. In particular, angiotensin-converting enzyme (ACE) inhibitors and/or other classes of renin–angiotensin system (RAS) antagonists have been found to protect kidney function in both nondiabetic (Wright et al., 2002) and diabetic patients (see Chapter 13). Addition of diuretics is particularly useful because they help control edema and prevent hyperkalemia from RAS blockers. The National Kidney Foundation recommends restricting dietary salt and protein. A decrease in albuminuria with therapy usually portends an improved prognosis (see Chapter 12).

CASE STUDY 3.1 CONCLUDED

Because this patient has only mild proteinuria and is normotensive, RAS blockers are not started at this time. The patient is followed in renal clinic to monitor for the possible development of worsening proteinuria, hypertension, or renal impairment.

VIGNETTE 1

3

A 55-year-old woman with diabetes mellitus presents for a routine clinic visit. She has been following the dietician's recommendations and eating a low-carbohydrate diet and low-fat diet with a high content of lean protein, fiber, fruits, and vegetables. She has been walking to the park every day, which takes about 45 minutes round trip. Her ophthalmologist has told her that she does not have retinopathy, and she has no foot ulcers. Her BP measured at the local pharmacy has been around 145/95 mm Hg. Medications include insulin, hydrochlorothiazide, aspirin, and simvastatin. Physical examination reveals that she does not have distress; her BP is 150/90 mm Hg, and she is obese.

Blood chemistry:
Sodium: 134 mmol/L
Potassium: 3.4 mmol/L
Chloride: 106 mmol/L
Total CO_2: 22 mmol/L
Urea nitrogen: 26 mg/dL (urea: 9.3 mmol/L)
Creatinine: 2.0 mg/dL (177 mcmol/L)
Glucose: 185 mg/dL (10.3 mmol/L)
Glycated hemoglobin: 8.2%

Complete blood count:
WBC: 4,200/mm³
Hemoglobin: 11.0 g/dL (110 g/L)
Hematocrit: 38%
Platelets: 299,000/mm³

Urinalysis:
Specific gravity: 1.025
pH: 5.5
Protein: 1+
Blood: 1+
Glucose: 2+
Ketones: negative
Bilirubin: negative
Urobilinogen: negative
Leukocyte esterase: negative
Nitrite: negative
WBC: 2/hpf
RBC: 0/hpf
Granular casts: few
Microalbumin screen:
UACR: 200 mg/g (22.6 mg/mmol)

Q: Which of the following interventions is not indicated?

1. Control diabetes
2. Control BP
3. Add an ACE inhibitor
4. Renal ultrasound
5. Protein restriction of 0.6 g/kg/day

A: First, we need to establish the etiology of the renal disease. The plasma creatinine is elevated, presumably indicating chronic kidney disease (CKD) (although a previous or follow-up level is needed to be certain). A renal ultrasound is indicated because of the presence of azotemia to evaluate renal anatomy and exclude obstruction. Microalbuminuria is urinary albumin excretion between 30 and 300 mg/day (or 30–300 mg/g creatinine [3.4–34 mg/mmol] or 20–200 mcg/min) and, if persistent, suggests the presence of glomerular disease. A UACR allows estimation of 24-hour albuminuria from a random sample of urine. This patient has 200 mg/g (22.6 mg/mmol), which is in the microalbuminuric range. It is imperative to bring the diabetes under control and control the BP to prevent progression of CKD (see Chapters 12 and 13). An ACE inhibitor or angiotensin-receptor blocker is warranted in all diabetic patients with microalbuminuria. Protein restriction of 0.8 to 1.0 g/kg may be useful in early CKD, but a protein restriction of 0.6 g/kg could lead to protein malnutrition and would be inappropriate in this setting.

3

A 70-year-old woman with chronic anemia, hyperlipidemia, and a recent left hip fracture is admitted for fever and hypotension. She complains of rib pain, back pain, and pain and numbness in the lower extremities. She also describes chronic fatigue, nausea, vomiting, constipation, frequent urination, depression, and memory loss.

Medications include ferrous sulfate, vitamin B_{12}, and simvastatin. Physical examination reveals her to be moderately febrile (T 38°C) and hypotensive (BP 90/75 mm Hg). She appears chronically ill. There is diffuse abdominal guarding and diffuse bony tenderness. There are no focal neurologic findings.

Blood chemistry:
Sodium: 147 mmol/L
Potassium: 4.2 mmol/L
Chloride: 104 mmol/L
Total CO_2: 23 mmol/L
Urea nitrogen: 50 mg/dL (urea: 17.8 mmol/L)
Creatinine: 2.5 mg/dL (221 mcmol/L)
Total calcium: 12.0 mg/dL (3 mmol/L)
Albumin: 4.0 g/dL (40 g/L)
Aspartate transaminase (AST): 60 U/L
Alanine transaminase (ALT): 65 U/L
Alkaline phosphatase: 100 U/L
Total bilirubin: 2.0 mg/dL (34 mcmol/L)

Complete blood count:
WBC: 4,000/mm^3
Hemoglobin: 7 g/dL (70 g/L)
Hematocrit: 25%
Platelets: 115,000/mm^3

Urinalysis:
Specific gravity: 1.005
pH: 5.0
Protein: 1+

Blood: 1+
Glucose: negative
Ketones: 1+
Bilirubin: negative
Urobilinogen: negative
Leukocyte esterase: negative
Nitrite: negative
WBC: 2/hpf
RBC: 0/hpf
Bacteria: few

Microalbumin Screen:
UACR: 60 mg/g (6.8 mg/mmol)
UPCR: 2,000 mg/g (226 mg/mmol)
Blood cultures × 2: no growth 48 hours
Intact parathyroid hormone (PTH): 5 pg/mL (normal 10–65)
Thyroid-stimulating hormone (TSH): 2.0 mIU/L (normal)
Serum protein electrophoresis, monoclonal immunoglobulin G (IgG) spike
Urine protein electrophoresis, monoclonal IgG spike, free light chains
Chest X-ray, clear lungs; rib fractures
Skull films, diffuse lytic lesions

Q: What type of proteinuria does this patient have?

1. Functional glomerular proteinuria
2. Pathologic glomerular proteinuria
3. Tubular proteinuria
4. Overflow proteinuria

A: This patient is admitted for acute renal failure and possible sepsis. However, her chest X-ray, blood cultures, and urinalysis do not provide any evidence of an infection. She has hypercalcemia, which may explain the inappropriately low urine specific gravity in the face of hypernatremia (nephrogenic diabetes insipidus). Intact PTH is appropriately low in the face of hypercalcemia, so primary hyperparathyroidism is excluded. The rib fracture and lytic bony lesions, coupled with anemia, hypercalcemia, proteinuria without substantial albuminuria, and a monoclonal gammopathy, lead us to the diagnosis of multiple myeloma, which is later confirmed by bone marrow biopsy.

Recall that the urinalysis reveals only 1+ proteinuria with minimal albuminuria despite the large amount of total protein in the urine. The dipstick primarily detects albumin. In this case, the excess urinary protein consists of paraproteins, predominantly light chains (Bence Jones proteins).

Overflow proteinuria occurs in situations in which large concentrations of small proteins (such as light chains, hemoglobin, or myoglobin), which are freely filtered at the glomerulus, overwhelm the reabsorptive capacity of the renal tubules. Albumin is too large to freely pass in large quantities through the normal glomerular basement membrane into the urine and that which does cross the glomerular barrier is normally mostly reabsorbed by the tubules. Therefore, albuminuria is a sign that the glomeruli are damaged and is called glomerular proteinuria. Glomerular proteinuria can be functional if it results from increased hydrostatic pressure or variables such as exercise or fever, in which case it is transient. Persistent glomerular proteinuria is pathologic. Tubular proteinuria is usually caused by the failure of damaged tubules to reabsorb small molecular weight, freely filtered proteins; in some cases, the damaged tubular cells also leak proteins into the urine.

Incidentally, the acute renal failure is probably due to multiple myeloma (light chain cast nephrotoxicity) as there are free light chains in the urine.

References

Adler AI, Stevens RJ, Manley SE, et al. Development and progression of nephropathy in type 2 diabetes. The United Kingdom Prospective Diabetes Study (UKPDS 64). *Kidney Int.* 63:225–232, 2003.

Bigazzi R, Bianchi S, Baldari D, et al. Microalbuminuria predicts cardiovascular events and renal insufficiency in patients with essential hypertension. *J Hypertens.* 16:1325–1333, 1998.

Klag MJ, Whelton PK, Randall BL, et al. End-stage renal disease in African-American and white men: 16-year MRFIT findings. *JAMA.* 277:1293–1298, 1997.

Leehey DJ, Kramer HJ, Daoud TM, et al. Progression of kidney disease in type 2 diabetes: beyond blood pressure control—an observational study. *BMC Nephrol.* 6:8, 2005.

Leischner MP, Naratadam GO, Hou SH, et al. Evaluation of proteinuria in healthy live kidney donor candidates. *Transplant Proc.* 38(9):2796–2797, 2006.

Mogensen CE. Combined high blood pressure and glucose in type 2 diabetes: double jeopardy. British trial shows clear effects of treatment, especially blood pressure reduction. *BMJ.* 317(7160):693–694, 1998.

Peterson JC, Adler S, Burkart JM, et al. Blood pressure control, proteinuria, and the progression of renal disease—the Modification of Diet in Renal Disease study. *Ann Intern Med.* 123:754–762, 1995.

Poortmans JR, Brauman H, Staroukine M, et al. Indirect evidence of glomerular/tubular mixed-type postexercise proteinuria in healthy humans. *Am J Physiol.* 254(2, pt 2):F277–F283, 1988.

UK Prospective Diabetes Study (UKPDS) Group. Intensive blood glucose control with sulphonylureas or insulin compared with conventional treatment and risk of complications in patients with type 2 diabetes (UKPDS 33). *Lancet.* 352:837–853, 1998.

Wright JT Jr, Bakris G, Greene T, et al. Effect of blood pressure lowering and antihypertensive drug class on progression of hypertensive kidney disease. Results from the AASK trial. *JAMA.* 288:2421–2431, 2002.

Hematuria

Hematuria is the presence of red blood cells (RBCs) in the urine. In microscopic hematuria (Thompson, 1987), RBCs can be demonstrated only by examination with a microscope. In gross hematuria, the urine is visibly red (more likely urologic bleeding) or the color of cola (more likely of renal origin).

- Distinguish red urine (negative dipstick) from myoglobin/hemoglobin (positive dipstick) versus hematuria (+RBCs and +dipstick) (see Chapter 1).
- Coexistent hematuria and proteinuria suggests glomerular disease (Richards, 1991) (see Chapter 10).
- Presence of RBC casts in urine indicates glomerular hematuria (see Chapter 1). Dysmorphic RBCs (Offringa & Benbassat, 1992) are also suggestive of a glomerular origin.

CASE STUDY 4.1

A 48-year-old healthy Caucasian female presents for evaluation for kidney donation. Her past medical history is significant only for irritable bowel syndrome that has been well controlled over the past few years. The patient has been evaluated before for possible kidney donation but was turned down after she was found to have isolated microscopic hematuria. She has never experienced gross hematuria.

Urinalysis:
Color: yellow
Specific gravity: 1.002
pH: 7.0
Protein: negative
Blood: small
Glucose: negative
Ketones: negative

Bilirubin: negative
Urobilinogen: negative
Nitrite: negative
Leukocyte esterase: negative
RBC: 5 to 10/hpf
WBC: 1 to 3/hpf
Bacteria: none
Epithelial cells: occasional

Question 4.1.1: What is the differential diagnosis for isolated microscopic hematuria?

CAUSES OF ISOLATED HEMATURIA (See Table 4.1) (Mariani et al., 1989; Ritchie et al., 1986)

- Transient hematuria
  - Exercise

Most Likely Diagnoses Based on History, Physical Examination, and Laboratory Findings

	Dysuria	Trauma/heavy exercise	Flank pain	Male with voiding difficulties	Upper respiratory symptoms	Family history of hematuria and/or kidney disease	Congestive heart failure/atrial fibrillation	History and physical negative
Findings	Dysuria Usually abnormal urinalysis (+leucocyte esterase, nitrite, WBC, bacteria) Sexually active Urethral discharge		Costovertebral angle tenderness	Suprapubic fullness				
Diagnoses	UTI prostatitis (in males) Urethritis	Traumatic/exercise-induced hematuria	Nephrolithiasis Loin pain/hematuria syndrome Sickle cell trait (if African American)	Urethral stricture BPH Prostate cancer	IgA nephritis	IgA nephritis, Alport syndrome, or thin basement membrane disease Polycystic kidney disease	Renal embolism/infarction	Exclude cancer (prostate, bladder, renal), especially in smokers Crystalluria (calcium, uric acid)

BPH, benign prostatic hypertrophy; UTI, urinary tract infection.

- Trauma
- Menstruation
- Sexual intercourse
- Viral illness
- Anticoagulant toxicity
■ Persistent hematuria
  ■ Urologic causes (more common)
    • Cystitis/urethritis
    • Trauma (including Foley catheter)
    • Kidney stones (can be detected on renal ultrasound, computed tomography [CT] scan without contrast) (Teichman, 2004)
    • Benign prostatic hypertrophy (BPH), prostatitis, or prostate cancer
    • Bladder, ureteral, or renal cancer (most common in male smokers) (Mulholland & Stefanelli, 1990)
  ■ Nephrologic causes
    • Glomerulonephritis (GN)—differential diagnosis of isolated glomerular hematuria is immunoglobulin A (IgA) nephropathy (Tanaka et al., 1996), Alport disease, or thin basement membrane disease
    • Sickle cell disease/trait (sickling in kidney medulla leading to infarction)
    • Vascular (arteriovenous malformation, renal infarct)
    • Cystic disease (e.g., polycystic kidney disease)
    • Medullary sponge kidney
    • Hypercalciuria/hyperuricosuria ($\pm$ stones)

Question 4.1.2: What is the differential diagnosis in this patient?

CASE STUDY 4.1 CONTINUED

The patient denies a history of frequent urinary tract infections. She is not sexually active and does not have any abnormal vaginal discharge. She has not suffered any trauma. She has never passed a kidney stone. She denies use of nonsteroidal anti-inflammatory drugs (NSAIDs). She has no vision or hearing issues. There is no family history of renal failure, deafness, or ocular problems. She is physically active and engages in bike rides of up to 20 to 30 miles. She does not smoke. She does not have loin pain.

EVALUATION OF ISOLATED HEMATURIA

The steps for evaluation of isolated hematuria are presented in Figure 4.1.

EVALUATION OF HEMATURIA/PROTEINURIA (SEE FIG. 4.2)

■ Suspect GN or renal vasculitis (see Chapter 10)

Isolated Hematuria[1]

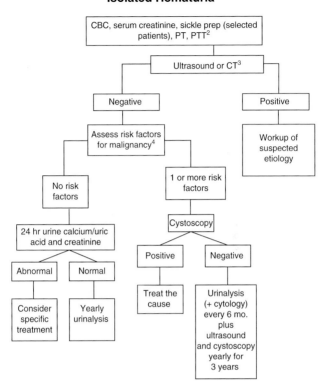

1. Hematuria > 3 RBC/hpf on two out of three urinalyses or;
   > 100 RBC/hpf on 1 urine sample or;
   1 episode of gross hematuria
   No dipstick proteinuria
2. Most recommend further evaluation for hematuria in presence of coagulopathy since 30% to 50% of patients have underlying pathology.
3. CT without contrast recommended for detection of stone disease and CT with contrast recommended for detection of tumors
4. Risk factors for malignancy
   Age > 50
   Heavy smoking
   Exposure to certain dyes and rubber compounds
   History of analgesic abuse
   History of pelvic irradiation
   Cyclophosphamide exposure

FIGURE 4.1. Evaluation of isolated hematuria. CBC, complete blood count; CT, computed tomography; PT, prothrombin time; PTT, partial thromboplastin time.

CASE STUDY 4.1 CONTINUED

Renal ultrasound does not show any kidney stones, cysts, or masses. CT abdomen with and without contrast is also negative for kidney stones, cysts, or masses. She has also been seen by urology and has a negative workup including cystoscopy, CT urogram, and cytology.

Hematuria/Proteinuria

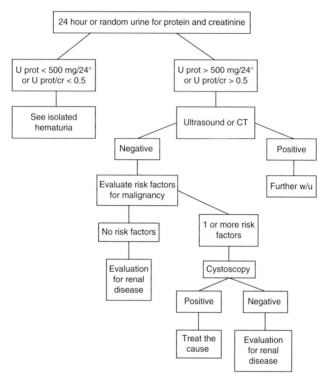

FIGURE 4.2. Evaluation of hematuria/proteinuria. CT, computed tomography.

Question 4.1.3: **What is the differential diagnosis at this point?**

Isolated hematuria of nephrologic origin is usually due to IgA nephropathy, Alport syndrome, or thin basement membrane disease. Crystalluria also remains in the differential.

CASE 4.1 CONCLUDED

24-hour urine:
Uric acid: 0.7 g/day (normal <0.75 g/day in females)
Calcium: 100 mg/day (normal <200 mg/day in females)
A renal biopsy showed thin basement membrane disease.

Question 4.1.4: **Is this patient an acceptable kidney donor?**

Thin basement membrane disease is generally a benign disease, but its risk for renal transplant recipients and donors is unknown. Selected patients, that is, otherwise healthy patients without proteinuria, hypertension, or renal impairment, may undergo kidney donation and recipients generally do well.

4

A 60-year-old white male with a history of a seizure disorder for the past 40 years presents for evaluation of the new-onset asymptomatic microscopic hematuria. He denies trauma, pain/burning with urination, or recent exertion/exercise. He has no abdominal pain. His urinary stream is strong, and there is no nocturia. His prostate-specific antigen (PSA) 6 months ago was normal. He denies sore throat, viral syndrome, or recent bacterial infection. He has no history of kidney disease. His only medication is phenytoin. His physical examination is significant only for an enlarged prostate on rectal examination.

Blood chemistry:
Sodium: 138 mmol/L
Potassium: 4.2 mmol/L
Chloride: 104 mmol/L
Total CO_2: 24 mmol/L
Urea nitrogen: 18 mg/dL
   (urea: 6.4 mmol/L)
Creatinine: 1.1 mg/dL (97 mcmol/L)
Glucose: 120 mg/dL (6.7 mmol/L)
Complete blood count:
WBC: 14,000/mm^3
Hemoglobin: 13 g/dL (130 g/L)
Hematocrit: 40%
Platelets: 250,000/mm^3

Coagulation profile:
Prothrombin time: 13 seconds
   (INR: 1.2)

Partial thromboplastin time:
   25 seconds

Urinalysis:
Color: yellow
Specific gravity: 1.025
pH: 6
Protein: negative
Blood: negative
Glucose: negative
Ketones: negative
Bilirubin: negative
Urobilinogen: negative
Leukocyte esterase: negative
Nitrate: negative
RBC: 10/hpf
WBC: 3/hpf
Bacteria: none
No cellular casts

Q: What is the next best step?

1. Urology referral for enlarged prostate
2. Administer an alpha blocker
3. Discontinue phenytoin
4. Repeat urinalysis in 2 weeks
5. Give amoxicillin for pharyngitis

A: The history helps one to exclude most of the etiologies of hematuria. Lack of trauma excludes traumatic hematuria. Lack of pain/burning with urination argues against urinary infection. In addition, hematuria is not due to exertion/exercise. He has no symptoms of prostatism, and the normal PSA argues against prostate cancer. The absence of sore throat, viral syndrome, or recent bacterial infection makes postinfectious GN or IgA nephropathy unlikely.

The physical examination reveals an enlarged prostate. His renal function is normal. There is no coagulopathy. The absence of proteinuria and cellular casts on urinalysis makes GN unlikely, and there is no suggestion of infection (no pyuria or bacteriuria). So the differential at this point includes bladder cancer, BPH, and, possibly (though unlikely), GN. Should we consult the urology for bladder cancer or BPH? Or should we just start an alpha blocker? Should we discontinue the phenytoin? Might a short course of amoxicillin help? Since this is the first time microscopic hematuria is evident, the most appropriate next step in management is to determine whether the hematuria is persistent. Only persistent microscopic hematuria (>3 RBC/hpf on two of three urinalyses or >100 RBC/hpf) or gross hematuria requires evaluation.

VIGNETTE 2

A 55-year-old African American male presents for evaluation of persistent microscopic hematuria. Hematuria was initially discovered on a routine urinalysis done at his workplace 2 years ago, and this was confirmed on two additional urine samples obtained during the next year. He denies gross blood in his urine. He leads a sedentary lifestyle and does not exercise. He is a heavy smoker. He is sexually active. He has no pain or burning with urination. He takes no regular medications. He had a cystoscopy 1 year ago, which was normal, and urine cytology revealed no malignant cells. He is a textile factory worker and states he works with dyes. His family history is positive for prostate cancer (father and paternal uncle). On physical examination, a left nostril polyp is noted, and scattered wheezes are heard on lung auscultation.

Blood chemistry:
Sodium: 138 mmol/L
Potassium: 5.0 mmol/L
Chloride: 104 mmol/L
Total CO_2: 24 mmol/L
Urea nitrogen: 20 mg/dL (urea: 7.1 mmol/L)
Creatinine: 1.1 mg/dL (97 mcmol/L)
Glucose: 100 mg/dL (5.6 mmol/L)

Complete blood count:
WBC: 4,100/mm^3
Hemoglobin: 12 g/dL (120 g/L)
Hematocrit: 40%
Platelets: 200,000/mm^3

Urinalysis:
Color: yellow
pH: 5.5
Specific gravity: 1.015
Protein: negative
Blood: 2+
Glucose: negative
Ketones: negative
Bilirubin: negative
Urobilinogen: negative
Leukocyte esterase: negative
Nitrite: negative
RBC: 10/hpf
WBC: 2/hpf

Bacteria: none
RBC casts: not seen
Dysmorphic RBCs: present
Peripheral smear: no sickle cells
    or spherocytes

PSA: 2.0 ng/mL (normal)
Chest X-ray: negative
Renal CT with contrast: negative

Q: What is the most likely cause of hematuria?

1. Bladder cancer
2. Prostate cancer
3. BPH
4. Sickle cell trait
5. IgA nephropathy
6. Thin basement membrane disease

A: Persistent asymptomatic hematuria should be evaluated. Renal causes should be investigated by evaluation of the urinalysis for proteinuria, RBC casts, and dysmorphic RBCs (i.e., RBCs that have undergone transformation during transit through the nephron), and blood chemistry for azotemia. In our patient, isolated renal hematuria is suggested by the presence of dysmorphic RBCs, although RBC casts were not seen and there is no proteinuria. IgA nephropathy is the most common renal cause of isolated hematuria. Other possibilities are thin basement membrane disease and hereditary nephritis. In an African American, sickle cell trait should also be considered (hematuria occurs because of sickling of RBCs in the hypoxic hypertonic environment of the renal papillae).

IgA nephropathy is characterized by immunoglobulin A deposition in the mesangium with mesangial proliferation. It is postulated that abnormal galactosylation of IgA leads to decreased clearance by the liver, autoantibody formation, and mesangial deposition. Thin basement membrane disease and hereditary nephritis are familial causes of isolated hematuria (IgA nephropathy can also be familial in some cases).

Bladder cancer should always be considered in the presence of risk factors such as smoking, age >40, occupational exposure to chemicals or dyes, or exposure to cyclophosphamide. African American men have the highest risk of this disease. Our patient is a middle-aged African American male with a long history of heavy smoking and exposure to textile dyes, both of which are major risk factors for bladder cancer. Moreover, even though his PSA is normal, he has a strong family history of prostate cancer, which could be another reason for urologic evaluation. Although he did not have bladder or prostate cancer 1 year ago, he should undergo repeat yearly cystoscopy for the next 2 years.

If no urologic cause for hematuria is found, a renal biopsy could be considered for diagnosis of suspected glomerular disease. However, because there is no specific treatment for any of the renal causes of isolated hematuria, biopsy is optional.

References

Mariani AJ, Mariani MC, Macchioni C, et al. The significance of adult hematuria: 1000 hematuria evaluations including a risk-benefit ratio and cost-effectiveness analysis. *J Urol.* 141:350–355, 1989.

Mulholland SG, Stefanelli JL. Genitourinary cancer in the elderly. *Am J Kidney Dis.* 16(4):324–328, 1990.

Offringa M, Benbassat J. The value of urinary red cell shape in the diagnosis of glomerular and post-glomerular hematuria. A meta-analysis. *Postgrad Med J.* 68:648–654, 1992.

Richards J. Acute post-streptococcal glomerulonephritis. *W V Med J.* 87:61–65, 1991.

Ritchie CD, Bevan EA, Collier SJ. Importance of occult hematuria found at screening. *BMJ.* 292:681–683, 1986.

Tanaka H, Kim S-T, Takasugi M, et al. Isolated hematuria in adults: IgA nephropathy is a predominant cause of hematuria compared with thin glomerular basement membrane nephropathy. *Am J Nephrol.* 16:412–416, 1996.

Teichman JM. Acute renal colic from ureteral calculus. *N Engl J Med.* 350:684–693, 2004.

Thompson IM. The evaluation of microscopic hematuria: a population-based study. *J Urol.* 138:1189–1190, 1987.

Disorders of Plasma Sodium Concentration

DEFINITIONS

- Hyponatremia is defined as a plasma sodium concentration ([Na^+]) of <135 mmol/L. Hypernatremia is defined as a plasma sodium concentration ([Na^+]) of >145 mmol/L.
- Disorders of sodium concentration (dysnatremic states) usually reflect a disorder in water balance rather than sodium balance.
  - In the steady state, water intake equals water output.
  - Water excess without a change in total body sodium content leads to hyponatremia.
  - Water deficit without a change in total body sodium content leads to hypernatremia.

PHYSIOLOGIC REGULATION OF PLASMA SODIUM CONCENTRATION [NA$^+$]

- $\uparrow$ water intake $\rightarrow \downarrow$ plasma [Na^+] $\rightarrow \downarrow$ antidiuretic hormone (ADH) release and thirst $\rightarrow \uparrow$ renal water excretion and $\downarrow$ water intake $\rightarrow$ normalization of plasma [Na^+]
- $\downarrow$ water intake $\rightarrow \uparrow$ plasma [Na^+] $\rightarrow \uparrow$ ADH and thirst $\rightarrow \downarrow$ renal water excretion and $\uparrow$ water intake $\rightarrow$ normalization of plasma [Na^+]
- Both thirst and ADH are triggered at a plasma osmolality of about 285 mmol/kg ("osmotic threshold") and shut off at lower plasma osmolality.
- Ability to excrete water depends on the following:
  - Glomerular filtration of solute
  - Delivery of solute to the distal nephron (main solutes are sodium, potassium, accompanying anions, and urea [which is generated from protein])
  - Impermeability to water in the collecting duct (when ADH is suppressed)

REGULATION OF ADH

- ADH is arginine vasopressin (AVP), an octapeptide synthesized by the supraoptic and paraventricular nuclei in the hypothalamus and stored and secreted by the posterior pituitary.
- ADH acts on the collecting duct to increase water reabsorption and thus decrease renal water excretion. In the presence of substantial amounts of ADH, the urine will be concentrated, that is, urine osmolality (U_{osm}) > plasma osmolality (P_{osm}).

- ADH secretion is physiologically regulated by osmotic and non-osmotic factors (Robertson & Athar, 1976). A small (1%–2%) increase in effective osmolality ([Na$^+$] + [glucose]) will increase ADH release. A large (~10%) decrease in blood volume or blood pressure will also increase ADH release and can override the effect of osmolality. ADH release can also be affected by other nonosmotic stimuli (e.g., drugs, pain, stress).
- Assuming normal renal response to its effects, when ADH is completely suppressed, urine osmolality is very low (<150 to ~50 mmol/kg); when maximally active, urine osmolality is high (>700 to ~1,200 mmol/kg).

HYPONATREMIA

Etiology of Hyponatremia
- Pseudohyponatremia (plasma sodium is low, but plasma osmolality is normal)
  - Plasma normally consists of 93% water and 7% nonaqueous material (proteins and lipids). Pseudohyponatremia is an exaggeration of the physiologic dilution of plasma water sodium by an increase in nonaqueous material in the plasma (i.e., severe hyperproteinemia or hyperlipidemia).
  - Many clinical laboratories measure sodium using an indirect ion-selective electrode (ISE), which involves diluting the plasma sample and measuring plasma sodium based on the assumption that the sample is composed of 93% of water. If the plasma water is <93% of the plasma volume (owing an increase in the percentage of nonaqueous material), this leads to a spurious underestimation of the plasma sodium concentration. However, the sodium concentration of the aqueous portion of a plasma sample, as determined by a direct ISE in undiluted serum or plasma, is normal.
  - Not all patients with isotonic hyponatremia have pseudohyponatremia. Since calculated $P_{osm} = 2 \times$ Na (mmol/L) + glucose (mg/dL)/18 + urea nitrogen (mg/dL)/2.8, measured plasma osmolality can be normal despite hyponatremia if either plasma urea nitrogen or glucose is high. Using SI units, $P_{osm} = 2 \times$ Na (mmol/L) + glucose (mmol/L) + urea (mmol/L).
- **Hypertonic hyponatremia** (plasma osmolality is high)
  - Hyperglycemia. Elevated glucose in plasma osmotically draws water from cells, thus lowering the plasma [Na$^+$]. Corrected [Na$^+$] = [Na$^+$] + (1.6 × [(glucose/100) − 1]) (where glucose concentration is expressed as mg/dL). Since every 100 mg/dL (5.6 mmol/L) increase in plasma glucose lowers the plasma sodium by only 1.6 mmol/L, plasma osmolality will progressively increase as plasma glucose increases. Note that the correction factor is larger (up to 4) when there is extreme hyperglycemia.
  - Exogenous solutes (e.g., hypertonic mannitol that is used to treat cerebral edema). The mechanism is the same as for hyperglycemia.
- **Hyponatremia with variable osmolality**
  - Addition of an isosmotic but non–sodium-containing fluid to the extracellular space, such as glycine or sorbitol used as

endoscopic irrigant solutions in transurethral resection of the prostate (TURP), hysteroscopy, or laparoscopic surgery, can occasionally result in severe hyponatremia. The plasma osmolality is variable and can be normal because of the presence of glycine or sorbitol in the plasma, in which case there will be a large osmolal gap (measured osmolality minus calculated osmolality). Glycine and/or sorbitol metabolism and urinary excretion lead to gradual improvement in hyponatremia and normalization of the osmolal gap.

- **Hypotonic hyponatremia** (plasma osmolality is low)
  - Hypotonic (or hypoosmolal) hyponatremia can be further subdivided into euvolemic, hypovolemic, and hypervolemic types based on clinical and laboratory assessment of plasma/extracellular volume. Most hyponatremia falls into this category.

CASE STUDY

A 55-year-old male with a history of subarachnoid hemorrhage 10 days previously presents for evaluation of dizziness, muscle cramps, and weakness.

Physical examination:
Vitals: pulse 115 beats/min; respiratory rate 20 breaths/min; blood pressure 100/60 mm Hg; temperature 98°F; oxygen saturation 96%
Chest: clear
Heart: regular rate and rhythm (RRR), tachycardic, weak pulses
Abdomen: soft with normoactive bowel sounds
Skin: decreased skin turgor
Neurologic: no focal findings

Blood chemistry:
Sodium: 125 mmol/L
Potassium: 4.0 mmol/L
Chloride: 90 mmol/L
Total CO_2: 24 mmol/L
Urea nitrogen: 30 mg/dL (urea: 10.8 mmol/L)
Creatinine: 1.0 mg/dL (88.4 mcmol/L)
Glucose: 200 mg/dL (11.2 mmol/L)
Osmolality (measured): 275 mmol/kg
Osmolality (calculated): 272 mmol/kg
Uric acid: 2.5 mg/dL (149 mcmol/L)

Urine chemistry:
Osmolality: 300 mmol/kg
Sodium: 50 mmol/L
Creatinine: 20 mg/dL (1,768 mcmol/L)

Complete blood count:
WBC: 4,500/mm³
Hemoglobin: 16 g/dL (160 g/L)
Hematocrit: 50%
Platelets: 250,000/mm³

Lipid profile:
Total cholesterol: 200 mg/dL (5.2 mmol/L)
Triglycerides: 450 mg/dL (5.1 mmol/L)

Computed tomography (CT) of the head shows stable subarachnoid hemorrhage with no extension of bleed.

Question 5.1.1: What are the initial steps in evaluating the hyponatremia?

The initial steps in evaluating hyponatremia are to (1) determine whether hyponatremia is acute or chronic, (2) assess the severity of hyponatremia, and (3) determine whether it is symptomatic or asymptomatic.

1. The duration of hyponatremia, in this case, is uncertain and should be assumed to be chronic. Chronic hyponatremia should be corrected slowly; acute hyponatremia should be corrected rapidly, especially when symptomatic (see section on Treatment of Hyponatremia after Question 5.1.8).
2. Mild hyponatremia is defined as plasma $[Na^+]$ between 130 and 135 mmol/L; moderate hyponatremia as plasma $[Na^+]$ between 120 and 129 mmol/L; and severe hyponatremia as plasma $[Na^+]$ <120 mmol/L. With acute hyponatremia, even moderate hyponatremia may be symptomatic, whereas chronic severe hyponatremia may be associated with few or any symptoms.
3. Mild-to-moderate symptoms of hyponatremia include headache, nausea, vomiting, fatigue, gait disturbances, and confusion; these are relatively nonspecific. Severe symptoms of hyponatremia include seizures, obtundation, coma, and respiratory arrest.

CASE STUDY 5.1 CONTINUED

In this case, the patient has moderate hyponatremia and is mildly to moderately symptomatic, though most of his symptoms are probably because of volume depletion rather than hyponatremia per se (see Question 5.1.4).

Question 5.1.2: What other laboratory tests are useful in characterizing the hyponatremia?

1. Consider the plasma glucose.

   When plasma glucose is elevated, there is osmotic shift of water from the intracellular to the extracellular space, thus lowering the plasma $[Na^+]$. A number of formulae have been devised to predict the effect of hyperglycemia on plasma sodium concentration. A commonly used one (using US laboratory units) is:

   $$\text{Corrected } [Na^+] = [Na^+] + (1.6 \times [(\text{glucose}/100) - 1])$$

   Since the plasma glucose was 200 mg/dL, the corrected blood sodium is 126.6, which is not substantially higher than the measured plasma sodium.

2. Determine the plasma osmolality.

In most clinical conditions, hyponatremia will be accompanied by hypoosmolality (hypoosmolal or hypotonic hyponatremia). However, occasionally, the plasma osmolality will be normal or even high in the face of hyponatremia (see above).

CASE STUDY 5.1 CONTINUED

In this patient, the measured plasma osmolality is 272 mmol/kg, confirming hypoosmolal hyponatremia.

Question 5.1.3: What causes hypoosmolal hyponatremia?

Pathogenesis of Hypotonic Hyponatremia

- Plasma sodium concentration $[Na^+]$ reflects the relationship between total body cations (sodium plus potassium) $(TBNa^+ + TBK^+)$ and total body water (TBW), that is, $[Na^+] = \alpha (Na_e^+ + K_e^+)/TBW + \beta$, where Na_e^+ = isotopically measured exchangeable sodium, K_e^+ = isotopically measured exchangeable potassium (Edelman et al., 1958).

- Why is potassium important? The answer is that sodium is essentially confined to the extracellular fluid (ECF), whereas potassium is mostly in the intracellular fluid (ICF). Administration of sodium will increase the content of sodium in the ECF; the increase in ECF $[Na^+]$ will then draw water out of the ICF by osmosis. The change in plasma $[Na^+]$ will thus depend on the amount of sodium administered and the sum of ECF and ICF volume, that is, TBW. On the other hand, administration of potassium will increase the content of potassium in the ICF; the increase in ICF $[K^+]$ will draw water into the cells, thus increasing the plasma $[Na^+]$. Since ECF $[Na^+]$ is approximately equal to ICF $[K^+]$: plasma $[Na^+] \approx (TBNa^+ + TBK^+)/TBW$.

- Thus, plasma $[Na^+]$ only gives an indication of the relative amount of total body cations and TBW and not the absolute amount of either.

- In the absence of severe potassium depletion, plasma $[Na^+]$ reflects the ratio of $TBNa^+$ and TBW.

- Hyponatremia = excess of TBW relative to $TBNa^+$. Some examples are as follows:

  - ↑ TBW with normal $TBNa^+$. This typically occurs when there is an inappropriate increase in ADH secretion, that is, syndrome of inappropriate antidiuretic hormone (SIADH). For example, if a tumor is secreting ADH, ADH secretion is not being regulated by the plasma sodium concentration, and if water is ingested, it will be retained, causing persistent hyponatremia.

  - ↓ TBW with ↓↓ $TBNa^+$. This usually occurs when there are sodium and water losses, with replacement of water but not sodium. For example, some patients taking diuretics (which cause renal loss of sodium and water) will ingest a large amount of water, possibly because of stimulation of thirst by volume depletion; volume depletion, if severe, can also (appropriately) cause ADH release, which contributes to hyponatremia.

- ↑↑ TBW with normal or ↑ TBNa$^+$. This may occur in edematous disorders, that is, congestive heart failure (CHF), liver cirrhosis, nephrotic syndrome, and renal failure (Schrier, 1988a, b). For example, in severe CHF, there is a decrease in "effective blood volume" or "effective circulatory volume" owing to impaired cardiac output; because there is decreased renal perfusion, the kidney perceives volume depletion and retains sodium and water. ADH release is increased because of the decrease in effective blood volume and blood pressure, which contributes to hyponatremia.

- It should be obvious that the plasma sodium concentration per se gives no information about the TBNa$^+$. Because sodium is in the ECF, estimation of TBNa$^+$ means assessing the ECF volume. Signs of low TBNa$^+$ (ECF volume) are flat neck veins, decreased skin turgor, dry mucous membranes, absence of edema, and orthostatic changes in pulse and blood pressure. The principal sign of high TBNa$^+$ (ECF volume) is edema (see Question 5.1.4).

- Normal kidneys can excrete a large amount of water because of the great ability of the kidneys to form dilute urine. In the absence of ADH, urine osmolality can be as low as 50 mmol/kg. The daily solute load is generally 600 to 1,200 mmol/day. Even if urine osmole excretion is 600 mmol/day, 12 L of dilute urine can be excreted. Because sustained fluid intake in excess of 12 L/day is decidedly uncommon, hyponatremia resulting from fluid ingestion alone is very rare. Therefore, hyponatremia usually indicates impaired renal water excretion due to the following:

  - Decreased solute excretion. If osmole (solute) excretion is lower than normal, hyponatremia may ensue as a result of smaller fluid intakes. This has been described in beer drinkers, who ingest much fluid but very little (i.e., 100–200 mmol/day) solute (beer drinker's potomania).

  - Impaired urinary dilution, due to the following:
    - Excess ADH production (either appropriate, i.e., in response to a physiologic stimulus, or inappropriate).
    - Intrarenal factors (independent of ADH). Normal renal ability to excrete water depends on three factors: (1) filtration of solute by the glomeruli, (2) delivery of solute to distal (diluting) nephron sites, and (3) water impermeability of diluting nephron sites, which occurs providing ADH is absent. Thus, intrarenal factors that impair water excretion include (1) renal failure (which decreases glomerular filtration rate [GFR] and thus filtration of solute), (2) decreased delivery of solute to distal (diluting) segments of the nephron because of solute avidity at proximal nephron sites (e.g., with CHF), and (3) diuretics (which impair generation of dilute urine by preventing solute reabsorption in water-impermeable nephron segments).

Question 5.1.4: How should the patient's volume status be assessed?

This is accomplished by clinical examination (examination of neck veins, skin turgor, mucous membranes, orthostatic changes in pulse and/or blood pressure, and the presence or absence of edema) that is on occasion supplemented by volume and/or pressure measurements (such as central venous pressure and ultrasound of inferior vena cava). Hypoosmolal hyponatremia then can be further subdivided into euvolemic, hypovolemic, and hypervolemic subtypes.

Etiology of Hypotonic (Hypoosmolar) Hyponatremia (Table 5.1)

- **Hypovolemic hyponatremia** indicates a decrease in $TBNa^+$, which can be because of either renal or extrarenal sodium losses.
  - Renal sodium losses—diuretics (Ashraf et al., 1981); primary adrenal insufficiency (Addison disease), isolated mineralocorticoid deficiency, salt-wasting nephropathies

TABLE 5.1   Hypotonic Hyponatremia

Hypovolemic		Euvolemic	Hypervolemic	
$FENa < 1$; $U_{osm} > P_{osm}$	$FENa > 1$; $U_{osm} \sim$ or $> P_{osm}$	$FENa$ usually >1; $U_{osm} > P_{osm}$ except $< P_{osm}$ in reset osmostat, psychogenic polydipsia, and beer drinker's syndrome	$FENa < 1$; $U_{osm} > P_{osm}$	$FENa > 1$; $U_{osm} \sim P_{osm}$
Gastrointestinal or sweat losses	Salt-losing nephropathy	SIADH/reset osmostat/ NSIAD	CHF	Renal failure
	Adrenal insufficiency/ isolated mineralocorticoid deficiency	Psychogenic polydipsia	Cirrhosis	
	Diuretics	Beer drinker's syndrome	Nephrotic syndrome	
		Exercise hyponatremia		
		Postoperative hyponatremia		
		Drugs either stimulating ADH secretion or increasing its action		
		Hypothyroidism		

ADH, antidiuretic hormone; CHF, congestive heart failure; NSIAD, nephrogenic syndrome of inappropriate antidiuresis; SIADH, syndrome of inappropriate antidiuretic hormone.

- Salt-wasting nephropathies
  - Proximal tubule (PT)
    - Fanconi syndrome
    - Cerebral salt wasting (CSW) (see below)
  - Thick ascending limb (TAL)
    - Bartter syndrome (defective sodium potassium 2-chloride [NKCC2] transporter, calcium-sensitive receptor [CaSR], or renal outer medullary potassium [ROMK] channel)
  - Distal convoluted tubule (DCT)
    - Gitelman syndrome (defective sodium chloride channel [NCC])
  - Cortical collecting duct (CCD)
    - Congenital adrenal hyperplasia (21-hydroxylase deficiency leads to decreased glucocorticoid and mineralocorticoid production)
    - Pseudohypoaldosteronism type 1 (PHA-1) (mutation in the mineralocorticoid receptor or defective epithelial sodium channel [ENaC])
  - Extrarenal sodium losses—diarrhea, vomiting, excessive sweating
- **Euvolemic hyponatremia** implies normal or near-normal TBNa$^+$. Examples include the following:
  - SIADH (Bartter & Schwartz, 1967)—most commonly due to (1) tumor, (2) pulmonary disease, and (3) central nervous system (CNS) disease. In some cases, the set point for ADH secretion is altered ("reset osmostat").
  - Nephrogenic syndrome of inappropriate antidiuresis (NSIAD). Looks similar to SIADH except that ADH levels are unmeasurable. ADH receptors are mutated and constitutively activated (Feldman et al., 2005)
  - Severe hypothyroidism (may be because of decreased cardiac output and GFR)
  - Psychogenic polydipsia (increased water intake) (Hariprasad et al., 1980)
  - Beer drinker's potomania (decreased solute intake)
  - Exercise hyponatremia (increased water intake plus ADH release)
  - Postoperative hyponatremia (increased hypotonic fluid administration plus ADH release)
- **Hypervolemic hyponatremia** indicates increased TBNa$^+$. Examples include the following:
  - CHF
  - Liver cirrhosis
  - Nephrotic syndrome
  - Renal failure

CASE STUDY 5.1 CONTINUED

This patient is clinically hypovolemic as evidenced by relative hypotension, decreased skin turgor, increased hematocrit, and increased plasma urea nitrogen to creatinine ratio.

Question 5.1.5: Is hypovolemic hyponatremia due to a renal or extrarenal cause?

CASE STUDY 5.1 CONTINUED

The urine sodium concentration is 50 mmol/L, and urine osmolality is 300 mmol/kg. The patient does not complain of diarrhea or vomiting and is not sweating excessively, which are the usual causes of extrarenal salt losses. Because urine sodium is elevated (>20 mmol/L), this suggests a renal salt-wasting disorder.

Question 5.1.6: What is the differential diagnosis?

In a patient with subarachnoid hemorrhage, one should consider either the SIADH or CSW (Rahman & Friedman, 2009). Both conditions are associated with elevated urine sodium concentration and inappropriate antidiuresis. Note that even though the urine is not overtly concentrated, the urine osmolality is inappropriately elevated in view of the low plasma osmolality. Although SIADH is euvolemic and CSW is hypovolemic, these two conditions can be difficult to distinguish in practice.

- Cerebral salt wasting
  - Occurs in the setting of subarachnoid hemorrhage or other CNS disease
  - Typical onset is within 10 days of CNS event, but up to 1 month has been reported
  - CSW closely mimics SIADH except that the patient is hypovolemic (not euvolemic)
  - Typical laboratory data are the same as in SIADH: plasma sodium (PNa) < 135 mmol/L; U_{osm} > 100 mmol/kg (usually >300 mmol/kg); urine sodium (UNa) > 40 mmol/L; low plasma uric acid (usually <3 mg/dL)
  - Mechanism of hyponatremia: volume depletion stimulates baroreceptors, leading to nonosmotic ADH release and subsequent inability to make dilute urine
  - Mechanism of salt wasting: poorly understood
    - The sympathetic nervous system (SNS) normally promotes sodium, uric acid, and water reabsorption in the PT as well as renin release; CNS disease leads to removal of the SNS stimulus
    - Brain natriuretic peptide (BNP) is released causing:
      - Decreased Na reabsorption
      - Inhibition of renin release
      - Decreased autonomic outflow
    - Volume depletion from salt wasting may limit increases in intracranial pressure (ICP)
  - Diagnosis: volume repletion with isotonic saline leads to removal of the hypovolemic stimulus to ADH release, resulting in water diuresis and correction of hyponatremia. This is the opposite of SIADH, in which isotonic saline worsens hyponatremia (see below).
  - Hypouricemia and high fractional excretion of uric acid (FE uric acid > 10%) do not normalize with water restriction. This is different from SIADH, in which water restriction normalizes the slightly elevated plasma volume, normalizing reabsorption of

uric acid in the PT. The mechanism of persistent hypouricemia in CSW is not understood.

- CSW can coexist with SIADH in some cases.
- Treatment of CSW:
  - Fluid restriction without saline administration will lead to further volume depletion and may increase the risk of cerebral infarction in CSW.
  - Acute management is based on the severity of hyponatremia and the clinical condition of the patient. General guidelines are as follows:
    - Plasma [Na^+] <120 mmol/L—3% saline
    - Plasma [Na^+] = 120 to 135 and ICP <10 mm Hg or no ICP monitoring possible — 0.9% saline
    - Plasma [Na^+] = 120 to 135 and ICP >10 mm Hg — 3% saline
  - If persistent, CSW can be managed with salt tablets and/or mineralocorticoids (fludrocortisone).
  - CSW usually resolves in 3 to 4 weeks; long-term treatment is usually not necessary.
- SIADH (Bartter & Schwartz, 1967)
  There are four types of SIADH:
  A: Unregulated secretion of ADH (this is the most common)
  B: Increased basal secretion of ADH with normal regulation
  C: Reset osmostat (see below)
  D: Undetectable ADH
  - NSIAD. Looks similar to SIADH except that ADH levels are unmeasurable. ADH receptors are mutated and constitutively activated (Feldman et al., 2005)
  - Postreceptor defect or abnormal control of aquaporin-2 channels leading to ADH-independent antidiuresis
  - Antidiuretic principle other than AVP
- Characterized by ADH secretion despite low plasma osmolality, and absence of nonosmotic stimulus to ADH release (such as volume depletion, decreased cardiac output, decreased systemic vascular resistance, and hypotension)
- ADH secretion leads to water retention, increased TBW, and hypotonic hyponatremia
- SIADH is characterized by euvolemic hyponatremia because there is no sodium retention (i.e., no edema)
- Plasma volume expansion because of water retention results in increased excretion of sodium in the urine; this results in euvolemia but also worsens hyponatremia
- Conditions necessary for the diagnosis of SIADH:
  - Hypoosmolality
  - Less than maximally dilute urine (urine osmolality > 100 mmol/kg; often urine osmolality > plasma osmolality, but this is not always seen)
  - Euvolemia
  - Absence of heart, liver, or kidney disease
  - Normal thyroid function
  - Normal adrenal function
  - No recent diuretic use

- Other typical features of SIADH:
  - Low plasma uric acid (usually <3 mg/dL with FE uric acid >10% increased plasma volume leads to uricosuria)
  - UNa > 40 mmol/L and FENa >1% (increased plasma volume leads to natriuresis)
  - FEurea > 55% (increased plasma volume decreases urea reabsorption)
  - Failure to correct hyponatremia with isotonic saline; sodium is excreted and water is retained, and thus worsening hyponatremia can ensue.
  - Correction of hyponatremia with fluid restriction
  - Elevated plasma ADH despite hypotonicity and euvolemia
- Causes of SIADH:
  - Cancer
  - Lung disease
  - CNS disease
  - Surgery (pain, stress)
  - Hereditary (NSIAD)
  - Idiopathic (usually in elderly patients)
  - Drugs. Many drugs have been reported to cause SIADH. They usually fall into one of the following categories:
    - Antiepileptic (e.g., carbamazepine)
    - Antipsychotic (e.g., selective serotonin reuptake inhibitors)
    - Chemotherapeutic (e.g., cyclophosphamide)
    - Thiazides—cause volume contraction with subsequent reabsorption of salt and water at the PT and decreased delivery of water to the collecting duct (Fichman et al., 1971).
    - Drugs that enhance ADH action (nonsteroidal anti-inflammatory drugs [NSAIDs], chlorpropamide)
- Treatment of SIADH:
  - Fluid restriction
  - Salt tablets
  - Demeclocycline 300 to 600 mg daily in divided doses (blocks effect of ADH)
  - Vasopressin receptor type 2 (V2) antagonists (e.g., tolvaptan 15–60 mg daily). Vaptans are only recommended for SIADH with chronic hyponatremia with plasma sodium between 120 and 132 mmol/L because they can potentially lead to rapid correction with more severe hyponatremia and can lead to transaminitis/liver toxicity. They are also very expensive.
  - Loop diuretics such as furosemide (Lasix) can cause net excretion of water and can be used in addition to fluid restriction.
  - Normal saline should generally not be used because it often leads to worsening of hyponatremia owing to excretion of administered sodium coupled with retention of water. Normal saline has 150 mmol/L NaCl with an osmolality of approximately 300 mmol/kg. The urine osmolality will generally be greater than the plasma osmolality due to the effect of ADH. If 1 liter of saline is administered, the sodium will be excreted but some of the water will be retained. For example, if the urine osmolality is 600 mmol/kg, half of the administered water is retained and hyponatremia will worsen.

Administration of loop diuretics such as furosemide to lower the urine osmolality to about 300 mmol/kg should prevent worsening hyponatremia if saline needs to be administered.

- Hypertonic (3%) saline may be necessary in symptomatic patients (see Question 5.1.8).

Question 5.1.7: What are the typical laboratory abnormalities in hyponatremia?

Laboratory Evaluation of Hyponatremia

- Plasma osmolality (low in hypotonic hyponatremia; see above)
- Urine osmolality (urine should be maximally dilute, i.e., $U_{osm} \sim 50$ mmol/L in the presence of hypoosmolality; however, generally urine is inappropriately concentrated, except in psychogenic polydipsia, reset osmostat, and beer drinker's syndrome).
- Low UNa (<10 mmol/L) or FENa $<1\%$ suggests extrarenal loss of sodium or an edematous disorder (in which kidneys are sodium avid, and thus causing edema, usually owing to a decrease in effective circulatory volume); "normal" UNa (>40 mmol/L) or FENa $>1\%$ suggests renal loss of sodium or excess ADH in the absence of renal sodium avidity, as in SIADH.
- Plasma urea nitrogen levels are typically increased in hypovolemic or hypervolemic hyponatremia (owing to increased PT urea reabsorption) and low or normal in euvolemic hyponatremia.
- Plasma uric acid levels are typically reduced in SIADH and CSW but elevated in most patients with hypovolemic or hypervolemic hyponatremia (owing to increased PT urate reabsorption).
- Thyroid-stimulating hormone (TSH) and plasma cortisol levels may indicate hypothyroidism or hypoadrenalism, respectively.
- CT of the head and radiography of the chest can be helpful if SIADH or CSW is suspected.

Question 5.1.8: How rapidly should the plasma sodium concentration be corrected?

The rate of correction of plasma sodium depends on the presence or absence of symptoms attributed to hyponatremia.

Symptoms of Hyponatremia

- With decreased sodium in the extracellular compartment, water moves into the cells and, in severe cases, causes cellular swelling.
- Because the calvarium cannot expand, brain swelling can be very symptomatic. Fatigue, headache, irritability, restlessness, loss of appetite, cramps, weakness, nausea, vomiting, confusion, decreased consciousness, hallucinations, convulsions, and coma may result.

Treatment of Hyponatremia

- Rate of correction is dependent on severity of problem, that is, whether hyponatremia is deemed to be acute or chronic.
- Hypovolemic hyponatremia is generally treated with isotonic saline.
- Hypervolemic hyponatremia is generally treated with fluid restriction and diuretics.
- Euvolemic hyponatremia (e.g., SIADH) is treated as follows:

- Mild asymptomatic hyponatremia should be considered a diagnostic clue but does not mandate treatment.
- More severe asymptomatic hyponatremia (i.e., plasma sodium < 125 mmol/L) should be treated with water restriction, salt tablets, and/or loop diuretics.
- Vasopressin receptor antagonists (vaptans) can be used for the treatment of euvolemic (and hypervolemic) hyponatremia (with the caveats given above). Conivaptan is currently available for intravenous (IV) treatment and tolvaptan for oral treatment in the United States.
- Symptomatic hyponatremia (confusion, seizures, coma due to hyponatremia) is considered a medical emergency. The optimal treatment has been the source of much controversy and a host of articles in the medical literature. However, it can be summarized as follows:
  - Initial treatment with hypertonic (3%) saline (513 mmol/L) is appropriate. However, the magnitude of correction should not exceed 10 mmol/L from baseline (e.g., from 100 to 110 mmol/L). The rate of correction should not exceed 2 mmol/L/h (some recommend slower rates of correction).
  - In the absence of overt volume depletion, a loop diuretic, such as furosemide, may be administered to "fix" urinary sodium concentration, usually at about 75 mmol/L. Theoretically, the patient will then lose more water than sodium in the urine, and the sodium lost can be replaced by hypertonic saline. This is particularly useful in patients with SIADH, in whom urine sodium losses will otherwise be very high during hypertonic saline administration (Hantman et al., 1973).
  - Greater acute increases in plasma sodium concentration must be strictly avoided to avoid the complication of osmotic demyelination syndrome (ODS) (Sterns et al., 1986), which is frequently fatal (see below). ODS has been associated with rapid correction or overcorrection of hyponatremia and is due to cerebral dehydration. Remember that even in symptomatic hyponatremia, the amount of excess brain water cannot exceed 10% above normal because of the limited ability of the brain to swell in the cranial cavity. Therefore, ~10% increase in plasma sodium and plasma osmolality should restore brain water to the normal range.
  - In patients in whom hyponatremia is known to be chronic and who have only mild symptoms, a rate of correction should not exceed 0.5 mmol/L/h (Sterns et al., 1986) and should not exceed 8 mmoL/L over 24 hours.

Important Points to Remember
- Hyponatremia usually indicates impaired urinary dilution, because of either high ADH or ADH-independent intrarenal mechanisms. Rarely, diluting ability is normal, as in psychogenic polydipsia, reset osmostat, and decreased solute excretion (beer drinker's syndrome).
- In hypovolemic hyponatremia, osmoreceptors and volume receptors receive opposing stimuli (low osmolality and low

volume, respectively). This causes the osmoreceptors to lower their set point. Thus, ADH is secreted even in the presence of hypoosmolality.

■ In edematous disorders, both sodium and water retention occur. In CHF, the aortic and carotid sinus baroreceptors sense decreased effective blood volume (because of decreased cardiac output) and stimulate ADH release (Quillen et al., 1988). In cirrhosis, there is decreased effective blood volume and enhanced ADH release because of systemic vasodilation and decreased intrathoracic blood volume. In addition, hypoalbuminemia and third-spacing may decrease plasma volume and stimulate ADH release. In nephrotic syndrome, hypoalbuminemia-induced intravascular volume contraction may occur and stimulate ADH release. Intrarenal mechanisms may also be operative. In renal failure, hyponatremia may occur because of a decrease in free water clearance coupled with increased fluid intake.

CASE STUDY 5.1 CONCLUDED

The final diagnosis is CSW. The patient is treated with physiologic (0.9%) saline, and plasma [Na$^+$] increases to 133 mmol/L over 24 hours. He is then started on salt tablets, and the plasma [Na$^+$] remains in the 135 range. Two weeks later, salt tablets are discontinued and hyponatremia does not recur.

CASE STUDY

A 54-year-old male with liver cirrhosis and ischemic heart disease presents with nausea, vomiting, heartburn, chest pain, and muscle cramps. He smokes 1 ppd and admits to heavy ethanol intake. He denies other drug use and is single and not sexually active. He is not taking any medications.

Physical examination:
Vitals: pulse 86 beats/min; respiratory rate 20 breaths/min; blood pressure 116/74 mm Hg; temperature 98°F, weight 66.7 kg
Chest: clear
Heart: S1 and S2 no murmurs
Abdomen: soft; no shifting dullness
Lower extremities: no edema
Skin: normal
Neurologic: no focal findings

Blood chemistry:
Sodium: 120 mmol/L
Potassium: 1.6 mmol/L
Chloride: 82 mmol/L
Total CO_2: 35 mmol/L
Urea nitrogen: 6 mg/dL (urea: 2.1 mmol/L)
Creatinine: 1.0 mg/dL (88.4 mcmol/L)
Glucose: 90 mg/dL (5 mmol/L)
Calcium: 6.2 mg/dL (1.55 mmol/L)
Magnesium: 1.0 mg/dL (0.41 mmol/L)
Osmolality (measured): 250 mmol/kg
Osmolality (calculated): 246 mmol/kg

Urine chemistry:
Osmolality: 80 mmol/kg
Sodium: 15 mmol/L
Potassium: 5 mmol/L

Complete blood count:
WBC: 8,500/mm^3
Hemoglobin: 11 g/dL (160 g/L)
Hematocrit: 33%
Platelets: 125,000/mm^3

Lipid Profile:
Total cholesterol: 200 mg/dL (5.2 mmol/L)
Triglycerides: 450 mg/dL (5.1 mmol/L)
Troponin $\times$ 3, negative
EKG, normal sinus rhythm, no ischemic changes
CT head, negative
CT chest, negative for pulmonary embolism

Question 5.2.1: What is the differential diagnosis?

CASE STUDY 5.2 CONTINUED

Similar to the first patient, this patient also has hypoosmolar hyponatremia. On clinical examination, however, he appears euvolemic (jugular venous pressure is normal, no orthostasis, no edema). Also, as opposed to the first patient, both plasma and urine osmolality are low. Therefore, he does not have inappropriate antidiuresis, i.e., he is forming an appropriately dilute urine.

Question 5.2.2: What is the most likely diagnosis?

- There are three conditions that can result in hyponatremia with appropriately dilute urine: (1) psychogenic polydipsia, (2) beer drinker's potomania (also known as "tea-and-toast" hyponatremia), and (3) reset osmostat.
- **Psychogenic Polydipsia:**
  - Psychogenic polydipsia (increased water intake) (Hariprasad et al., 1980)—this is rare, because if urinary diluting ability is normal, up to 20 L daily water intake can normally be excreted.
  - Therefore, do NOT use 3% saline in psychogenic polydipsia even if hyponatremia is symptomatic because there will be a rapid increase in plasma sodium concentration with fluid restriction alone.
- **Beer drinker's syndrome ("potomania")**
  - A healthy person ingesting a usual diet typically has an osmole excretion of 600 to 900 mmol/day. These osmoles come from dietary electrolytes and protein (10 g of protein produces ~50 mmol urea). In this case, with normal urine dilution, >12 to 18 L of water must be ingested to overwhelm the capacity of the kidney to excrete water (this is what occurs in psychogenic polydipsia).
  - Beer has very little sodium and has no protein. Moreover, it has some caloric content that prevents protein breakdown from occurring. In patients subsisting on beer alone, obligatory daily

solute excretion is very low (e.g., 200 mmol/day). Even with maximal urinary dilution ($U_{osm} \sim 50$ mmol/kg), fluid intake >4 L leads to hyponatremia.

- Typical presentation:
  - Excessive beer drinking
  - Often, there is a history of recent binge drinking or illness, which may precipitate a rapid drop in plasma [Na^+], leading to neurologic symptoms such as confusion, altered mental status, or gait disturbance.
  - Hypokalemia (because of decreased potassium intake)
  - Low plasma urea nitrogen (because of low protein intake)
  - Brisk diuresis if solute intake is increased
  - Low urine [Na^+] and osmolality
- Pathophysiology:
  - ADH is low
  - Brisk diuresis with solute intake (recommendation is to keep NPO for 24 hours)
  - Brisk diuresis also occurs with isotonic saline
  - Rapid rise in plasma sodium can occur and the risk of ODS is very high (see below for further discussion of ODS)

- **Reset Osmostat**
  - This is a variant of SIADH in which the threshold for ADH secretion is reset such that ADH is secreted at a plasma osmolality lower than 280 to 285 mmol/kg, which is the usual threshold for ADH release. The kidney retains the ability to appropriately concentrate and dilute the urine.
  - Causes include chronic illness, malnutrition, epilepsy, quadriplegia (Leehey et al., 1988), neurologic disorders, pregnancy, and malignancy.
  - Reset osmostat should be suspected if SIADH seems like the likely diagnosis, but there is little or no response to fluid restriction. In such a case, a water loading test can aid in the diagnosis.
  - Water loading test:
    - A water load consisting of 20 mL/kg is administered
    - If >80% of the water load is excreted within 4 hours and the urine osmolality decreases to <100 mmol/kg, reset osmostat is the likely diagnosis

CASE STUDY 5.2 CONTINUED

Hyponatremia, hypokalemia, hypocalcemia, hypoalbuminemia, and hypomagnesemia point to beer drinker's syndrome. Although a similar constellation of laboratory abnormalities can be seen in proximal tubulopathy (Fanconi syndrome), urinary loss rather than decreased intake is responsible for the electrolyte disturbances in that disorder. The low urine sodium and potassium in our patient point to decreased intake.

Clinical course: The patient is given IV potassium, calcium, and magnesium. In addition, fluid restriction of 1.8 L/day is instituted. He is given a regular diet. At 8 hours, the plasma sodium concentration has increased to 125 mmol/L.

When the duration of hyponatremia is unknown, the hyponatremia should be assumed to be chronic. In chronic hyponatremia, the goal is an increase in plasma sodium of no more than 8 mmol/L in 24 hours at a rate of no more than 0.5 mmol/L/h. In this case, the plasma sodium has already increased by 5 mmol/L in only 8 hours, exceeding the desired rate of correction. Because the urine is very dilute, it is appropriate to start 5% dextrose in water (D5W) to match the urine output and monitor the plasma sodium every 2 hours.

Question 5.2.3: What should be done next?

CASE STUDY 5.2 CONTINUED

Despite D5W, the plasma sodium continues to increase to 130 mmol/L at 10 hours after presentation. He becomes obtunded and is noted to have brisk reflexes, dysarthria, and inability to chew or speak.

Question 5.2.4: What is the reason for worsening clinical status?

- **Osmotic demyelination syndrome (ODS)**
  - In acute symptomatic hyponatremia, movement of water into brain cells leads to brain edema. However, in chronic hyponatremia, brain cell adaptation to hypotonicity of ECF occurs; the mechanism involves efflux of electrolytes and intracellular organic osmoles from cells
  - Rapid correction of hyponatremia increases extracellular osmolality, resulting in movement of water out of the brain and cell shrinkage. Although this is beneficial in restoring normal brain cell volume in acute hyponatremia, it is deleterious if brain cell volume is normal or near-normal in chronic hyponatremia
  - Oligodendrocytes are very sensitive to osmotic stress, resulting in ODS
  - Clinical presentation
    - Neurologic findings include upper motor neuron deficits, pseudobulbar palsy, spastic quadriparesis, confusion, and coma
    - May not present until 2 to 3 days after correction of plasma sodium
    - Can be biphasic with initial improvement of mental status after raising plasma sodium followed by subsequent decline
  - Diagnosis
    - Magnetic resonance imaging (MRI) shows hyperintense lesions on T2-weighted images in central pons, medulla oblongata, and mesencephalon
  - Treatment
    - Reverse overcorrection of hyponatremia with D5W and/or desmopressin.

Question 5.2.5: What should one do if a patient develops ODS?

Overcorrection of plasma sodium not adequately responsive to D5W, especially when it is accompanied by clinical findings of ODS, requires immediate lowering of the plasma sodium with desmopressin.

Indications for desmopressin include the following: (1) diuresis occurs at an excessive rate (i.e., unable to be matched by D5W); (2) 24-hour goal for change in plasma sodium has been exceeded or is predicted to do so despite D5W; and (3) symptoms of ODS develop (Sanghvi et al., 2007).

CASE STUDY 5.2 CONCLUDED

Clinical course: Desmopressin 2 mcg IV q8h is started.
At 14 hours, plasma sodium has decreased again to 125 mmol/L, which is finally at goal.
At 24 hours, plasma sodium is 128 mmol/L, and desmopressin and D5W are stopped. Fortunately, the neurologic symptoms improve.

Question 5.2.6: **What is the ideal way to treat beer drinker's potomania?**

Patients undergoing a water diuresis may have a rapid increase in plasma sodium. In acute hyponatremia, this will not pose a clinical problem, but in chronic hyponatremia (such as malnourished patients with low solute intake), there is a high risk of ODS.
- Prevention of ODS in high-risk patients:
  - NPO except medications for 24 hours
  - NO IV saline if possible
  - Check plasma sodium every 2 hours
  - Goals: plasma [Na$^+$] increase <8 mmol/L in first 24 hours and any subsequent 24-hour period. Avoid overcorrection!
  - Relower plasma sodium levels if necessary
  - If caloric intake is needed, use D5W

CASE STUDY

A 40-year-old healthy male weighing 70 kg runs a marathon for the first time. The ambient temperature was 77°F and the humidity was 45%. He later relates that he experienced thirst, nausea, shakiness, leg cramps, and dizziness during the last hour of the marathon. He also estimates that he drank about 10 L of fluid during the marathon, of which half was Gatorade and half bottled water. He did not urinate during the marathon. Shortly after crossing the finish line, he has a seizure and is attended by paramedics on the scene. He is given 100 mL of 3% saline (sodium concentration 513 mmol/L) and is sent by ambulance to the nearest emergency room (ER).

Physical examination (in ER):

Vitals: pulse 115 beats/min; respiratory rate 24 breaths/min; blood pressure 110/70 mm Hg; temperature 98°F; oxygen saturation 96%

HEENT: normal extraocular movements
Chest: clear
Heart: tachycardic, RRR
Abdomen: soft, nontender

Skin: diaphoretic
Neurologic: obtunded, no
    focal findings

Blood chemistry:
Sodium: 125 mmol/L
Potassium: 3.0 mmol/L
Chloride: 85 mmol/L
Total CO_2: 20 mmol/L
Urea nitrogen: 6 mg/dL
    (urea: 2.1 mmol/L)
Creatinine: 1.0 mg/dL (88.4
    mcmol/L)

Glucose: 90 mg/dL (5 mmol/L)
Osmolality (measured): 260
    mmol/kg
Osmolality (calculated): 256
    mmol/kg
Creatinine kinase (CK): 2,000
    U/L (20 mckat/L)

Urine chemistry:
Osmolality: 80 mmol/kg
Sodium: 15 mmol/L
Potassium: 5 mmol/L
CT head, negative

Question 5.3.1: What is the cause of his neurologic symptoms?

- **Exercise-induced hyponatremia (EAH)**
    This patient has developed acute hyponatremia during marathon running. This is primarily due to nonosmotic ADH release (possibly because of exercise itself or other nonosmotic stimuli such as pain, stress, and nausea) coupled with fluid intake in excess of what he can excrete through sweat and respiration (Siegel, 2015). Gatorade has been developed to replace sweat losses and thus contains amounts of electrolytes (sodium plus potassium of 23 mmol/L) designed to be sufficient to prevent electrolyte depletion from sweating. However, this patient also drinks ~5 L of additional electrolyte-free water, which can explain the hyponatremia.

    The degree of hyponatremia can be predicted from the following equation:

    Initial plasma sodium concentration (Na_i) × initial total body water (TBW_i) = final plasma sodium concentration (Na_f) × final total body water (TBW_f)

    In this patient, assuming he lost 5 L of sweat during the race but drank 10 L of fluid:

    $$TBW_i = (0.6 \times 70 \text{ kg}) = 42 \text{ L}$$

    $$TBW_f = TBW_i + 5 \text{ L} = 47 \text{ L}$$

    $$Na_i = 140 \text{ mmol/L}$$

    Therefore, $Na_f = (Na_i \times TBW_i)/TBW_f = (140 \times 42)/47 = 125$ mmol/L

    When a patient presents with hyponatremia, use the free water excess (deficit) formula, which is based on the same equation:

    Free water excess = ($TBW_f - TBW_i$) = [($Na_i \times TBW_i$)/Na_f] − $TBW_i = TBW_i$ [(Na_i/Na_f) − 1]

    In this case, free water excess = 42 [(140/125) − 1] = 5 L

    The urine osmolality is appropriately dilute, indicating that ADH is now suppressed (though it may have been elevated during the race).

Question 5.3.2: How aggressively should you treat the hyponatremia?

CASE STUDY 5.3 CONTINUED

This is a case of acute, symptomatic hyponatremia that requires rapid correction. Neurologic symptoms are as a result of water movement into the brain cells resulting in brain swelling and increased ICP. The patient receives appropriate treatment on the scene, but he is still hyponatremic and obtunded and, therefore, should receive additional 3% saline. As opposed to the previous patient, there is no concern about the development of ODS because this is acute hyponatremia and there was no time for brain adaptation (solute egress from brain cells) to occur.

It is elected to administer 3% saline by infusion until the plasma sodium is normalized (135 mmol/L).

Question 5.3.3: How much 3% saline would you predict would be needed?

In this case, we want to calculate the effect of administered sodium on the plasma sodium concentration. For simplicity, we will disregard the small volume of fluid administered and assume that there are no fluid and/or electrolyte losses during the infusion:

When sodium is administered, it enters the ECF. However, fluid movement from the ICF to the ECF (because of increase in osmolality in the ECF) will occur. Therefore, we need to think of sodium as moving into TBW. If we assume TBW is still 47 L and want to raise the plasma sodium by 10 to 135 mmol/L, the amount of sodium that will need to be administered is 470 mmol. Since 3% saline contains 513 mmol/L, this would be ~900 mL of 3% saline.

Based on this calculation, one would expect that it would be necessary to administer 3% saline at 150 mL/h for 6 hours, measuring plasma sodium every 2 hours. A quick "rule of thumb" when deciding how much hypertonic saline to administer is that 1 mL/kg of 3% saline is expected to increase plasma sodium by about 1 mmol/L.

Because in real life things are more complicated (the above patient would be expected to have ongoing insensible water losses and urinary water losses), it would be prudent to administer 3% saline at a somewhat slower rate and measure plasma sodium every 1 to 2 hours to guide therapy. It is also important to recognize that any potassium administered to correct the hypokalemia will also increase total body electrolyte content and thus plasma sodium concentration. This is because the administered potassium will enter the ICF leading to water movement into cells.

CASE STUDY 5.3 CONCLUDED

Clinical course: A 500 mL bag of 3% saline containing 40 mEq/L potassium is administered at 100 mL/h. After 5 hours, the plasma sodium concentration has increased from 125 to 135 mmol/L and the patient's mental status becomes normal. The infusion is stopped, and he is discharged from the ER and advised to limit free water ingestion during future marathon running.

Question 5.3.4: How much water should one drink in a marathon?

Adhere to the following guidelines:

A: Do practice runs

B: Weight yourself every hour

C: Drink 16 oz for every 1lb weight loss OR drink 400-800 mL/hr (14-27 fl oz/h)

D: Don't force fluid consumption

E: No NSAIDs

F: Drink less if stomach becomes queasy/sloshy

G: Drink sports drinks (although it isn't proven that they are better than water)

H: Don't drink immediately after a marathon

I: Risk factors for hyponatremia are: weight gain, run > 4h, and small or large BMI

HYPERNATREMIA

Etiology of Hypernatremia (Table 5.2)

- Sodium is the primary determinant of plasma osmolality; hypernatremia is thus always a hypertonic or hyperosmolar condition. Plasma osmolality = $2 \times$ Na (mmol/L) + urea nitrogen (mg/dL)/2.8 + glucose (mg/dL)/18. Alternatively, $2 \times$ Na (mmol/L) + urea (mmol/L) + glucose (mmol/L).

- Hypernatremia occurs only when hyperosmolality is accompanied by an impaired thirst mechanism (Zerbe & Robertson, 1983) or when water ingestion is restricted.

- In response to hypernatremia, water moves out of cells with a resulting decrease in brain volume. The brain responds by

TABLE 5.2	Hypernatremia		
	Hypovolemic	**Euvolemic**	**Hypervolemic**
$FENa < 1$; $U_{osm} > P_{osm}$	$FENa > 1$; $U_{osm} \sim P_{osm}$	$FENa$ usually <1; $U_{osm} < P_{osm}$ in DI; U_{osm} usually $> P_{osm}$ in other conditions	$FENa > 1$; $U_{osm} > P_{osm}$
Gastrointestinal or sweat losses	Osmotic diuresis	DI	Primary aldosteronism
	Diuretics	Partial DI	Hypertonic fluids
	Postobstruction	Nephrogenic DI	Salt-water drowning/salt poisoning
	Salt-wasting nephropathy	Hypodipsia	
		Respiratory or sweat (insensible) loss	

DI, diabetes insipidus.

intracellular uptake of electrolytes, amino acids, and other organic solutes. Therefore, rapid hydration can cause cerebral edema.

Pathogenesis of Hypernatremia

- Hypernatremia = increased $[Na^+]$ = decrease in TBW relative to $TBNa^+$. Some examples are as follows:
  - ↓ TBW with normal $TBNa^+$. This is typical of two clinical conditions: (1) patients in nursing homes with decreased thirst or inability to drink water; (2) diabetes insipidus (DI), in which ADH release is impaired or absent (central DI or CDI) or the kidney does not respond to ADH (nephrogenic DI or NDI).
  - ↓↓ TBW with ↓ $TBNa^+$. This can occur when water losses exceed sodium losses from sweat, gastrointestinal (GI) tract, or kidneys.
  - Normal TBW with ↑ $TBNa^+$. This is usually iatrogenic owing to administration of hypertonic fluids or isotonic fluids in the setting of renal water losses (i.e., concentration of sodium in administered fluid is greater than urinary concentration).
  - Again, it should be obvious that the plasma sodium concentration per se gives no information about the $TBNa^+$.

- In the presence of ADH, normal kidneys can concentrate urine to a urine osmolality of 1,200 mmol/kg (in older patients, urine osmolality generally will increase only to the 700–1,000 mmol/kg range). Thus, if the daily solute load is 600 mmol/day, urine output can be as low as 500 mL/day (with lesser daily solute loads, daily urine output can be theoretically even lower when maximally concentrated). These low urinary volumes will minimize renal water loss if water intake is impaired. However, remember that insensible water loss (primarily via respiration) is about 500 to 700 mL/day. Therefore, even when there is maximum antidiuresis, total cessation of water intake will lead to hypernatremia over a period of hours to a few days (desert animals such as the kangaroo rat can concentrate urine to >5,000 mmol/kg and thus can live without water for much longer than can humans!)

CASE STUDY

5.4

A 35-year-old female with juvenile rheumatoid arthritis (JRA) treated with NSAIDs presents with complaints of 1 week of nausea and fatigue. She denies vomiting. She feels malaise, fatigue, and diffuse body pain and feels sleepy all day. She has had persistent low-grade fever. The patient thinks this is typical of her rheumatoid flares. During hospitalization, she develops headaches, nuchal rigidity, photophobia, and encephalopathy.

Physical examination:

Vitals: pulse 110 beats/min; respiratory rate 20 breaths/min; blood pressure 100/60 mm Hg; temperature 101°F; oxygen saturation 94%

HEENT: no abnormalities

Heart: RRR, no murmurs/rubs/gallops, jugular veins flat
Lungs: clear
Abdomen: soft, nontender
Extremities: no edema
Skin: decreased skin turgor
Neurologic: drowsy, no focal findings
Workup for infectious etiology of fever and obtundation is nega-
   tive. Despite copious IV fluids and multiple antibiotics, fever
   of unknown origin persists. Subsequently, it is noted that the
   patient is excreting in excess of 300 mL of urine per hour.

Blood chemistry:
Sodium: 150 mmol/L
Potassium: 4.0 mmol/L
Chloride: 116 mmol/L
Total CO_2: 24 mmol/L
Urea nitrogen: 6 mg/dL (urea: 2.1 mmol/L)
Creatinine: 0.5 mg/dL (44.2 mcmol/L)
Glucose: 90 mg/dL (5 mmol/L)
Total calcium: 7.8 mg/dL (1.9 mmol/L)
Albumin: 1.5 g/dL (15 g/L)
Ionized calcium: 1.2 mmol/L
Osmolality (measured): 310 mmol/kg
Osmolality (calculated): 306 mmol/kg

Complete blood count:
WBC: 17,000/mm^3
Hemoglobin: 8.6 g/dL (86 g/L)
Hematocrit: 27%
Platelets: 236,000/mm^{3}CT head, negative
Urinalysis: specific gravity 1.005, pH 7.0, protein negative, RBC
   none, WBC <1/hpf, no bacteria
A nephrology consult is placed for hypernatremia and polyuria.

Question 5.4.1:   **What kind of hypernatremia is present in this patient?**

Hypernatremia is always associated with hyperosmolality. As with
hyponatremia, hypernatremia can be divided into hypovolemic, euvolemic, and hypervolemic types based on clinical evaluation (examination of neck veins, skin turgor, mucous membranes, orthostatic
changes in pulse and/or blood pressure, presence or absence of edema).

- **Hypovolemic hypernatremia** implies a decrease in TBNa$^+$ be-
  cause of either of the following:
  - Renal Na$^+$ losses—diuretics (with inadequate water intake),
    osmotic diuresis (due to hyperglycemia, mannitol, urea, or so-
    dium chloride), postobstructive diuresis, tubular injury (recov-
    ery phase of acute tubular necrosis [ATN])
  - Extrarenal Na$^+$ losses—sweating, diarrhea, vomiting (with inad-
    equate water intake)
- **Euvolemic hypernatremia** implies pure water loss with normal
  or near-normal TBNa$^+$
  - CDI (trauma, brain injury, space-occupying lesions, infections,
    mutations in the *AVP* gene, idiopathic tumor)

- ■ NDI (congenital, drugs, hypercalcemia, tubular disease) (Morello & Bichet, 2001) (see below)
- ■ Decreased water intake ("nursing home syndrome")
- ■ **Hypervolemic hypernatremia** implies hypertonic water gain
  - ■ Iatrogenic administration of hypertonic fluid (hypertonic saline, bicarbonate, etc.)
  - ■ Mineralocorticoid excess states (e.g., hyperaldosteronism)—causes mild hypernatremia
  - ■ Salt poisoning (and seawater ingestion)

CASE STUDY 5.4 CONTINUED

This patient appears hypovolemic on examination (flat neck veins, decreased skin turgor). She does not appear to have had extrarenal water losses as she was not sweating profusely and there is no history of diarrhea or vomiting, though she has nausea. The observation that she is profoundly polyuric speaks to renal water loss leading to a decrease in TBW relative to total body sodium as the mechanism of hypernatremia. She has not taken diuretics, there is no evidence of tubular injury, and there is no reason to suspect partial obstruction to urine flow.

Urine chemistry:
Sodium: 80 mmol/L
Potassium: 20 mmol/L
Osmolality: 290 mmol/L

Question 5.4.2: What further laboratory evaluation is needed?

Urine electrolytes and osmolality are needed to determine the cause of polyuria and to calculate the electrolyte-free water clearance (CeH_2O),

$$CeH_2O = V\,[1 - ((UNa + UK)/PNa)]$$

What is the electrolyte-free water clearance and how is the formula derived?

Over 50 years ago, Homer Smith (1952) introduced the concept that the urine flow could be thought of as two separate compartments: one component containing osmotically active particles (osmoles) at the same concentration as that present in the plasma, and the other component consisting of either free water excreted (when the kidney is forming dilute urine) or free water reabsorbed (when the kidney is forming concentrated urine). Thus,

$$V = C_{osm} + CH_2O$$

where V is urine flow, C_{osm} is osmolal clearance, and CH_2O is free water clearance.

The volume of plasma that is cleared of osmoles per unit time (C_{osm}) × plasma osmolality (P_{osm}) is equal to the urinary excretion of osmoles (urine osmolality [U_{osm}] × urine flow). In mathematical form,

$$C_{osm} \times P_{osm} = U_{osm} \times V$$

$$C_{osm} = (U_{osm} \times V)/P_{osm}$$

Therefore,

$$CH_2O = V - C_{osm} = V - (U_{osm} \times V/P_{osm}) = V(1 - U_{osm}/P_{osm})$$

Electrolyte-free water clearance (CeH_2O) is the clearance of water free of electrolytes (sodium, potassium, and accompanying anions) but not other solutes. Urine contains many other osmotically active particles, such as urea and ammonium, in addition to electrolytes. Excretion of these substances does not aid in predicting the response to fluid management in dysnatremic states.

To derive the formula for CeH_2O, one substitutes electrolyte clearance (approximated by the clearance of the sum of sodium and potassium) for C_{osm}. Thus, the term C_{osm} is replaced by $C(Na + K)$. This results in:

$$CeH_2O = V[1 - ((UNa + UK)/PNa)]$$

Another calculation we will want is the urinary total solute (UTS) excretion, which is simply: $U_{osm} \times V$. This is very helpful in the evaluation of polyuria.

Polyuria can result from water diuresis, solute diuresis, or mixed diuresis.

■ In water diuresis, $U_{osm} < 150$ mmol/kg, that is, urine is dilute.
■ In solute diuresis, the concentrating and diluting abilities of the kidney are both compromised, resulting in a tendency toward isosmotic urine (~300 mmol/kg).
■ In a mixed diuresis, U_{osm} will be in the 150 to 299 mmol/kg range.

CASE STUDY 5.4 CONTINUED

In our case, U_{osm} is 290, suggesting a mixed diuresis.

The 24-hour urine volume in this patient is 7.2 L (300 mL/h)

$$UTS = U_{osm} \times V = 290 \text{ mmol/kg} \times 7.2 \text{ L} = 2,088 \text{ mOsm}$$

A UTS >1,400 indicates a solute diuresis (Oster et al., 1997). In "real life", a UTS >1000 is suggestive of a solute diuresis.

$$CeH_2O = V[1 - ((UNa + UK)/PNa)] = 7.2[1 - ((80 + 20)/150)] = 2.4 \text{ L/day}$$

This means that the kidney is excreting over 2 L of electrolyte-free water daily. Therefore, there is also an electrolyte-free water diuresis in addition to the solute diuresis. Solute diuresis causes medullary washout leading to inability to concentrate the urine in response to ADH; hence, an acquired NDI.

Question 5.4.3: **What is the cause of the solute diuresis?**

One must establish whether this is an electrolyte or nonelectrolyte diuresis.

The most common causative electrolytes are Na, K, Cl, and bicarbonate. The most common causative nonelectrolytes are glucose, urea, and mannitol.

To distinguish between electrolyte and nonelectrolyte diuresis, one must calculate the urinary electrolyte (UE) and urinary nonelectrolyte (UNE) content.

$$UE = (2[UNa + UK]) \times \text{urine volume (V)}$$

UE >600 mOsm/day suggests electrolyte diuresis

$$UNE = UTS - UE$$

UNE >600 mOsm/day suggests nonelectrolyte diuresis

CASE STUDY 5.4 CONCLUDED

In our patient,

$$UE = 2\,(80+20) \times 7.2 = 1{,}440 \text{ mmol}$$

$$UNE = UTS - UE = 2{,}088 - 1{,}440 = 648 \text{ mmol}$$

Therefore, this is both an electrolyte and nonelectrolyte diuresis, though predominantly an electrolyte diuresis. The electrolyte diuresis was as a result of IV saline administration and the nonelectrolyte diuresis probably due to fever and catabolic state resulting in increased urea generation.

IV fluids and antibiotics are discontinued and the patient is allowed to drink to thirst. Fevers resolved on their own, and she has made an uneventful recovery and is subsequently discharged.

CASE STUDY

A 60-year-old female presents with bitemporal hemianopsia due to a pituitary tumor and undergoes resection of a prolactinoma. Postoperatively, she develops polyuria and hypernatremia.

Physical Examination:
Vitals: pulse 70 beats/min; respiratory rate 16 breaths/min; blood pressure 130/80 mm Hg; temperature 99°F; oxygen saturation 99% on room air
HEENT: no abnormalities
Heart: RRR, no murmurs
Lungs: clear to auscultation
Abdomen: soft, nontender
Extremities: no edema
Neurologic: no visual deficits
Skin: normal turgor

Blood Chemistry:
Sodium: 150 mmol/L
Potassium: 4.0 mmol/L
Chloride: 116 mmol/L
Total CO_2: 24 mmol/L
Urea nitrogen: 24 mg/dL (urea: 8.6 mmol/L)
Creatinine: 0.5 mg/dL (44.2 mcmol/L)

Glucose: 90 mg/dL (5 mmol/L)
Osmolality (measured): 310 mmol/kg
Osmolality (calculated): 306 mmol/kg

Urine Chemistry:
Osmolality: 100 mmol/kg
Sodium: 15 mmol/L
Potassium, 10 mmol/L
The 24-hour urine volume is 6 L

Question 5.5.1: What kind of hypernatremia is present?

Clinically, the patient is euvolemic (normal vitals and skin turgor with no edema).

- Euvolemic hypernatremia implies pure water loss with normal or near-normal TBNa$^+$
- CDI (trauma, brain injury, space-occupying lesions, infections, mutations in the *AVP* gene)
- NDI (congenital, drugs, hypercalcemia, tubular disease) (Morello & Bichet, 2001) (see below)
- Decreased water intake ("nursing home syndrome")

Question 5.5.2: Is this a water diuresis, a solute diuresis, or a mixed diuresis?

UTS = $100 \times 6 = 600$ mmol. Thus, there is no evidence of a solute diuresis.

$$CeH_2O = 6\,[1 - (15 + 10)/150)] = 5 \text{ L}$$

Since $U_{osm} << P_{osm}$, with $U_{osm} < 150$ mmol/kg, this is a pure water diuresis, and the patient has DI.

Question 5.5.3: How do you distinguish CDI from NDI?

- Differentiating between CDI and NDI in polyuric patients
  - Differential diagnosis of polyuria:
    - Primary polydipsia (low or low-normal plasma sodium and osmolality)
    - CDI (high or high-normal plasma sodium and osmolality)
    - NDI (high or high-normal plasma sodium and osmolality)
  - Water restriction test and administration of desmopressin can usually differentiate between CDI and NDI
  - Water restriction test
    - Measure urine volume and osmolality hourly and plasma sodium and osmolality every 2 hours beginning 2 hours after restricting water
    - $U_{osm} > 600$ mmol/kg in the face of hypernatremia is normal
    - U_{osm} consistently <600 mmol/kg with $P_{osm} > 295$ mmol/kg and/or PNa > 145 mmol/L suggests DI
    - Obtain plasma sample for AVP, then administer 4 mcg of desmopressin
      - In NDI, plasma AVP is high and there will be little or no response to DDAVP

- In CDI, plasma AVP is low and there will be a marked response to DDAVP
- Measurement of copeptin, the C-terminal glycoprotein moiety of pro-AVP. A baseline copeptin level >21.4 pmol/L is diagnostic of NDI (Timper et al., 2015). A recent study suggests that hypertonic saline–stimulated plasma copeptin is superior to the water deprivation test in the diagnosis of DI (Fenske et al., 2018)

CASE STUDY 5.5 CONTINUED

Clinical course: In this patient, a water deprivation test is unnecessary since P_{osm} > 295 mmol/kg and P[Na^+] >145 mmol/L, so an AVP level and DDAVP (desmopressin) challenge are performed. After DDAVP, U_{osm} has increased to 600 mmol/kg. Plasma AVP later appears as undetectable, consistent with CDI.

Question 5.5.4: **What is the etiology of CDI in this case?**

CDI is due to disruption of the hypothalamic pituitary axis resulting in AVP secretion arrest on postoperative day 1.

CASE STUDY 5.5 CONTINUED

Clinical course: The patient is started on intranasal DDAVP two sprays twice daily; each spray is 0.1 mL, which is equivalent to 10 mcg DDAVP. On day 7, the plasma sodium is 125 mmol/L and plasma osmolality is 262 mmol/L. The urine osmolality has increased to 350 mmol/kg.

Question 5.5.5: **What is the reason for the development of hyponatremia?**

Typically, a week after pituitary surgery, there is neuronal degeneration leading to large amounts of AVP being released.

CASE STUDY 5.5 CONCLUDED

Clinical course: Exogenous DDAVP is discontinued. The patient is placed on fluid restriction. Over the next week, plasma sodium stabilizes at 135 mmol/L. The patient ultimately requires DDAVP but at a lower dose than before (10 mcg twice daily).

Question 5.5.6: **What if there is no response to DDAVP?**

This means that the collecting ducts are not responding to DDAVP or are resistant to DDAVP. This is known as nephrogenic diabetes insipidus (NDI).

- Nephrogenic diabetes insipidus (NDI)
  - Etiology: tubular dysfunction leading to decreased sensitivity to ADH
  - Causes:
    - Acute kidney injury (AKI), chronic kidney disease (CKD)
    - Hydronephrosis

- Electrolyte disorders: hypercalcemia, hypokalemia
- Medications: lithium, foscarnet, amphotericin, vaptans, demeclocycline
- Loss of function mutations: *V2R* gene, *Aquaporin-2* gene, *Aquaporin-1* gene
- Lithium-induced NDI
    - Lithium enters the principal cell through ENaC channels; amiloride, which blocks ENaC channels, can be used to treat lithium-induced NDI
    - Lithium causes tubulointerstitial nephritis and CKD, both of which can cause NDI
    - Lithium inhibits glycogen-synthase kinase 3, which is required for principal cells to respond to AVP
    - Lithium induces cyclooxygenase-2 (COX-2), which produces prostaglandins that inhibit AVP-stimulated salt transport in TAL and water transport in CD. However, it is not recommended to use NSAIDs to treat NDI.

CASE STUDY

A 90-year-old female is admitted from a nursing home with obtundation. She has not been eating and drinking for the past week. There is no history of vomiting or diarrhea. She was reported to weigh 60 kg and had a plasma sodium concentration of 140 mmol/L 1 week ago.

Physical examination:
Vitals: pulse 70 beats/min; respiratory rate 16 breaths/min; blood pressure 110/70 mm Hg; temperature 98°F; oxygen saturation 99% on room air
HEENT: atraumatic
Chest: clear
Heart: soft systolic ejection murmurs
Abdomen: soft, nontender
Skin: normal turgor
Neurologic: no focal findings

Blood chemistry:
Sodium: 160 mmol/L
Potassium: 4.0 mmol/L
Chloride: 126 mmol/L
Total CO_2: 24 mmol/L
Urea nitrogen: 24 mg/dL (urea: 8.6 mmol/L)
Creatinine: 0.5 mg/dL (44.2 mcmol/L)
Glucose: 90 mg/dL (5 mmol/L)
Osmolality (measured): 310 mmol/kg
Osmolality (calculated): 306 mmol/kg

Urine chemistry:
Sodium: 10 mmol/L
Potassium: 20 mmol/L
Osmolality: 600 mmol/kg

Question 5.6.1: What is the cause of the hypernatremia?

CASE STUDY 5.6 CONTINUED

This patient is clinically euvolemic despite marked hypernatremia. She has not been eating and drinking, but her kidneys have been able to conserve sodium to the extent that she has not become hypovolemic and she has had no extrarenal sodium losses. Her urine is concentrated, which has limited but not eliminated free water loss, and she has continued to have insensible water losses, leading to hypernatremia.

Question 5.6.2: What is the most appropriate management?

CASE STUDY 5.6 CONTINUED

As she is hemodynamically stable and is dehydrated but not clinically sodium (volume) depleted, administration of D5W is appropriate.

The first step is to calculate free water deficit.

The degree of hypernatremia can be predicted from the following equation:

Initial plasma sodium concentration (Na_i) × initial total body water (TBW_i) = final plasma sodium concentration (Na_f) × final total body water (TBW_f)

$$TBW_f = (0.5 \times 60 \text{ kg}) = 30 \text{ L}$$

$$Na_i = 140 \text{ mmol/L}$$

$$Na_f = 160 \text{ mmol/L}$$

Therefore, $TBW_i = (Na_f \times TBW_f)/Na_i = (140 \times 30)/160 = 26.25 \text{ L}$ and she has a 3.75 L water deficit.

The free water deficit formula is based on the same equation:

$$\text{Free water deficit} = (TBW_f - TBW_i) = [(Na_i \times TBW_i)/Na_f] - TBW_i = TBW_i [(Na_i/Na_f) - 1]$$

Since TBW_i is 26.25, free water deficit = $26.25 \times [160/140 - 1]$ = 3.75 L

Assuming no ongoing water losses, what would be an appropriate rate of fluid administration?

The goal is to correct the plasma sodium by no more than 0.5 mmol/L/h. You decide to correct to a plasma sodium of 150 mmol/L over the first 24 hours. This will require administration of ~2 L of D5W (83 mL/h × 24 hours).

However, ongoing water losses are expected. How is this handled?

For simplicity, let us assume that there are no extrarenal losses. The amount of ongoing water loss that must be replaced in addition to the existing water deficit can be calculated using the electrolyte-free water clearance formula:

$$CeH_2O = V [1 - ((UNa + UK)/PNa)]$$

Because this patient's kidneys are very salt-avid, most of the osmoles in the urine are nonelectrolyte (predominantly urea). Assuming the patient excretes 1 L of urine in the first 24 hours of IV D5W administration, urine electrolyte concentrations do not change, and an average plasma sodium concentration of 155 mmol/L.

$$CeH_2O = 1\,[1 - 30/155] = 0.8\ L.$$

Thus, this patient has excreted an additional 800 mL of electrolyte-free water. This is why hypernatremia will not usually correct as rapidly as would be predicted by calculation of free water deficit alone. If one adds in 500 mL/day of insensible loss, one can see that the expected change in plasma sodium is less than half of that predicted by the free water deficit formula.

Treatment of Hypernatremia
- Hypovolemic hypernatremia is generally treated with hypotonic fluids.
- Use isotonic saline if there is hemodynamic instability, followed by hypotonic fluids. Hemodynamically stable patients should receive hypotonic fluids.
- Euvolemic hypernatremia is treated with water administration (plus ADH in CDI).
- Hypervolemic hypernatremia can be problematic. If severe, it may require both water administration and either diuretics or dialysis to remove the excess sodium. Use of a distal acting diuretic such as metolazone with or without loop diuretics may be particularly useful, though this has not been well studied.
- Calculation of water deficit:
  - Calculate free water deficit (see Case Study 5.6); correct the free water deficit over 48 hours.
  - Ongoing water losses need to be replaced.
  - Stool/sweat losses are usually about 30 to 40 mL/h and should also be replaced.
  - Urinary water losses can be calculated using the electrolyte-free water loss formula.
  - Rate of correction should generally not exceed 0.5 mmol/L/h, as with chronic hypernatremia (i.e., developing over days), because the brain has adapted by accumulating "idiogenic osmoles." In this setting, too rapid a reduction in plasma sodium and osmolality may result in shift of water into the brain, causing brain edema. Acute hypernatremia is very rare, so caution in rate of correction is usually in order. However, if hypernatremia is known to have occurred over a period of minutes to hours (e.g., salt poisoning), more rapid correction is indicated. This is because the brain has not had time to accumulate idiogenic osmoles, and therefore, there is a little risk of development of brain edema with more rapid correction of hypernatremia (Lien et al., 1990).

Important Points to Remember
- Hypernatremia is always associated with hyperosmolality. The normal renal response is stimulation of ADH release leading to concentrated urine to limit urinary water losses. If the urine is not appropriately concentrated, this indicates the absence of or decreased ADH response owing to either CDI or NDI.

- In the past, most patients with hypernatremia have been dehydrated and thus has low TBW as the etiology and are appropriately treated by administration of water. However, hypernatremia has now become common in the ICU setting, where the mechanism is sodium gain resulting from large volume IV saline administration. In this setting, treatment must include measures to decrease TBNa$^+$ (diuretics and/or dialysis) coupled with administration of water.
- An initial estimate of the amount of water to administer to correct hypernatremia can be made by calculating the free water deficit. However, many patients will have ongoing water losses that must be replaced in order to effectively correct hypernatremia.

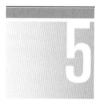

VIGNETTE 1

HYPONATREMIA

A 45-year-old male with hypertension and hyperlipidemia presents for evaluation of shortness of breath and cough for the past month. He takes hydrochlorothiazide for blood pressure control. He denies chest pain or palpitations. He has what he thinks are migraines twice a week, which resolve with ibuprofen. He has smoked 1/2 ppd for the past 25 years. On a recent visit to the ER, he has noted to have hyponatremia. Vital signs and physical examination are normal.

Blood chemistry:
Sodium: 125 mmol/L
Potassium: 4.0 mmol/L
Chloride: 104 mmol/L
Total CO$_2$: 24 mmol/L
Urea nitrogen: 10 mg/dL (Urea: 3.6 mmol/L)
Creatinine: 1.2 mg/dL (106 mcmol/L)
Glucose: 100 mg/dL (5.6 mmol/L)
Plasma osmolality (measured): 260 mmol/kg
Plasma osmolality (calculated): 263 mmol/kg

Urine chemistry:
Osmolality: 900 mmol/kg
Sodium: 60 mmol/L
Creatinine: 20 mg/dL (urea: 1,768 mcmol/L)

Complete blood count:
WBC: 4,500/mm^3
Hemoglobin: 12 g/dL (120 g/L)
Hematocrit: 40%
Platelets: 250,000/mm^3

Lipid profile:
Total cholesterol: 200 mg/dL (5.2 mmol/L)
Triglycerides: 450 mg/dL (5.1 mmol/L)
Chest X-ray: 2-cm lung in right upper lobe nodule
MRI head with and without (1,768 mcmol/L) FENa: 2.9%
Plasma ADH: undetectable
TSH: 2.0 mIU/L (normal)
Fasting AM cortisol: 10 mcg/dL (276 nmol/L) (normal)

Q: What is the next step?

1. Fluid restriction
2. Lung nodule biopsy
3. Stop ibuprofen
4. Stop hydrochlorothiazide
5. Administer gemfibrozil
6. Give IV isotonic saline
7. Give IV hypertonic saline

A: After the history and physical examination, the first step in the evaluation of hyponatremia is to obtain a plasma osmolality, urine osmolality, and urine electrolytes. He is clinically euvolemic, and plasma hypoosmolality, coupled with high urine sodium and high urine osmolality, suggests SIADH. The plasma sodium is not extremely low and he is asymptomatic, so emergent IV isotonic or hypertonic saline is not necessary. The FENa may be elevated because of the thiazide diuretic. Thiazides have also been implicated in SIADH as well as impaired urinary dilution because of ADH-independent effects of the drug (impairment of urinary dilution). The triglycerides are high, but pseudohyponatremia is not present because plasma osmolality is low. The lung nodule is concerning for an ADH-secreting malignant tumor; however, the plasma ADH is undetectable. Hence, we have an SIADH picture without ADH, which is consistent with NSIAD. NSIAD is usually caused by a mutated ADH (V_2) receptor, which is constitutively active ("gain-of-function mutation"). It is usually diagnosed in infants, but can present for the first time in adulthood. It is treated with fluid restriction and, if necessary, oral urea. Incidentally, the patient later undergoes a needle biopsy of the lung nodule, which reveals a benign hamartoma.

VIGNETTE **2**

5

HYPONATREMIA

A 65-year-old male with CHF, diabetes mellitus (DM), and a recent subdural hematoma presents for evaluation of new-onset seizures. Currently, he is tired and has a headache. He complains of nausea and has vomited once. His family reports that he drinks a lot of water. Medications include furosemide 20 mg daily, lisinopril 10 mg daily, aspirin 81 mg daily, and insulin. He does not smoke or use alcohol or illicit drugs. Vitals are normal except for a mild fever of 38°C. Physical examination is significant for irritability and restlessness. There is no papilledema, but there is mild nuchal rigidity. He does not have peripheral edema, jugular venous distension, or rales on pulmonary auscultation. He weighs 100 kg.

Blood chemistry:
Sodium: 105 mmol/L
Potassium: 4.0 mmol/L
Chloride: 71 mmol/L
Total CO_2: 24 mmol/L
Urea nitrogen: 10 mg/dL (urea: 3.6 mmol/L)
Creatinine: 1.2 mg/dL (106 mcmol/L)
Glucose: 100 mg/dL (5.6 mmol/L)
Plasma osmolality: 220 mmol/kg

Urine chemistry:
Osmolality: pending
Sodium: pending
Drug screen: negative
Complete blood count:

WBC: 4,500/mm^3
Hemoglobin: 12 g/dL (120 g/L)
Hematocrit: 40%
Platelets: 250,000/mm^3

Lipid profile:
Total cholesterol: 200 mg/dL (5.2 mmol/L)
Triglycerides: 210 mg/dL (5.1 mmol/L)
Chest X-ray: normal
CT of the head: stable subdural hematoma (similar to CT done 2 weeks ago)
Lumbar puncture: normal
TSH: 2.0 mIU/L (normal)
Fasting AM cortisol: 10 mcg/dL (276 nmol/L) (normal)

Q: What is the next step in treatment?

1. Fluid restriction 2 L/day
2. Stop furosemide and lisinopril
3. Give isotonic saline 2.5 L over 5 hours
4. Give 3% hypertonic saline 1.2 L over 5 hours

A: The patient's primary problem is new-onset seizures. His history of subdural hematoma prompts us to evaluate him for intracranial pathology. His CT of the head is negative for worsening of subdural hematoma or other intracranial lesions. He has mild fever, but lumbar puncture findings are normal. There is no evidence of toxic ingestion, and he is not hypoglycemic or hypoxic. His mental status changes and seizures are attributed to severe hyponatremia. He appears euvolemic because he has neither lower extremity edema nor jugular venous distension or pulmonary rales. Even without urine osmolality and urine electrolytes, it seems likely that SIADH is the cause of the hyponatremia. This can be further delineated by the laboratory findings when available (high urine sodium and osmolality are expected). However, without dwelling on etiology, it is imperative to acutely raise the plasma sodium. Because he is very symptomatic, raising the plasma sodium to ~115 mmol/L at a rate of 2 mmol/L/h is indicated. The amount of sodium required to bring the plasma sodium from 105 to 115 is calculated to be 600 mmol [$(115 - 105) \times 100$ kg $\times 0.6$]. Administration of 1.2 L of 3% hypertonic saline (which contains ~500 mmol/L of sodium) over 5 hours is reasonable. However, one should monitor plasma sodium every 1 to 2 hours to assure an appropriate rate and magnitude of correction. For instance, if the urine osmolality is unexpectedly low, or the stimulus for ADH release wanes and the urine becomes dilute during treatment, spontaneous water excretion may lead to a more rapid increase in plasma sodium level than predicted on the basis of the above formula. It is especially important not to overcorrect the plasma sodium because of the risk of ODS. Because >8% to 10% acute increase in brain water will lead to herniation and death, there is a limit to the amount of brain edema that can occur. Therefore, it is unnecessary and potentially dangerous to acutely raise the plasma sodium level >8% to 10% even in severe symptomatic hyponatremia. In SIADH, isotonic saline is ineffective because administered sodium will be excreted and some of the administered water retained because of high ADH levels.

VIGNETTE 3

HYPERNATREMIA

A 92-year-old man with multi-infarct dementia, coronary artery disease, prostate cancer, benign prostatic hypertrophy, and DM presents from a nursing home with decreased oral intake, decreased urination, and increasing confusion. He has also had generalized weakness, dizziness, and palpitations. He now does not recognize his son, who visits every day. Medications include glyburide 10 mg daily, aspirin 81 mg daily, metoprolol 25 mg bid, lisinopril 10 mg daily, and tamsulosin (Flomax) 0.4 mg daily. Vitals are as follows: pulse, 120 beats/min; blood pressure, 90/70 mm Hg; respiratory rate, 22 breaths/min; temperature, 35°C. Physical examination is significant for confusion, irritability, and lack of cooperation. There is decreased turgor of the skin, dry oral mucosae, and weakness in all extremities. There are no neurologic deficits.

Blood chemistry:
Sodium: 150 mmol/L
Potassium: 4.5 mmol/L
Chloride: 115 mmol/L
Total CO_2: 25 mmol/L
Urea nitrogen: 60 mg/dL (urea: 21 mol/L)
Creatinine: 2.0 mg/dL (177 mcmol/L)
Glucose: 110 mg/dL (6.1 mmol/L)
Osmolality: 330 mmol/kg
Creatine kinase: 100 U/L
TSH: 2.3 mIU/L

Urine chemistry:
Osmolality: 800 mmol/kg

Sodium: 5 mmol/L
Potassium: 20 mmol/L
Chloride: 10 mmol/L
Complete blood count:
WBC: 4,000/mm^3
Hemoglobin: 16 g/dL (160 g/L)
Hematocrit: 50%
Platelets: 300,000/mm^3

Urinalysis:
Color: dark yellow
pH: 6
Specific gravity: 1.025
Protein: negative
Blood: negative
Glucose: negative
Ketones: 2+

Bilirubin: negative
Urobilinogen: negative
Leukocyte esterase: negative
Nitrite: negative
WBC: 2/hpf
RBC: 0/hpf
Bacteria: rare

CT of the head: generalized cortical atrophy
MRI brain: cortical atrophy with multiple cerebral infarcts and a hypothalamic infarct, age undetermined

Q: Which of the following is least likely to be contributing to hypernatremia?

1. Dementia
2. Altered thirst sensation
3. Decreased access to water
4. CDI

A: In any case of altered mental status, acute intracranial abnormalities should be excluded. In the elderly, especially with underlying dementia, hypoxia, hypotension, and sepsis should be considered. Electrolyte disorders, especially hyponatremia and hypernatremia, need to be excluded, and one should test thyroid, kidney, and liver function. Vitamin deficiencies (such as deficiency in vitamin B_{12}, thiamine, or niacin) and psychiatric conditions should be considered.

This patient has multi-infarct dementia and has decreased oral intake at the nursing home. Both altered thirst sensation and decreased access to water are common underlying factors resulting in decreased water intake and hypernatremia in such patients. The physical examination (tachycardia, hypotension, decreased skin turgor, and dry mucosae) is consistent with volume depletion. Hypernatremia and acute prerenal failure (low urinary sodium, concentrated urine) are the important laboratory findings. Starvation ketosis resulting in ketonuria is also present.

This patient thus has evidence of volume depletion (based on physical examination, prerenal failure, and hemoconcentration) as well as dehydration (based on hypernatremia). Both plasma and urine osmolalities (as well as urine specific gravity) are high, indicating appropriate ADH release, because hyperosmolality, hypovolemia, and hypotension are all stimuli for the secretion of ADH. ADH causes the insertion of water channels in the collecting duct, which allows for the conservation of water. Though this patient has had a hypothalamic stroke, raising the possibility of CDI, ADH production is appropriate, as reflected by the appropriately high urine specific gravity and osmolality.

5

HYPERNATREMIA

A 51-year-old female with dilated cardiomyopathy and chronic obstructive pulmonary disease presents for evaluation of shortness of breath. She quit smoking 3 months ago. She has been using her albuterol nebulizer four times a day as opposed to her usual usage of once per day or less. She thinks her lower extremity edema is worse. She also reports three pillow orthopnea and daily paroxysmal nocturnal dyspnea. She denies excess sodium intake. She denies fever, chills, or dysuria. She does have cough with yellow sputum. Medications include bupropion, prednisone (started 1 week ago by her primary physician), Combivent (ipratropium/albuterol), Flovent (fluticasone), albuterol via nebulizer prn, furosemide, lisinopril, carvedilol, baby aspirin, and simvastatin. Vitals are as follows: pulse, 90 beats/min; blood, 115/85 mm Hg; respiratory rate, 20 breaths/min; temperature, 36.5°C. Positive findings on physical examination include jugular venous distension, a third heart sound (S3), and bibasilar rales halfway up the lungs. There is also shifting dullness on abdominal percussion and 3+ edema in the lower extremity. The neurologic examination is normal.

Blood chemistry:
Sodium: 150 mmol/L
Potassium: 5.5 mmol/L
Chloride: 115 mmol/L
Total CO_2: 25 mmol/L
Urea nitrogen: 30 mg/dL (urea: 10.7 mmol/L)
Creatinine: 1.7 mg/dL (150 mcmol/L)
Glucose: 133 mg/dL (7.4 mmol/L)
Osmolality: 320 mmol/kg

Urine chemistry:
Osmolality: 350 mmol/kg

Sodium: 40 mmol/L
Potassium: 10 mmol/L
Chloride: 60 mmol/L

Complete blood count:
WBC: 4,000/mm^3
Hemoglobin: 12 g/dL (120 g/L)
Hematocrit: 36%
Platelets: 220,000/mm^3
Chest X-ray: enlarged heart, pulmonary edema
D-Dimer: 1.0 mcg/L
CT scan chest: no pulmonary embolus, pulmonary edema, pleural effusions

Q: Which of the following is not a potential treatment for the hypernatremia?

1. D5W
2. Loop diuretics
3. Dialysis
4. Isotonic saline

A: The history indicates a dyspneic patient who is not getting relief through nebulizer treatments and who complains of orthopnea and paroxysmal nocturnal dyspnea. In addition, the patient has recently started prednisone, which probably caused worsening of fluid overload because of renal sodium retention. Jugular venous distension, the presence of an S3, diffuse rales on lung auscultation, and lower extremity edema as well as possible ascites on abdominal percussion all confirm hypervolemia. Hypernatremia indicates that total body sodium is in excess of TBW, probably because of the effects of prednisone (renal sodium retention) and furosemide (renal water loss in excess of renal sodium loss). Plasma osmolality is high; although urine osmolality is higher than plasma osmolality, it should be higher than this degree of hyperosmolar hypernatremia. This is probably due to diuretics (which limit urinary concentrating ability). There is no evidence for an acute myocardial infarction (MI) or pulmonary embolism. Treatment of hypervolemic hypernatremia is often problematic. This patient needs diuretics to treat the pulmonary edema (the cause of the initial presentation, i.e., dyspnea), but this can lead to further worsening of hypernatremia. Isotonic D5W can be used simultaneously to dilute the plasma sodium; however, it should not be given until hypervolemia is improved. If the kidneys fail to diurese, dialysis should be implemented. Isotonic saline is not appropriate for hypervolemic hypernatremia.

References

Ashraf N, Locksley R, Arieff AI. Thiazide-induced hyponatremia associated with death or neurologic damage in outpatients. *Am J Med.* 70(6):1163–1168, 1981.

Bartter FE, Schwartz WB. The syndrome of inappropriate secretion of antidiuretic hormone. *Am J Med.* 42:790–806, 1967.

Edelman IS, Liebman J, O'Meara MP, et al. Interrelations between serum sodium concentration, serum osmolarity and total exchangeable sodium, total exchangeable potassium and total body water. *J Clin Invest.* 37(9):1236–1256, 1958.

Feldman BJ, Rosenthal SM, Vargas GA, et al. Nephrogenic syndrome of inappropriate antidiuresis. *N Engl J Med.* 352:1884–1690, 2005.

Fenske W, Refardt J, Chifu I, et al. A copeptin-based approach in the diagnosis of diabetes insipidus. *N Engl J Med.* 379(5):428–439, 2018.

Fichman MP, Vorherr H, Kleeman CR, et al. Diuretic induced hyponatremia. *Ann Intern Med.* 75:853–863, 1971.

Hantman D, Rossier B, Zohlman R, et al. Rapid correction of hyponatremia in the syndrome of inappropriate secretion of antidiuretic hormone. An alternative treatment to hypertonic saline. *Ann Intern Med.* 78(6):870–875, 1973.

Hariprasad MK, Eisinger RP, Nadler IM, et al. Hyponatremia in psychogenic polydipsia. *Arch Intern Med.* 140:1639–1642, 1980.

Leehey DJ, Picache AA, Robertson GL. Hyponatraemia in quadriplegic patients. *Clin Sci (Lond).* 75(4):441–444, 1988.

Lien YH, Shapiro JI, Chan L. Effects of hypernatremia on organic brain osmoles. *J Clin Invest.* 85:1427–1435, 1990.

Morello JP, Bichet DG. Nephrogenic diabetes insipidus. *Ann Rev Physiol.* 63:607–630, 2001.

Oster JR, Singer I, Thatte L, et al. The polyuria of solute diuresis. *Arch Intern Med.* 157:721–729, 1997.

Quillen EW, Reid IA, Keil LC. Carotid and arterial baroreceptor influences on plasma vasopressin and drinking. In Cowley AW Jr, Liard JF, Ausiello DA, eds. *Vasopressin: Cellular and Integrative Functions.* New York, NY: Raven Press; 1988:405–411.

Rahman M, Friedman WA. Hyponatremia in neurosurgical patients: clinical guidelines development. *Neurosurgery.* 65(5):925–935, 2009.

Robertson GL, Athar S. The interaction of blood osmolality and blood volume in regulating plasma vasopressin in man. *J Clin Endocrinol Metab.* 42:613–620, 1976.

Sanghvi SR, Kellerman PS, Nanovic L. Beer potomania: an unusual cause of hyponatremia at high risk of complications from rapid correction. *Am J Kidney Dis.* 50(4):673–680, 2007.

Schrier RW. Pathogenesis of sodium and water retention in high-output and low output cardiac failure, nephrotic syndrome, cirrhosis, and pregnancy. *N Engl J Med.* 319:1065–1072, 1988a.

Schrier RW. Pathogenesis of sodium and water retention in high-output and low output cardiac failure, nephrotic syndrome, cirrhosis, and pregnancy. *N Engl J Med.* 319:1127–1134, 1988b.

Siegel AJ. Fatal water intoxication and cardiac arrest in runners during marathons: Prevention and treatment based on updated clinical paradigms. *Am J Med.* 128:1070–1075, 2015.

Smith HW. Renal excretion of sodium and water. *Fed Proc.* 11:701–705, 1952.

Sterns RH, Riggs JE, Schochet SS. Osmotic demyelination syndrome following correction of hyponatremia. *N Engl J Med.* 314:1535–1542, 1986.

Timper K, Fenske W, Kühn F, et al. Diagnostic accuracy of copeptin in the differential diagnosis of the polyuria-polydipsia syndrome: a prospective multicenter study. *J Clin Endocrinol Metab.* 2015;100(6):2268–2274.

Zerbe RL, Robertson GL. Osmoregulation of thirst and vasopressin secretion in human subjects: effect of various solutes. *Am J Physiol.* 244:E607–E614, 1983.

6

Disorders of Potassium Homeostasis

TOTAL BODY POTASSIUM AND ITS DISTRIBUTION

- Most abundant cation in humans—~50 mmol/kg (mEq/kg)—mostly intracellular—only ~1 mmol/kg extracellular. Plasma (or serum) potassium concentration $[K^+]$ depends on total body potassium (external potassium balance) as well as distribution of K^+ between extracellular fluid (ECF) and intracellular fluid (internal potassium balance) (Fig. 6.1).
- External potassium balance—normal dietary K^+ intake ~80 to 100 mmol/day—varies according to diet—in the steady state, excretion of potassium equals intake and occurs primarily via the kidneys and, to a lesser extent, by the gut. Urinary potassium concentration can vary between 5 and >100 mmol/L.
- Internal potassium balance—a variety of factors affect distribution of potassium between cells and ECF, the most important being insulin and catecholamines (increase cell uptake of K^+) and acid–base status.

RENAL HANDLING OF POTASSIUM (Giebisch et al., 2007)

- Glomerular filtration—filtered potassium = glomerular filtration rate × plasma $[K^+]$ = 180 L/day × 4 mmol/L = 720 mmol/day
- Proximal tubule—~50% of filtered potassium reabsorbed by proximal convoluted tubule

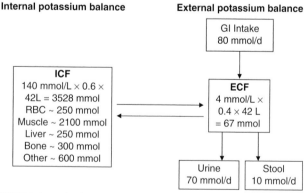

Internal potassium balance

External potassium balance

| GI Intake |
| 80 mmol/d |

ICF
140 mmol/L × 0.6 ×
42L = 3528 mmol
RBC ~ 250 mmol
Muscle ~ 2100 mmol
Liver ~ 250 mmol
Bone ~ 300 mmol
Other ~ 600 mmol

ECF
4 mmol/L ×
0.4 × 42 L
= 67 mmol

| Urine | | Stool |
| 70 mmol/d | | 10 mmol/d |

FIGURE 6.1. Internal and external potassium balance. The figure depicts typical potassium balance in a 70-kg man with a total body water of 42 L. ECF, extracellular fluid; ICF, intracellular fluid; GI, gastrointestinal.

- Loop of Henle—reabsorbs 40% to 50% of filtered potassium—thick ascending limb (TAL) has a furosemide-sensitive Na–K–Cl cotransporter that reabsorbs one sodium ion, one potassium ion, and two chloride ions
- Distal tubule—changes in urinary potassium excretion usually reflect the amount of potassium secretion by this nephron segment—<10% of filtered potassium reaches the distal convoluted tubule, but fraction of filtered K^+ leaving late distal tubule is 20%, indicating active secretion into distal tubule
- Cortical collecting tubule—secretes K^+ in response to active Na^+ uptake (site of aldosterone action)
- Medullary collecting tubule and duct—in response to K^+ excess, secretion of K^+ into the lumen can occur—usually no net K^+ flux

FACTORS INFLUENCING RENAL POTASSIUM EXCRETION

- Mineralocorticoid hormone (aldosterone)—enhances active transport of K^+ from blood to distal tubular cell and increases Na^+ permeability of luminal membrane, thus increasing K^+ secretion
- Acid–base balance—acute metabolic acidosis decreases intracellular K^+ and K^+ excretion; acute metabolic alkalosis increases intracellular K^+ and K^+ excretion; however, both chronic metabolic acidosis and alkalosis are associated with increased K^+ excretion (Adrogué & Madias, 1981)
- Anion effects—nonchloride anions stimulate K^+ secretion
- Tubular flow rate—increases in urinary flow increase K^+ excretion independent of sodium delivery—antidiuretic hormone increases K^+ excretion; this effect helps to maintain external K^+ balance under conditions of antidiuresis
- Sodium intake—increased Na^+ intake increases K^+ excretion; decreased Na^+ intake decreases K^+ excretion
- Potassium intake—K^+ loading causes decreased reabsorption by TAL and increased K^+ secretion by distal nephron segments
- Intracellular and plasma potassium concentration—increases in plasma (extracellular) $[K^+]$ result in increased K^+ excretion
- Diuretics—osmotic diuretics (urea, glucose, mannitol), thiazides, carbonic anhydrase inhibitors, and loop diuretics all increase K^+ excretion by increasing fluid delivery to distal tubule; loop diuretics also block K^+ reabsorption by TAL. Spironolactone (aldosterone antagonist), triamterene, and amiloride all decrease K^+ excretion at the level of distal tubule
- Magnesium—a decrease in intracellular magnesium, caused by magnesium deficiency, decreases the magnesium-mediated inhibition of renal outer medullary potassium (ROMK) channels and increases potassium secretion

GASTROINTESTINAL HANDLING OF POTASSIUM

- No role in normal potassium homeostasis
- In chronic renal failure and potassium loading, fecal excretion of K^+ increases several-fold owing to active colonic K^+ secretion, at least part of which is aldosterone dependent

CONTROL OF INTERNAL POTASSIUM BALANCE

- Insulin—physiologic regulator of plasma [K$^+$]—stimulates uptake of K$^+$ into cells (primarily muscle and liver)—effect mediated by Na$^+$–K$^+$ pump and can be blocked by ouabain
  - Clinical significance: insulinopenia is associated with hyperkalemia (e.g., diabetic ketoacidosis); insulin is useful in emergency treatment of hyperkalemia
- Catecholamines—alpha-receptor stimulation increases plasma K$^+$; β_2 agonists decrease plasma K$^+$ (no effect of β_1 agonists)
  - Clinical significance: conditions associated with increased circulating catecholamines (myocardial ischemia, pheochromocytoma) are associated with hypokalemia; β_2 agonists can be used to treat hyperkalemia
- Hypertonicity—infusion of hypertonic solutions results in water and K$^+$ movement out of cells
  - Clinical significance: uncertain, though hypertonic glucose (given for diabetic coma) may result in hyperkalemia
- Acid–base balance—K$^+$ distribution affected by pH, with acidosis causing K$^+$ shift out of cells and alkalosis shifting K$^+$ into cells (Adrogué & Madias, 1981). However, relationship between acidemia and hyperkalemia complex—in inorganic metabolic acidosis (e.g., renal failure), HCl administration or H$^+$–K$^+$ exchange leads to hyperkalemia, whereas in organic metabolic acidosis (e.g., lactic acidosis, ketoacidosis), when H$^+$ ions move into cells, they are accompanied by organic anions. Because electroneutrality is maintained, there is no need for K$^+$ to exit from cells; thus, little or no increase in plasma [K$^+$]
  - Clinical significance: hyperkalemia associated with organic acidosis probably not because of acidosis per se but secondary to associated events (e.g., tissue breakdown, renal failure, insulinopenia)

HYPOKALEMIA

CASE STUDY 6.1 A 35-year-old male with no previous medical history was admitted 5 days ago for *Pseudomonas* sepsis and was treated with piperacillin/tazobactam and gentamicin. Over the past 24 hours, sepsis has been resolving, but he has developed muscle cramps in his arms and legs, severe fatigue, anorexia, and polyuria. There is no nausea, vomiting, or constipation, and no nonsteroidal anti-inflammatory drug (NSAID) use. He has not received diuretics.

Physical Examination:

Vitals: pulse 100 beats/min (supine and standing); respiratory rate 20 breaths/min, blood pressure (BP) 120/70 mm Hg (supine) and 105/60 mm Hg (standing); temperature 99°F; oxygen saturation 96% on room air

General: alert and oriented to time, place, and person

Skin: poor skin turgor

Heart: normal S1/S2, no murmurs/rubs/gallops
Lungs: clear
Abdomen: soft, no guarding/rebound
Neurology: no focal findings
Extremities: no edema

Blood chemistry:
Sodium: 135 mmol/L
Potassium: 2.5 mmol/L
Chloride: 100 mmol/L
Total CO_2: 32 mmol/L
Urea nitrogen: 30 mg/dL (urea: 10.7 mmol/L)
Creatinine: 1.0 mg/dL (88.4 mcmol/L)
Glucose: 90 mg/dL (5 mmol/L)
Calcium: 9.0 mg/dL (2.25 mmol/L)
Magnesium: 1.0 mg/dL (0.41 mmol/L)

Urine chemistry:
Urine sodium: 45 mmol/L
Urine potassium: 50 mmol/L
Urine chloride: 45 mmol/L
Urine calcium: 10 mg/dL (2.5 mmol/L)
Urine magnesium: 12 mg/dL (4.9 mmol/L)
Urine creatinine: 120 mg/dL (10.6 mmol/L)
Urine osmolality: 450 mmol/kg
Fractional excretion of magnesium (FEMg): 14%

Question 6.1.1: What is the initial approach to hypokalemia?

The initial step is to determine the etiology of hypokalemia, that is, whether is it due to decreased intake or increased extrarenal or renal loss.

A urine potassium concentration <20 mmol/L supports either poor intake or extrarenal potassium losses, whether it is because of compartment shifts (shift into cells) or gastrointestinal losses. A urine potassium concentration >20 mmol/L (in particular, when >40 mmol/L) indicates hypokalemia is due to renal loss of potassium. However, spot urine potassium can be misleading in two conditions: (a) the cause of renal potassium wasting has resolved or (b) the patient is polyuric. A urine K:Cr ratio is not affected by urine volume; a urine K:Cr ratio <22 mmol/g supports poor intake or extrarenal potassium losses and >22 mmol/g supports renal losses. Similarly, a 24-hour urine K <20 mmol/d supports poor intake or extrarenal potassium losses and >20 mmol/d renal losses; however, getting a 24-hour urine is often impractical. In the setting of vomiting, urine K is often high due to secondary aldosteronism (from chloride depletion) and bicarbonaturia.

Etiologies of Hypokalemia (Table 6.1)
- Hypokalemia resulting from transcellular redistribution (increased K^+ uptake into cells with total body potassium usually normal)
  - Alkalemia—increased H^+ exit and K^+ uptake by cells
  - Periodic paralysis—weakness during hypokalemia that usually lasts 3 to 4 hours but may last up to 24 hours

TABLE 6.1 Etiologies of Hypokalemi

Hypokalemia

Renal potassium loss (Urine K > 20 mmol/L or urine K:Cr >22 mmol/g creatinine [2.5 mmol/mmol creatinine])				Decreased potassium intake, extrarenal potassium loss, or increased cellular uptake (Urine K < 20 mmol/L or urine K:Cr <22 mmol/g creatinine [2.5 mmol/mmol creatinine])
High renin High aldosterone (secondary aldosteronism)	Low renin High aldosterone	Low renin Low aldosterone	Variable renin and aldosterone	Variable renin and aldosterone

Malignant hypertension
Renin-secreting tumor
Pheochromocytoma
Renovascular hypertension
Vomiting
Bartter syndrome
Gitelman syndrome
Diuretics
	Primary aldosteronism
	Glucocorticoid-remediable hyperaldosteronism (GRH)
	Low renin hypertension (aldosterone is usually normal but functionally too high in setting of salt-sensitive hypertension)
		Congenital adrenal hyperplasia (CAH)
		Apparent mineralocorticoid excess (AME)
		Licorice ingestion
		Liddle syndrome
		Cushing syndrome
		Exogenous steroid use
			Proximal or distal renal tubular acidosis (RTA) (see chapter 7)	Diarrhea
				Laxatives
				Low-potassium diet
				Increased cellular potassium uptake:
				  Insulin
				  Bicarbonate
				  Periodic paralysis

- Hereditary form—attacks may be precipitated by high carbohydrate meals (increased insulin release) or exercise (increased circulating catecholamines) (voltage-gated channel gene mutation)
- Acquired form—associated with thyrotoxicosis (thyroid hormone–sensitive K^+ transporter mutation). Resolves with treatment of thyrotoxicosis
- Administration of insulin or β_2 adrenergic agonists (or increased endogenous secretion)—shift K^+ into cells

■ Hypokalemia with low total body potassium
  ■ Decreased intake—inadequate K^+ in diet (e.g., in elderly and alcoholic patients)
  ■ Gastrointestinal potassium losses—vomiting, diarrhea, laxative abuse, villous adenoma
  ■ Renal potassium losses
    - Associated with hypertension—Conn syndrome (primary mineralocorticoid excess) (Blumenfeld et al., 1994; Conn et al., 1985), renovascular hypertension (secondary mineralocorticoid excess), Cushing disease or iatrogenic steroids (glucocorticoid excess), licorice abuse (increases mineralocorticoid effect of cortisol), diuretics (increase fluid delivery to distal tubule)
    - Associated with normal BP—renal tubular acidosis (RTA) (covered in Acid/Base chapter), osmotic diuresis, diuretics, antibiotics (increased anion delivery to distal tubule), Bartter syndrome (defect in ion transport in the loop of Henle), Gitelman syndrome (defect in ion transport at distal tubule) (Gladziwa et al., 1995), leukemia (associated with lysozymuria), magnesium depletion (increases renal potassium excretion) (Whang et al., 1985). Vomiting also causes renal potassium wasting because of a combination of volume/chloride depletion leading to renin and aldosterone secretion (secondary aldosteronism) and bicarbonaturia (obligating loss of accompanying cations sodium and potassium).

Consequences of Hypokalemia

■ Cardiovascular effects: electrocardiographic (EKG) changes (U-waves) (Fig. 6.2)

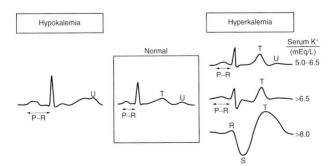

FIGURE 6.2. EKG changes in hypokalemia and hyperkalemia. EKG, electrocardiographic.

- Neuromuscular effects: weakness (even quadriparesis), rhabdomyolysis, ileus, encephalopathy (in patients with liver disease)
- Metabolic and hormonal effects: abnormal carbohydrate metabolism (decreased insulin release and peripheral effect), negative nitrogen balance, decreased aldosterone release
- Renal effects: polyuria, polydipsia (nephrogenic diabetes insipidus), increased renal NH_3 production (can cause hepatic encephalopathy)

Symptoms of Hypokalemia
- Muscle weakness, including respiratory muscles (impaired ventilation) and intestinal smooth muscle (ileus)—especially with plasma $[K^+] < 2.5$ mmol/L
- Muscle cramps
- Tetany
- Rhabdomyolysis and myoglobinuria

<hr>

Question 6.1.2: This patient has the constellation of hypokalemia; hypomagnesemia; metabolic alkalosis; mild orthostatic hypotension; and sodium, potassium, and magnesium wasting. What is the differential diagnosis?

CASE STUDY 6.1 CONTINUED

This patient has metabolic alkalosis, and thus RTA is excluded. There is no clinical history to support osmotic diuresis, and he has concentrated urine that does not suggest osmotic diuresis (see Sodium chapter). He does not receive either prescribed or surreptitious diuretics. There is no history of vomiting, and surreptitious vomiting is unlikely because the patient has been in an inpatient setting. Moreover, owing to chloride depletion, urinary chloride is low (<20 mmol/L) with vomiting.

Gitelman syndrome is an autosomal recessive disorder in which there is a genetic defect in the thiazide-sensitive Na–Cl cotransporter (NCC) in the distal tubule. It is also associated with renal magnesium wasting. The mechanism by which Gitelman syndrome causes hypomagnesemia involves reduction in activation of transient receptor potential cation channel subfamily M member 6 (TRPM6), a recently described magnesium transporter in the distal tubule (inhibition of NCC leads to inhibition of TRPM6). It can present in late adolescence or in adulthood. It is also associated with hypocalciuria (similar to blockade of the NCC with thiazide diuretics). The urine calcium to creatinine ratio is generally <44 mg/g (124 mmol/mol) in Gitelman syndrome (Matsunoshita et al., 2016; Viering et al., 2017), but in this patient, it is 83 mg/g. Bartter syndrome is also an autosomal recessive disorder but rarer than Gitelman syndrome (1:1,000,000 vs. 1:40,000). Bartter syndrome is diagnosed in childhood and is associated with growth retardation and mental retardation.

The patient has urinary magnesium wasting as reflected by an FEMg >> 2% in the face of hypomagnesemia, which also contributes to renal potassium wasting (hypomagnesemia increases potassium egress into the urine through luminal ROMK channels in the distal tubule). Both disorders are associated with stimulation of the renin–angiotensin–aldosterone system (RAAS) because of sodium chloride loss into the urine.

Whereas Gitelman syndrome appears to be always as a result of an NCC defect, Bartter syndrome is due to at least five different defects:

Type I—sodium/potassium/2-chloride cotransporter (NKCC2)
Type II—ROMK channel
Type III—basolateral chloride channel (CLCNKB)
Type IV—as in type III + sensorineural deafness
Type V—gain of function of calcium sensing receptor (CaSR)

Question 6.1.3: What is the final diagnosis?

Bartter-Like Syndrome Due to Aminoglycosides

Acquired Bartter syndrome (type V) can be caused by aminoglycosides, which stimulate the CaSR. Opening of ROMK channels leads to secretion of potassium into the apical tubular lumen, thereby allowing for potassium recycling and resultant sodium reabsorption via the NKCC2 channel in the TAL of the loop of Henle (TALH). The CaSR normally inhibits the ROMK channels, leading to decreased potassium secretion and decreased paracellular calcium absorption. Stimulation of the CaSR leads to opening up of the ROMK channels, increased potassium secretion, and hypokalemia. Hypercalcemia has also been reported to lead to a Bartter-like phenotype. There is a chloride channel (CLCNKB) on the apical luminal side that is important for chloride secretion and to overall function of the TALH. Injury, antibody to, or mutation in any of these channels can cause Bartter-like syndrome. Abnormal NaCl transport in the TAL alters the electrochemical gradient and increases calcium and magnesium excretion via the paracellular route (Fig. 6.3).

Acquired Gitelman syndrome can be caused by cisplatin-induced tubular injury predominantly in the distal convoluted tubule and collecting duct. Acquired Gitelman syndrome has also been described

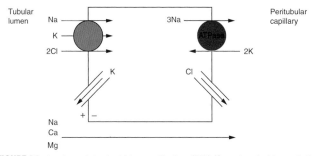

FIGURE 6.3. Ion channels in the thick ascending loop (TAL). (Reproduced with permission from Brater DC. Mechanism of action of diuretics. In: Post TW, ed. *UpToDate*. Waltham, MA: UpToDate. Accessed November 29, 2018. Copyright © 2018 UpToDate, Inc. For more information visit www.uptodate.com.)

due to antibodies to the NCC in Sjögren syndrome and other autoimmune diseases.

Although large doses of penicillins can cause hypokalemia and metabolic alkalosis by causing increased sodium delivery to the distal nephron and by acting as nonreabsorbable anions, this is no longer seen with doses currently used in clinical practice. Other medications that cause renal tubular injury frequently also cause hypokalemia. Amphotericin causes renal tubular toxicity, inhibition of H^+ secretion, magnesium depletion, and hypokalemia. Sirolimus can cause hypokalemia via tubular dysfunction. Methotrexate causes hypokalemia owing to an unknown mechanism. Tenofovir causes hypokalemia because of proximal tubular dysfunction.

> **Question 6.1.4:** How would you treat this patient?

Treatment of Hypokalemia

A rough estimate of potassium deficit can be obtained from plasma $[K^+]$; that is, each decrease in $[K^+]$ of 1 mmol/L represents an ~300-mmol total body deficit. Generally administered orally as potassium chloride (many preparations) or potassium citrate if coexisting metabolic acidosis. However, one must keep in mind that since most potassium is intracellular, the deficit must be replaced slowly to avoid hyperkalemia. A rule of thumb is to replace about half the deficit over 48 hours. This can generally be done by giving about 1 mEq/kg/day for the first 2 days. Further potassium needs depend on whether or not there are ongoing losses of potassium. In emergency or if po intake is impossible, give intravenous (IV) at 10 mmol/h (K rider). Higher rates (20–40 mmol/h) require cardiac monitoring in intensive care unit. Correction of magnesium deficiency is warranted. Continued potassium administration is needed if there are ongoing potassium losses (which is usually the case when there are renal potassium losses unless the underlying cause can be corrected).

CASE STUDY 6.1 CONCLUDED

IV fluids are continued. Potassium and magnesium are supplemented. Gentamicin is discontinued. Two weeks later, electrolyte abnormalities has resolved.

CASE STUDY A 55-year-old male with a previous cerebrovascular accident (CVA) at 45 years of age presents for evaluation of uncontrolled hypertension despite treatment with hydrochlorothiazide 25 mg daily, amlodipine 10 mg daily, lisinopril 40 mg daily, and metoprolol succinate 50 mg once daily. He denies blurred vision, chest pain, hematuria, abdominal pain, or intermittent claudication.

Physical Examination:
Vitals: pulse 55 beats/min, respiratory rate 20 breaths/min, BP 150/95, temperature 99°F
General: alert and oriented to time, place, and person, no Cushingoid features

Heart: normal S1/S2, no murmurs/rubs/gallops
Lungs: clear
Abdomen: soft, no guarding/rebound
Genitalia: normal
Neurology: no focal findings
Lower extremities: no edema

Blood chemistry:
Sodium: 142 mmol/L
Potassium: 3.0 mmol/L
Chloride: 100 mmol/L
Total CO_2: 28 mmol/L
Urea nitrogen: 18 mg/dL (urea: 6.4 mmol/L)
Creatinine: 1.0 mg/dL (88.4 mcmol/L)
Glucose: 90 mg/dL (5 mmol/L)
Calcium: 9.0 mg/dL (2.25 mmol/L)
Magnesium: 2.0 mg/dL (0.83 mmol/L)

Question 6.2.1: What is the differential diagnosis of hypertension in this patient?

CASE STUDY 6.2 CONTINUED

This patient has resistant hypertension, defined as uncontrolled BP (>140/90 mm Hg) despite appropriate doses of three antihypertensive medications. Essential hypertension is still possible. However, resistant hypertension associated with hypokalemia despite the use of a high-dose angiotensin-converting enzyme (ACE) inhibitor suggests the possibility of primary aldosteronism. Also in the differential of resistant hypertension with hypokalemia are hypercortisolism, renovascular hypertension (secondary aldosteronism as a result of renin secretion), sleep apnea (secondary aldosteronism), and pheochromocytoma (increased potassium shift into cells owing to hyperadrenergic state).

Question 6.2.2: What is the role of the RAAS in hypertension?

- Physiology of hypertension:
  - Mean arterial pressure (MAP) = Cardiac output × Total peripheral resistance (CO × TPR)
  - Hence, MAP is dependent on volume and vasoconstriction.
  - Volume (extracellular volume) is regulated by the kidneys via complex mechanisms involving both Starling forces and neurohormonal factors including the RAAS, sympathetic nervous system (SNS), and natriuretic peptides such as atrial natriuretic peptide (ANP) and brain natriuretic peptide (BNP). Because sodium content determines extracellular volume, volume is determined by sodium balance.
  - Vasoconstriction depends on neurohormonal activation by the RAAS and SNS as well as structural changes in arterioles.

- Renin is secreted from the juxtaglomerular apparatus (JGA) in response to several factors, including stretch (arterial BP), the SNS, sodium delivery to the macula densa, angiotensin II (Ang II), and vasodilatory prostaglandins
  - Decreased renal perfusion (such as with hypotension, renal artery stenosis, congestive heart failure, or cirrhosis) stimulates renin secretion.
  - Carotid baroreceptors are activated by a decrease in effective arterial volume (such as with hypovolemia or hypotension), stimulating the SNS, enhancing norepinephrine release that acts on beta-1 receptors on the JGA to cause renin secretion.
  - Decreased sodium delivery to the macula densa stimulates prostaglandin release that acts on the JGA to cause renin secretion. A high dietary sodium will increase distal sodium delivery and thus inhibits renin release.
  - Renin increases formation of Ang I from angiotensinogen; ACE causes conversion of Ang I to Ang II, which then acts on the AT1 receptors on the adrenal gland to cause aldosterone secretion. Ang II also directly inhibits renin release from vthe JGA.

Question 6.2.3: How is the activity of the RAAS measured and interpreted?

- Measurement of plasma renin activity (PRA) and plasma aldosterone concentration (PAC)
  - PRA is the capacity of renin to generate Ang I; this is still the most commonly used test but is labor intensive; it is difficult to measure renin at low levels; the assay is saturated at high levels and results in underestimation.
  - Plasma renin concentration (PRC) can be measured by immunosorbent assay but detects both prorenin and renin and is not used to determine the PAC/PRA ratio (see below)
  - Many medications have a lowering or elevating effect on renin. Beta-blockers suppress renin; RAAS inhibitors increase renin; calcium channel blockers and thiazides have lesser effects; there is a natural decline in renin with age.
  - PAC is influenced by Ang II levels, serum potassium, and medications. Spironolactone increases PAC; dihydropyridine calcium channel blockers and hypokalemia decrease PAC.
- Interpretation of PAC/PRA ratio
  - Primary aldosteronism increases PAC (because of increased adrenal secretion of aldosterone) and decreases PRA (because of volume-mediated inhibition of renin secretion), resulting in a marked increase in PAC/PRA; in secondary aldosteronism, a primary increase in PRA (owing to any stimulus that increases renin secretion) leads to an increase in PAC, and thus the ratio is not altered. Inhibition of renin secretion from any cause leads to low PRA and low PAC. Some causes of low PRA and low PAC are licorice ingestion (discussed below), some forms

of monogenic hypertension such as Liddle syndrome and apparent mineralocorticoid excess (AME) (discussed below), and ectopic adrenocorticotropic hormone (ACTH) secretion. Some patients with essential hypertension have low PRA and normal PAC (also discussed below).

■ The PAC/PRA ratio can generally be measured with the patient on his or her usual medications. However, it should be kept in mind that many drugs inhibit renin secretion and thus will elevate the ratio. These medications include beta-blockers, centrally acting alpha-agonists with sympatholytic action (clonidine, methyldopa), and NSAIDs. However, although the PAC/PRA ratio may be increased by these drugs, the PAC should not be elevated (i.e., will be <15 ng/dL). Other antihypertensive drugs increase renin secretion either by volume depletion (such as diuretics) or by preventing the negative feedback of Ang II on renin secretion (RAAS inhibitors) and thus lower the ratio. In this setting, an elevated PAC/PRA ratio despite these drugs is particularly suggestive of primary aldosteronism. Medications that have little effect on the ratio include verapamil, hydralazine, and alpha-blockers. These agents can be used to control BP if it desired to stop medications that affect the RAAS prior to PAC/PRA testing.

> **Question 6.2.4:** What are the clinical indications for PAC/PRA ratio determination (also called aldosterone to renin ratio or ARR)?

The ARR should be measured if there is a clinical suspicion of primary aldosteronism (Funder et al., 2016). One should suspect primary aldosteronism if one or more of the following are present:

1. Resistant hypertension (BP >140/90 mm Hg despite appropriate doses of three antihypertensive medications)
2. Severe hypertension (BP >160/100 mm Hg)
3. Hypertension associated with hypokalemia (spontaneous or caused by low-dose diuretic)
4. Hypertension associated with adrenal adenoma on computed tomography (CT) scan
5. Hypertension and a family history of hypertension or CVA at age < 40 years
6. Hypertension with a first degree relative with primary aldosteronism

■ Primary Aldosteronism
   ■ Usually due to unilateral adrenal adenoma (Conn syndrome) or bilateral adrenal hyperplasia
      • PRA/PAC ratio should be measured in the morning after the patient has been out of bed for ≥2 hours and after sitting 5 to 15 minutes; dietary salt intake should not be restricted; potassium should be normalized if possible (hypokalemia may result in a normal PAC)
      • A PAC of >15 combined with a PAC/PRA >20 suggests primary hyperaldosteronism
      • Suspect primary aldosteronism if PRA is low despite being on ACE inhibitor or Ang II receptor blocker (ARB)

- In most cases, aldosterone suppression testing is needed. This can be done either by oral or via IV salt loading
  - Oral Salt Loading:
    - High-sodium diet (>250 mEq/day × 3 days)
    - Measure 24-hour urine aldosterone, sodium, and creatinine on day 3 as well as PAC and PRA. The 24-hour urine **creatinine** is used to determine the completeness of the urine collection; the a 24-hour **urinary sodium** should be at least 200 mEq/day if salt loading is adequate. Urine aldosterone excretion >12 mcg/24 h in this setting is consistent with hyperaldosteronism.
  - IV Salt Loading:
    - 500 mL/h of isotonic sodium chloride solution is infused over 4 hours (total of 2 L of fluid volume). The PAC should decrease to <5 ng/dL in healthy subjects, and values that remain >10 mg/dL are consistent with primary aldosteronism.
- Treatment is with aldosterone antagonists or adrenalectomy. Adrenal venous sampling is necessary prior to consideration of surgery to assure unilateral secretion of aldosterone.
■ Familial Hyperaldosteronism (FH): three types (FH1, FH2, FH3)
  - FH1 (Glucocorticoid-Remediable Aldosteronism, GRA)
    - The enzyme CYP11B2 is present in the zona glomerulosa of the adrenal gland. It converts deoxycorticosterone to corticosterone. It also converts 18-OH-corticosterone to aldosterone.
    - The enzyme CYP11B1 is present in the zona fasciculata of the adrenal gland. It converts 11-deoxycortisol to cortisol. CYP11B1 is ACTH sensitive.
    - In GRA, there is a fusion of the CYP11B1 promoter with the coding sequences of CYP11B2. So ACTH activates CYP11B2 (aldosterone synthase) as well. This is insensitive to potassium loading.
    - Hypersecretion of aldosterone is reversed by physiologic doses of glucocorticoids.
    - Autosomal dominant
    - 18% have a history of CVA. 70% of the strokes are hemorrhagic.
    - Diagnosis is suggested by family history and history of stroke; dexamethasone suppression can be done; however, genetic testing is better. Urinary 18-OH-cortisol and 18-oxo-cortisol are elevated.
    - Treatment is with physiologic doses of a glucocorticoid (e.g., 7.5 mg prednisone daily). Mineralocorticoid antagonists are also useful. Treatment is indicated in normotensive individuals as well.
  - FH2—caused by an unknown mutation.
  - FH3—caused by mutations in potassium channel KCJN5.
    - FH2 can present with adrenal adenoma or hyperplasia; FH3 is associated with adrenal hyperplasia
    - Treat like Conn syndrome
    - Bilateral adrenalectomy may be needed in FH3.

Question 6.2.5: This patient had a normal PAC of 10 ng/dL and a low PRA of 1 ng/mL/h, giving an ARR of 10:1. How would you interpret this result?

The combination of low renin and low or normal aldosterone in a hypertensive patient can be seen in patients who have both corticosteroid and mineralocorticoid excess, such as exogenous steroids, Cushing syndrome, or congenital adrenal hyperplasia. Low renin and low aldosterone is typical of uncommon syndromes such as AME, licorice ingestion, ectopic ACTH secretion, and Liddle syndrome.

- Apparent Mineralocorticoid Excess:
  - Renal mineralocorticoid receptors (MRs) bind cortisol and aldosterone with similar affinity. However, activation of MR by cortisol is normally limited by conversion of cortisol to inactive cortisone by 11-beta-hydroxysteroid dehydrogenase 2 (11BHSD2).
  - This conversion is impaired in AME because of a mutation in the *11BHSD2* gene, resulting in activation of MR by cortisol. This is usually transmitted as an autosomal recessive trait.
  - AME can range from mild to severe. Usual manifestations are juvenile hypertension associated with low birth weight, failure to thrive, poor growth, hypokalemia, and metabolic alkalosis. Both PRA and PAC are low. Diagnosis can be made by an elevated urine cortisol to cortisone ratio. Genetic testing is also available. Adults can present with a milder late-onset syndrome.
  - Treatment consists of low-sodium diet, high-potassium diet, and blockade of mineralocorticoid effects (spironolactone, eplerenone, amiloride, or triamterene).
- Licorice Ingestion:
  - The pathogenesis is similar to AME. Licorice contains glycyrrhetinic acid, which inhibits 11BHSD2 in the kidney, preventing conversion of cortisol to inactive cortisone and activation of MR by cortisol.
  - Glycyrrhetinic acid is also present in snuff, diet substances, chewing tobacco, and grapefruit.
- Ectopic ACTH Syndrome:
  - Ectopic ACTH release (usually from small-cell lung cancer) results in very high cortisol levels, exceeding the metabolic capacity of 11BHSD2, and MR activation.
  - Patients typically present with weight loss and hypokalemic metabolic alkalosis. Cushingoid features may be absent. Marked elevation of serum ACTH and 24 hour urinary free cortisol are diagnostic.
- Liddle syndrome:
  - Autosomal dominant genetic disorder leading to gain-of-function mutation in the aldosterone-sensitive epithelial sodium channel (ENaC) in the distal tubule.
  - Clinical presentation is hypertension, hypokalemia, and metabolic alkalosis, similar to primary aldosteronism. However, there are reductions in both PAC and urinary aldosterone excretion. Genetic testing is available.

- Treatment is with amiloride or triamterene, which directly inhibit ENaC (spironolactone is ineffective).

Question 6.2.6: What is the most likely diagnosis?

CASE STUDY 6.2 CONTINUED

PAC <10 ng/dL excludes primary or secondary aldosteronism. There is no clinical evidence for exogenous steroids (no history), Cushing syndrome (not Cushingoid on physical examination), or congenital adrenal hyperplasia (no suggestive physical examination findings, e.g., the absence of secondary sexual characteristics or body hair). Low renin and low-to-normal aldosterone are typical of uncommon syndromes such as AME, licorice ingestion, ectopic ACTH, and Liddle syndrome. However, the most likely diagnosis is the much more common low renin hypertension, which is the most prevalent form of essential hypertension.

- Low renin hypertension:
  - Most frequent in African American and elderly patients.
  - There may be a gain of function in renal sodium channels with defective negative feedback of aldosterone release.
  - Aldosterone should be low in the face of low renin, so normal levels may indicate the presence of mineralocorticoid excess (Mackenzie & Brown, 2009).
  - Some patients with low renin hypertension have underlying mild primary aldosteronism. The prevalence of primary aldosteronism in different studies has varied from 0.05% to 2% to as high as 5% to 18% (Gyamlami et al., 2016). These differences likely reflect varied study populations and diagnostic criteria.
  - Dietary salt restriction is the cornerstone to treatment
  - Patients with low renin hypertension respond well to diuretics (thiazides, spironolactone, amiloride) and calcium channel blockers

CASE STUDY 6.2 CONCLUDED

The patient is treated with a combination of thiazide and spironolactone as well as amlodipine, a calcium channel blocker. BP decreases to 135/85 mm Hg and remains stable.

HYPERKALEMIA

CASE STUDY 6.3 An 18-year-old male with a family history of childhood hypertension in the father and brother presents with a history of developmental delay, dizziness, muscle weakness, and fatigue. He is not taking medications.

Vitals: pulse 65 beats/min, respiratory rate 20 breaths/min, BP 160/90 mm Hg, temperature 99°F.

Physical examination:
General: alert and oriented to time, place, and person, underweight.
Heart: normal S1/S2, no murmurs/rubs/gallops
Lungs: clear
Abdomen: soft, no guarding/rebound
Neurology: no focal findings
Lower extremities: no edema

Blood chemistry:
Sodium: 140 mmol/L
Potassium: 6.0 mmol/L
Chloride: 110 mmol/L
Total CO_2: 18 mmol/L
Urea nitrogen: 10 mg/dL (urea: 3.6 mmol/L)
Creatinine: 1.0 mg/dL (88.4 mcmol/L)
Glucose: 90 mg/dL (5 mmol/L)

Complete blood count:
WBC: 4,000/mm^3
Hemoglobin: 14 g/dL (140 g/L)
Hematocrit: 40%
Platelets: 200,000/mm^3
Urine potassium: 10 mmol/L
PRA: 1 ng/mL/h
Aldosterone: 10 ng/dL
Renal ultrasound: no hydronephrosis, no increased echogenicity, normal size

Question 6.3.1: What is the first step in the evaluation of hyperkalemia?

The first step in the evaluation of hyperkalemia when it occurs in a patient with normal renal function is to rule out spurious causes such as elevated white cell count and thrombocytosis (pseudohyperkalemia). Once that has been excluded, one needs to determine whether hyperkalemia is due to transcellular redistribution, decreased renal excretion, or increased intake or endogenous production.

Etiologies of Hyperkalemia (see Table 6.2)

- Pseudohyperkalemia—prolonged use of tourniquet, especially with concomitant fist clenching; hemolysis; increased WBC or platelet count (serum K^+ but not plasma K^+ increases due to clotting of blood with thrombocytosis). Most hospitals can now rapidly measure whole blood K^+; this will exclude most but not all cases of pseudohyperkalemia. Once pseudohyperkalemia is either excluded by being either clinically very unlikely or by retesting (as above), the etiology of hyperkalemia should be pursued.
- Hyperkalemia due to transcellular redistribution (impaired uptake of K^+ into cells or shift of K^+ out of cells with generally normal total body potassium):
  - Acidosis (inorganic metabolic acidosis) (increases H^+ uptake and K^+ exit by cells)
  - Hyperkalemic familial periodic paralysis (shift of K^+ out of cells; very rare)

Etiologies of Hyperkalemia (in the Absence of Severe AKI or CKD)

Hyperkalemia

Impaired Urinary Excretion Urine K < 20 mmol/L Fractional excretion of K (FEK) < 10%	Excessive Input Urine K > 20 mmol/L Fractional excretion of K (FEK) > 10%	Urine K Variable or Unknown
High renin Low aldosterone	High renin High aldosterone	Variable renin Variable aldosterone
High renin High aldosterone		
Normal renin High aldosterone		
Low renin Low aldosterone		

Impaired Urinary Excretion (Urine K < 20 mmol/L; FEK < 10%)

High renin / Low aldosterone
- Addison disease
- Primary hypoaldosteronism
- Congenital adrenal hyperplasia
- Direct renin inhibitors:
  - Aliskiren
  - ↑PRC, ↓PRA
- ACE inhibitors
- Angiotensin II receptor blockers
- Heparin

High renin / High aldosterone
- PHA-1
- Aldosterone resistance
- ENaC channel blockers:
  - Triamterene
  - Amiloride
  - Trimethoprim
  - Pentamidine
- Aldosterone receptor blockers (spironolactone, eplerenone)
- Calcineurin inhibitors:
  - Inhibit Na/K ATPase
  - Inhibit ROMK
  - Increase chloride reabsorption
  - Inhibit RAAS
  - Block ENaC channels
  - Cause aldosterone resistance

Normal renin / High aldosterone
- Chronic kidney disease

Low renin / Low aldosterone
- Renal tubular acidosis type 4
- Nonsteroidal anti-inflammatory drugs
- Acute interstitial nephritis (some cases)
- Obstruction (some cases)
- Gordon syndrome (PHA-2)
  - (Aldosterone can be low, high, or normal)

Excessive Input (Urine K > 20 mmol/L; FEK > 10%)

High renin / High aldosterone
- Tumor lysis syndrome
- Tissue necrosis
- Hemolysis
- Rhabdomyolysis
- Salt substitutes
- High-potassium foods:
  - White beans
  - Dark leafy greens
  - Potatoes
  - Yogurt
  - Salmon
  - Bananas
- Pica
- Intravenous penicillin
- Transfusions
- Potassium supplements

Urine K Variable or Unknown

Variable renin / Variable aldosterone
- Pseudohyperkalemia (spurious hyperkalemia)
  - Severe leukocytosis
  - Severe thrombocytosis
  - Fist clenching or prolonged use of tourniquet
- Compartment shifts
- Insulin deficiency
- Hyperglycemia
- Succinylcholine
- Inorganic (nonanion gap) metabolic acidosis
- Hyperosmolality
- Periodic paralysis
- Exercise
- Digoxin poisoning

ACE, angiotensin-converting enzyme; Cr, creatinine; ENaC, epithelial sodium channel; PHA-1, pseudohypoaldosteronism type 1; PRA, plasma renin activity; PRC, plasma aldosterone concentration; RAAS, renin–angiotensin–aldosterone system; ROMK, renal outer medullary potassium.

- Acute hypertonicity (osmolar water and K^+ shift out of cells)
- Insulin deficiency (decreased K^+ uptake into cells) (very common)
- Drugs—digitalis intoxication (blocks Na–K ATPase, increasing K^+ egress from cells)
- Beta-blockers (nonselective blockers impair K^+ uptake in response to β_2 receptor activation)
- Hyperkalemia due to decreased renal excretion:
  - Acute kidney impairment (AKI)/chronic kidney disease (CKD)
  - Drugs—potassium-sparing diuretics, RAAS inhibitors (block Ang II and aldosterone production or action), heparin (inhibits biosynthesis of aldosterone), NSAIDs (inhibit renin and aldosterone formation), cyclosporine, tacrolimus, trimethoprim, pentamidine (block tubular secretion)
  - Adrenal insufficiency—Addison disease, selective hypoaldosteronism (latter common in diabetics)
  - RTA
- Hyperkalemia due to increased intake or endogenous production (decreased renal excretion usually also present):
  - Increased intake: salt substitutes
  - Endogenous production: massive hemolysis, rhabdomyolysis, tumor lysis syndrome (Arrambide & Toto, 1993)

Question 6.3.2: How does one interpret urinary potassium concentration in the face of hyperkalemia?

Elevated urinary potassium (>20 mmol/L and usually >40 mmol/L) is the appropriate renal response to hyperkalemia. A 24-hour urine K >80 to 100 mmol/d supports increased potassium intake as the cause of hyperkalemia (usually in the setting of chronic kidney disease). A fractional excretion of potassium (FEK) >10% is practical and takes into account differences in urinary concentration. High FEK supports increased production (e.g., from cell breakdown), increased intake, compartment shifts, and certain medications, such as digoxin and succinylcholine.

The low urine potassium (<20 mmol/L) in this hyperkalemic patient indicates impaired renal excretion of potassium. An FEK <10% also indicates impaired renal excretion of potassium. The differential for decreased renal excretion of potassium includes CKD, obstructive uropathy, hyperkalemic RTA, and drugs that impair renal potassium excretion.

CASE STUDY 6.3 CONTINUED

This patient has no evidence of kidney disease, urinary obstruction, or hypoaldosteronism, and he is not taking drugs that decrease renal potassium excretion.

Question 6.3.3: What familial diseases can cause hyperkalemia due to decreased renal excretion?

Familial diseases that should be considered in hyperkalemia include pseudohypoaldosteronism type 1 (PHA-1) and pseudohypoaldosteronism type 2 (PHA-2, also called Gordon syndrome). These conditions are uncommon. Adrenal insufficiency (Addison disease) or selective hypoaldosteronism (i.e., with normal cortisol) should also be considered. Selective hypoaldosteronism is a common cause of hyperkalemic RTA (see Acid/Base chapter).

- PHA-1:
  - Autosomal dominant or autosomal recessive (systemic)
  - Characterized by aldosterone resistance because of a defect either in the ENaC or the MR
  - Plasma renin and aldosterone are both high
  - Treatment includes sodium administration, potassium restriction, and prostaglandin inhibitors to limit urinary sodium losses
- PHA-2 (Gordon syndrome):
  - Autosomal dominant disorder caused by abnormalities in WNK kinases
  - WNK1 activates NCC, which is present in the distal convoluted tubule, whereas WNK4 reduces trafficking of NCC to the plasma membrane
  - Absence of WNK kinase activity results in constitutive expression and activation of NCCs
  - Gordon syndrome is characterized by hyperkalemia, normal renal function, mild nonanion gap metabolic acidosis, low fractional excretion of sodium (FENa), hypercalciuria, hypertension, low PRA, and variable PAC
  - Treatment is with thiazide diuretics
- Hyporeninemic hypoaldosteronism
  - As opposed to hypoadrenalism (Addison disease), selective hypoaldosteronism is characterized by both diminished renin release and an adrenal defect in aldosterone production but normal cortisol production
  - Most common in patients with CKD due to diabetes or chronic interstitial disease or taking NSAIDs (inhibition of vasodilator prostaglandins inhibits renin release)
- Hyperreninemic hypoaldosteronism
  - Usually due to drug-induced inhibition of aldosterone production
    - RAAS inhibitors (interfere with stimulation of aldosterone by Ang II)
    - Heparin (inhibits biosynthesis of aldosterone) (Leehey et al., 1981)

Question 6.3.4: What are the clinical features of hypoaldosteronism?

Patients with hypoaldosteronism typically have a subclinical or moderate decrease in aldosterone release or resistance, and serum potassium is usually normal or mildly high. Overt hyperkalemia requires the presence of additional risk factors that further impair potassium excretion. These precipitating factors can include decrease in renal function or, more commonly, new medications. Medications that interfere with potassium handling include ENaC blockers (trimethoprim/sulfamethoxazole, amiloride, pentamidine), mineralocorticoid antagonists (spironolactone, eplerenone), ACE inhibitors, ARBs, or renin inhibitors.

Question 6.3.5: What are the consequences, symptoms and treatment principles of hyperkalemia?

Consequences of Hyperkalemia

- Cardiac effects: EKG changes (Fig. 6.2)—tall peaked T-waves, prolonged PR interval, widened QRS complex, disappearance of P-wave, "sine-wave" pattern
- Neuromuscular effects: weakness, paralysis
- Hormonal and renal effects: decreased NH_3 production, leading to impaired excretion of NH_4^+ and metabolic acidosis

Symptoms of Hyperkalemia

- Weakness, fatigue, muscle paralysis, palpitations, bradycardia, cardiac arrest

Treatment of Hyperkalemia

- Review diet and medications. Assure low K^+ diet (2 g/day) and discontinue any drugs that can cause hyperkalemia. Discontinue salt substitutes
- K-binding resins such as sodium polystyrene sulfonate (Kayexalate) useful to decrease total body K^+—1 g binds ~1 mmol of K^+ in the gut
- High-salt diet, loop diuretics—increase sodium delivery to distal tubule
- Mineralocorticoids (fludrocortisone or Florinef)—especially if aldosterone level is decreased
- In cases of life-threatening hyperkalemia (i.e., EKG changes and/or neuromuscular symptoms and signs), parenteral therapy is indicated: calcium gluconate or chloride (1 g) (antagonize electrical effects of potassium on cardiac tissue), insulin-glucose (10 U of insulin with 100 mL 50% dextrose), sodium bicarbonate (50–100 mmol) (both shift K^+ into cells). Hyperkalemia brings the activation potential closer to the resting potential, thereby facilitating depolarization; calcium reestablishes the distance between the resting potential and the activation potential

CASE STUDY 6.3 CONCLUDED

This patient is diagnosed with Gordon syndrome and is started on hydrochlorothiazide. Hyperkalemia, metabolic acidosis, and hypertension are resolved thereafter.

CASE STUDY 6.4

A 60-year-old female with type 2 diabetes mellitus treated with insulin presents for evaluation of CKD. She has retinopathy and macroalbuminuria. Three days previously, she was found to have a urinary tract infection (UTI) and started on an antibiotic. She is currently asymptomatic.

Physical examination is significant for hypertension (150/88 mm Hg) and lower extremity edema. The remainder of the examination is normal.

Blood chemistry:
Sodium: 140 mmol/L
Potassium: 6.5 mmol/L
Chloride: 105 mmol/L
Total CO_2: 20 mmol/L
Urea nitrogen: 30 mg/dL (urea: 10.7 mmol/L)
Creatinine: 2.2 mg/dL (195 mcmol/L)
Glucose: 100 mg/dL (5.6 mmol/L)
Osmolality: 300 mmol/kg

Urine chemistry:
pH: 5.0
Sodium: 30 mmol/L
Potassium: 15 mmol/L
Chloride: 20 mmol/L
Osmolality: 600 mmol/kg

Complete blood count:
WBC: 5,000/mm^3
Hemoglobin: 14 g/dL (140 g/L)
Hematocrit: 42%
Platelets: 200,000/mm^3
EKG: normal sinus rhythm; peaked T-waves

Question 6.4.1: **What is the etiology of hyperkalemia?**

Hyperkalemia can be due to compartment shift (from cells to ECF), excessive input or impaired secretion, or a combination of these factors. In this patient, the urine potassium concentration is low, indicating inability of the kidneys to excrete potassium despite hyperkalemia. Nonanion gap metabolic acidosis, coupled with a positive urine "net charge" (urine Na^+ plus K^+ > urine Cl^-), suggests RTA in this patient (see Acid/Base chapter). Low urine pH distinguishes hyperkalemic distal RTA type 4 from RTA type 1; RTA type 1 or distal RTA is characterized by inability to secrete protons into the urine (leading to inappropriately elevated urine pH) and hypokalemia.

Question 6.4.2: **What is the pathophysiology of RTA type 4?**

In diabetics, there is glycosylation of renin leading to hyporeninemic hypoaldosteronism. In addition, renal tubular damage may cause inadequate renin production, the adrenals may not produce adequate aldosterone, and/or the cortical collecting tubules may not respond to aldosterone.

Question 6.4.3: **How is RTA type 4 treated?**

It is treated with diuretics, oral bicarbonate, and, if necessary, potassium-binding resins or synthetic aldosterone (fludrocortisone).

Question 6.4.4: What precipitated RTA type 4 in this patient?

CASE STUDY 6.4 CONCLUDED

A phone call to the treating physician reveals that she has been given trimethoprim-sulfamethoxazole (Bactrim) one double-strength tablet twice daily to treat her UTI. Trimethoprim blocks ENaC, leading to decreased distal sodium delivery and decreased potassium secretion.

VIGNETTE 1

HYPOKALEMIA

A 44-year-old male with a history of transient ischemic attacks presents for evaluation of resistant hypertension. He denies chest pain, visual symptoms, hematuria, abdominal pain, nausea/vomiting, or headaches. Medications include metoprolol succinate 100 mg po qd, lisinopril 20 mg po qd, clonidine 0.3 mg po bid, and hydrochlorothiazide/triamterene 25/37.5 mg. He denies smoking, alcohol intake, or illicit drugs. Vitals are as follows: pulse 75 beats/min, respiratory rate 22 breaths/min, BP 177/110 mm Hg, temperature 37°C. He is not orthostatic, and his body mass index is normal. Funduscopic examination shows cotton wool spots. Cardiac examination demonstrates a prominent point of maximal impulse. The remainder of the examination is normal.

Blood chemistry:
Sodium: 146 mmol/L
Potassium: 3.0 mmol/L
Chloride: 106 mmol/L
Total CO_2: 30 mmol/L
Urea nitrogen: 15 mg/dL (urea: 5.4 mmol/L)
Creatinine: 1.0 mg/dL (88.4 mcmol/L)
Glucose: 133 mg/dL (7.4 mmol/L)

Urine chemistry:
Sodium: 50 mmol/L
Potassium: 45 mmol/L
Chloride: 60 mmol/L
Urinalysis : normal

Complete blood count:
WBC: 4,500/mm^3
Hemoglobin: 12 g/dL (120 g/L)
Hematocrit: 40%
Platelets: 300,000/mm^3
Chest X-ray: normal
Plasma aldosterone: 20 ng/dL (553 pmol/L)
PRA: 0.5 ng/mL/h

Q: What is the next step in the evaluation of the hypokalemia?

1. Renal Doppler ultrasound
2. 24-hour urine cortisol
3. 24-hour urine for metanephrines
4. 24-hour urine for aldosterone
5. CT of the adrenals

A: Resistant hypertension associated with hypokalemia with inappropriate kaliuresis, mild hypernatremia, and metabolic alkalosis suggests primary hyperaldosteronism. Hypokalemia despite use of triamterene and an ACE inhibitor is also suggestive of primary aldosteronism. The ratio of PAC to PRA is a good screening test for primary aldosteronism, with an elevated aldosterone level concomitant with suppressed PRA consistent with the diagnosis.

Also in the differential of resistant hypertension with hypokalemia are hypercortisolism, renovascular hypertension (secondary aldosteronism due to renin secretion), sleep apnea (secondary aldosteronism), and pheochromocytoma (increased potassium shift into cells due to hyperadrenergic state). A 24-hour urine cortisol could be useful to exclude hypercortisolism (Cushing syndrome), but there are no clinical manifestations to suggest this disorder, so it is not indicated. Renal Doppler ultrasound would be helpful in excluding renal artery stenosis, but there is no evidence for vascular disease on physical examination and hyperaldosteronism in renal artery stenosis would be secondary, that is, associated with elevated PRA. There is no clinical evidence of sleep apnea or pheochromocytoma. Also, hypernatremia is not expected with any of these alternative diagnoses.

Once the diagnosis of primary aldosteronism is confirmed by elevated 24-hour urine aldosterone excretion, the next step is to determine whether the disease process is caused by an adrenal adenoma or hyperplasia by a CT of the adrenals.

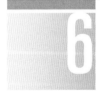

VIGNETTE 2

HYPOKALEMIA

A 26-year-old female with a history of depression, anxiety, and irritable bowel syndrome presents for evaluation of abdominal pain with associated symptoms of nausea, vomiting, and diarrhea. She denies hematemesis or hematochezia. She was at a party where contaminated food was served, and many of the people present at the party became sick with nausea, vomiting, diarrhea, and abdominal pain. She denies any recent new medications but takes Elavil (amitriptyline) and Xanax (alprazolam) for depression and anxiety on a daily basis. She denies smoking, alcohol abuse, or use of illicit drugs. Vitals are as follows: pulse 100 beats/min, BP 117/60 mm Hg (supine), pulse 120 beats/min, BP 90/55 mm Hg (standing), respiratory rate 20 breaths/min, temperature 37.5°C. There is some periumbilical tenderness, and bowel sounds are hyperactive. The remainder of the examination is normal.

Blood chemistry:
Sodium: 136 mmol/L
Potassium: 3.0 mmol/L
Chloride: 91 mmol/L
Total CO_2: 34 mmol/L
Urea nitrogen: 15 mg/dL (urea: 5.4 mmol/L)
Creatinine: 2.0 mg/dL (177 mcmol/L)
Glucose: 133 mg/dL (7.4 mmol/L)
Magnesium: 1.0 mg/dL (0.4 mmol/L)
Osmolality: 286 mmol/kg

Urine chemistry:
pH: 7
Sodium: 60 mmol/L
Potassium: 30 mmol/L
Chloride: 5 mmol/L
Osmolality: 500 mmol/kg
Creatinine: 60 mg/L (5,304 mcmol/L)
FENa: 1.5%

Complete blood count:
WBC: 4,500/mm^3
Hemoglobin: 14 g/dL (140 g/L)
Hematocrit: 42%
Platelets: 300,000/mm^3
Chest X-ray: no abnormalities

IV saline and potassium are administered, after which orthostasis resolves, the plasma urea nitrogen and creatinine normalize, and metabolic alkalosis resolves within 24 hours. Vomiting and diarrhea also completely resolve. However, a repeat plasma potassium level remains 3.0 mmol/L, and urine potassium is still 30 mmol/L.

Q: Which of the following actions should be taken?

1. Block aldosterone with spironolactone
2. Give additional IV potassium
3. Replace magnesium
4. 2 and 3 only
5. All of the above

A: The history and physical examination seem consistent with food poisoning. Laboratory studies indicate acute renal failure, hypokalemia, and metabolic alkalosis. The etiology of the renal failure is most certainly prerenal based on the history, examination, and improvement in renal function after fluid administration. The unexpectedly high FENa on admission is explained by excretion of sodium (as well as potassium) with bicarbonate by the kidney (the urine pH of 7 in the absence of infection indicates bicarbonate is present in the urine). Note that urine chloride is low owing to chloride and volume depletion. The low plasma urea nitrogen to creatinine ratio is probably because of poor oral intake and reduced urea generation.

What is the etiology of the initial hypokalemia, and why does it persist despite potassium administration and correction of metabolic alkalosis? The urine potassium of >20 mmol/L suggests that renal loss of potassium is the cause of hypokalemia. With active vomiting, bicarbonaturia and hypovolemia-induced secondary hyperaldosteronism in combination lead to urinary potassium loss, which explains the hypokalemia present on admission. However, even after vomiting has stopped and fluids and potassium repleted, there is still inappropriate renal potassium wasting in this patient.

The best answer is that hypomagnesemia must be corrected. Hypomagnesemia leads to renal potassium loss through activation of the ROMK channel. Therefore, the plasma potassium will not correct until the plasma magnesium is corrected. Additional IV potassium will be effective once magnesium is replaced. Aldosterone blockade is not indicated in the absence of hypertension or congestive heart failure.

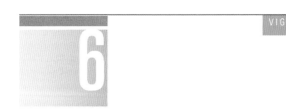

VIGNETTE 3

HYPERKALEMIA

A 60-year-old male with type 2 diabetes mellitus presents for evaluation of CKD. He has retinopathy and macroalbuminuria. He is going to be started on an ACE inhibitor when he is found to be hyperkalemic, so he is sent to the emergency room. He is asymptomatic otherwise. He takes metformin and glyburide. Physical examination is significant for hypertension (150/88 mm Hg) and 1+ lower extremity edema. The remainder of the examination is normal.

Blood chemistry:
Sodium: 140 mmol/L
Potassium: 6.5 mmol/L
Chloride: 105 mmol/L
Total CO_2: 20 mmol/L
Urea nitrogen: 30 mg/dL (urea: 10.7 mmol/L)
Creatinine: 2.2 mg/dL (195 mcmol/L)
Glucose: 100 mg/dL (5.6 mmol/L)
Osmolality: 300 mmol/kg

Urine chemistry:
pH: 5.0
Sodium: 30 mmol/L
Potassium: 26 mmol/L
Chloride: 18 mmol/L
Osmolality: 600 mmol/kg

Complete blood count:
WBC: 5,000/mm^3
Hemoglobin: 14 g/dL (140 g/L)
Hematocrit: 41%
Platelets: 200,000/mm^3
Fasting cortisol: 11 mcg/dL (303 nmol/L) (normal)
TTKG = (26/6.5)/(600/300) = 2
EKG: normal sinus rhythm, peaked T-waves

Q: In this patient, which of the following is not one of the mechanisms for hyperkalemia?

1. Renal tubular damage may cause inadequate renin production.
2. Adrenal dysfunction may cause inadequate aldosterone production.
3. Renal tubules are defective in the secretion of protons.
4. Principal cells of cortical collecting tubule may not respond to aldosterone.

A: In this patient with diabetes and CKD and EKG changes, hyperkalemia is truly present. However, in other circumstances, one should consider pseudohyperkalemia due to hemolysis, extreme thrombocytosis, or leukocytosis.

The urine potassium concentration is low, indicating inability of the kidneys to secrete potassium despite hyperkalemia. Nonanion gap metabolic acidosis, a positive urine net charge, and a low TTKG establish RTA in this patient. Low urine pH distinguishes RTA type 4 from RTA type 1; RTA type 1 or distal RTA is characterized by inability to secrete protons into the urine.

RTA type 4 or hyperkalemic RTA in diabetic patients is usually due to hyporeninemic hypoaldosteronism. Renal tubular damage may cause inadequate renin production, the adrenals may not produce adequate aldosterone, and/or the cortical collecting tubules may not respond to aldosterone. It is treated with diuretics, oral bicarbonate, and, if necessary, potassium-binding resins or synthetic aldosterone (fludrocortisone).

HYPERKALEMIA

A 60-year-old woman with polycystic kidney disease is seen by an outside physician for UTI. She is given an antibiotic and told to take it for 7 days. She does not remember the name of it. After finishing the antibiotic, she subsequently develops weakness and comes to the emergency room. On physical examination, her vital signs are normal. She has mild proximal muscle weakness in both upper and lower extremities, and reflexes are diffusely sluggish.

Blood chemistry:
Sodium: 140 mmol/L
Potassium: 6.5 mmol/L
Chloride: 105 mmol/L
Total CO_2: 20 mmol/L
Urea nitrogen: 30 mg/dL (urea: 10.7 nmol/L)
Creatinine: 2.2 mg/dL (195 mcmol/L)
Glucose: 100 mg/dL (5.6 mmol/L)
Osmolality: 300 mmol/kg

Urine chemistry:
pH: 5.0

Sodium: 30 mmol/L
Potassium: 26 mmol/L
Chloride: 18 mmol/L
Osmolality: 600 mmol/kg

Complete blood count:
WBC: 5,000/mm^3
Hemoglobin: 14 g/dL (140 g/L)
Hematocrit: 41%
Platelets: 200,000/mm^3
Fasting cortisol: 11 mcg/dL (303 nmol/L) (normal)
TTKG = (26/6.5)/(600/300) = 2
EKG: normal sinus rhythm, peaked T-waves

Q: What is the most likely diagnosis?

1. Hypoaldosteronism
2. Aldosterone resistance
3. Drug-induced hyperkalemia
4. Hyperkalemic distal RTA

A: One may observe that, by a strange coincidence, this patient has exactly the same laboratory data as the first patient. However, unlike the previous patient, this patient is not likely to have hypoaldosteronism because, as opposed to diabetes, this etiology of hyperkalemia is uncommon in polycystic kidney disease. A phone call to the treating physician reveals that she was given trimethoprim-sulfamethoxazole (Bactrim) one double-strength tablet twice daily. Trimethoprim has an amiloride-like effect on the distal tubule and blocks potassium secretion, which can lead to hyperkalemia in the setting of CKD. Note that a low TTKG in the face of hyperkalemia is not diagnostic of hypoaldosteronism; other etiologies need to be considered.

References

Adrogué HJ, Madias NE. Changes in plasma potassium concentration during acute acid-base disturbances. *Am J Med.* 71:456–467, 1981.

Arrambide K, Toto RD. Tumor lysis syndrome. *Semin Nephrol.* 13:273–280, 1993.

Blumenfeld JD, Sealey JE, Schlussel Y, et al. Diagnosis and treatment of primary hyper-aldosteronism. *Ann Intern Med.* 121:877–885, 1994.

Conn JW, Cohen EL, Rovner DR. Landmark article Oct 19, 1964: suppression of plasma renin activity in primary aldosteronism. Distinguishing primary from secondary aldosteronism in hypertensive disease. *JAMA.* 253(4):558–566, 1985.

Funder JW, Carey RM, Mantero F, et al. The management of primary aldosteronism: case detection, diagnosis, and treatment: an Endocrine Society Clinical Practice Guideline. *Clin Endocrinol Metab.* 101(5):1889–1916, 2016.

Giebisch G, Krapf R, Wagner C. Renal and extrarenal regulation of potassium. *Kidney Int.* 72:397–410, 2007.

Gladziwa U, Schwarz R, Gitter AH, et al. Chronic hypokalemia of adults: Gitelman's syndrome is frequent but classical Bartter's syndrome is rare. *Nephrol Dial Transplant.* 10:1607–1613, 1995.

Gyamlami G, Headley CM, Naseer A, et al. Primary Aldosteronism: diagnosis and management. *Am J Med Sci.* 352(4):391–398, 2016.

Leehey DJ, Gantt C, Lim VS. Heparin-induced hypoaldosteronism. *JAMA.* 246: 2189–2190, 1981.

Mackenzie IS, Brown MJ. Molecular and clinical investigations in patients with low-renin hypertension. *Clin Exp Nephrol.* 13(1):1–8, 2009.

Matsunoshita N, Nozu K, Shono A, et al. Differential diagnosis of Bartter syndrome, Gitelman syndrome, and pseudo-Bartter/Gitelman syndrome based on clinical characteristics. *Genet Med.* 18(2):180–188, 2016.

Viering DH, de Baaij JH, Walsh SB, et al. Genetic causes of hypomagnesemia, a clinical overview. *Pediatr Nephrol.* 32(7):1123–1135, 2017.

Whang R, Flink EB, Dyckner T, et al. Magnesium depletion as a cause of refractory potassium depletion. *Arch Intern Med.* 149:1686–1689, 1985.

7

Metabolic Acidosis and Alkalosis

INTRODUCTION

■ An acid is a compound capable of donating a proton (hydrogen ion), and a base is a compound capable of accepting a proton.
■ pH is defined as the negative logarithm of the hydrogen ion concentration [H⁺].

GENERAL CONCEPTS

■ Daily acid production
  ■ Volatile (CO_2 production—excreted by lungs)
  ■ Nonvolatile (acid production from intermediary metabolism, specifically catabolism of sulfur-containing amino acids in protein)
■ There are two main homeostatic mechanisms that are responsible for maintaining acid–base balance in response to nonvolatile acid production:
  ■ Internal buffer systems (neutralize acid)
  ■ Excretion of hydrogen ion (excrete acid)

METABOLIC ACIDOSIS

Metabolic acidosis is defined as a primary decrease in the bicarbonate concentration [HCO_3^-] of the plasma. It is normally accompanied by a decrease in partial pressure of carbon dioxide (pCO_2) (respiratory adaptation) to maintain near-normal pH.

Henderson and Henderson-Hasselbalch

Henderson and Henderson-Hasselbalch equations depict the relationship between the three determining variables in acid–base homeostasis.

Henderson   Henderson-Hasselbalch

$$[H+] = \frac{24pCO_2}{HCO_3^-} \quad \text{or} \quad pH = pK + \log\frac{HCO_3^-}{H_2CO_3}$$

pH	[H⁺] (nEq/L)
7.1	80
7.2	65
7.3	50
7.4	40
7.5	30
7.6	25
7.7	20

| | The Four Primary Acid–Base Disorders and Their Compensatory Responses | | |

Acid–Base Disorder	Primary Abnormality	Effect on [H⁺]	Compensatory Response
Metabolic acidosis	$\downarrow[HCO_3^-]$	Increase	$\downarrow pCO_2$
Metabolic alkalosis	$\uparrow[HCO_3^-]$	Decrease	$\uparrow pCO_2$
Respiratory acidosis	$\uparrow pCO_2$	Increase	$\uparrow[HCO_3^-]$
Respiratory alkalosis	$\downarrow pCO_2$	Decrease	$\downarrow[HCO_3^-]$

Acid–base homeostasis is dependent on the following reactions: $[H^+] + [HCO_3^-] \longleftrightarrow H_2CO_3 \longleftrightarrow H_2O + CO_2$ (excreted by lungs). A primary change in either $[HCO_3^-]$ or pCO_2 will produce an adaptive (compensatory) change in the other in the same direction, in an attempt to keep pH constant (Tables 7.1 and 7.2) (Javaheri et al., 1982; Madias, 2010; Pierce et al., 1970).

Renal Regulation of Acid–Base Balance

 Reabsorption of filtered bicarbonate. Most or all of bicarbonate filtered at the glomerulus is reabsorbed, primarily in the proximal tubule. Failure of this reabsorption mechanism leads to *proximal renal tubular acidosis (RTA)*.

| | Expected Compensation for Primary Acid–Base Disorders | | |

Type	Primary Change	Secondary Adaptation	Usual Limits of Adaptation
Metabolic acidosis	Decrease in $[HCO_3^-]$ of 1 mEq/L	Decrease in pCO_2 of 1.2 mm Hg; Alternatives: $pCO_2 = (1.5 \times [HCO_3^-]) + 8$ pCO_2 = last two digits of pH × 100	pCO_2 = 15 mm Hg (occasionally lower)
Metabolic alkalosis	Increase in $[HCO_3^-]$ of 1 mEq/L	Increase in pCO_2 of 0.7 mm Hg	pCO_2 = 55 mm Hg
Respiratory acidosis	Increase in pCO_2 of 10 mm Hg	Acute: increase in $[HCO_3^-]$ of 1.0 mEq/L; Chronic: increase in $[HCO_3^-]$ of 3.5 mEq/L	Acute: $[HCO_3^-]$ = 38 mEq/L; Chronic: $[HCO_3^-]$ = 45 mEq/L
Respiratory alkalosis	Decrease in pCO_2 of 10 mm Hg	Acute: decrease in $[HCO_3^-]$ of 2 mEq/L; Chronic: decrease in $[HCO_3^-]$ of 4–5 mEq/L	Acute: $[HCO_3^-]$ = 18 mEq/L; Chronic: $[HCO_3^-]$ = 15 mEq/L

Adapted from Emmett M. Diagnosis of simple and mixed disorders. In DuBose TD, Hamm LL, eds. *Acid-Base and Electrolyte Disorders: A Companion to Brenner and Rector's The Kidney.* Philadelphia, PA: WB Saunders; 2002:41–54.

- *Excretion of acid*. The kidney excretes acid in three fashions:
  - Free hydrogen ion (H^+) excretion (lowers urine pH)—this is quantitatively the least important mechanism
  - Titratable acid excretion (secreted H^+ combines with poorly re-absorbable anions such as phosphate)
  - Excretion of ammonium ion (NH_4^+). The kidney generates ammonia (NH_3) that combines with secreted H^+ and is excreted as ammonium ion.

  Failure of H^+ secretion and/or ammonia production/ammonium excretion results in *distal RTA*.

- High-anion gap (AG) acidosis

  The AG is a concept to give a clue as to the cause of metabolic acidosis (Gabow et al., 1980). Electroneutrality demands that the number of positive charges equals the number of negative charges (ions) in body fluids. Therefore, in plasma,

  $$Na^+ + K^+ + Ca^{2+} + Mg^{2+} = Cl^- + HCO_3^- + Alb^- + OA^- + PO_4^{-/=} + SO_4^=$$
  where OA = organic anions; Alb = albumin.

  Simplifying this equation to include only certain monovalent measured ions and calling the other ions unmeasured cations (UC) or unmeasured anions (UA):

  $$Na^+ + UC = Cl^- + HCO_3^- + UA$$
  $$AG = Na^+ - (Cl^- + HCO_3^-) = (UA - UC)$$
  $$UA - UC = AG = 10 \text{ to } 12 \text{ mEq/L}$$

  Overproduction of an endogenous organic acid (H^+A^-), where A^- is the acid anion, leads to high-AG metabolic acidosis (e.g., with lactic acidosis A^- = lactate). When lactic acid is produced, the H^+ is titrated by bicarbonate as follows:

  $$H^+A^- + HCO_3^- \rightarrow H_2CO_3 \rightarrow H_2O + CO_2 + A^-$$

  This reaction consumes 1 mol of bicarbonate for each mole of acid produced. If A^- is not excreted or metabolized, it will accumulate in plasma, resulting in an AG. Theoretically, with this type of acidosis, the increase in AG will equal the decrease in bicarbonate concentration (see Supplement for examples).

- Normal-AG (hyperchloremic) acidosis

  Metabolic acidosis can also occur because of decreased renal acid excretion leading to retention of acid (H^+ ions), which titrate extracellular bicarbonate, or it can be caused by loss of bicarbonate from the body. In either instance, the decrease in filtered bicarbonate results in decreased renal bicarbonate and increased renal chloride reabsorption (to maintain electroneutrality), resulting in a *hyperchloremic acidosis*. The plasma chloride rises to the same extent as the plasma bicarbonate falls, and the AG remains normal.

Causes of Metabolic Acidosis

- High-AG acidosis
  - Increased organic acid production (with organic anion shown in parenthesis)

- Lactic acidosis (lactate)
  - Type A lactic acidosis is due to tissue hypoperfusion
    - Most common etiology is sepsis but can occur with any cause of shock
    - Treat underlying cause; exogenous bicarbonate increases pCO_2 and may worsen intracellular acidosis; use only for very severe acidemia (pH < 7.1)
  - Type B lactic acidosis
    - No systemic hypoperfusion
    - Impairment of cellular metabolism
    - Metformin
      - Therapeutic metformin level < 2.5 mcg/mL
      - Hemodialysis is standard of care for severe intoxications
    - Malignancy
      - Increased anaerobic metabolism
      - Resolves with removal of tumor
    - Alcohol
    - HIV
    - Mitochondrial dysfunction
    - Nucleoside reverse transcriptase inhibitors
    - Propofol
    - Linezolid
    - Acquired
    - Congenital
  - Type D lactic acidosis
    - D-Lactate is a stereoisomer of L-lactate
    - Symptoms: confusion, cerebellar ataxia, slurred speech, memory loss (symptoms are not due to D-lactate but due to other toxins generated and absorbed in parallel with D-lactate)
    - Causes of D lactic acidosis
      - Diabetic ketoacidosis (DKA) (buildup of serum acetone)

        Acetone, dihydroxyacetone → methylglyoxal
        → D-lactic acid

      - Short bowel syndrome (intestinal bacteria, esp. *Lactobacilli*)
      - Malabsorption (intestinal bacteria)
      - Antibiotics can precipitate D-lactic acidosis by causing lactobacillus overgrowth
      - Propylene glycol (used as solvent for medications)
    - Treatment: bicarbonate (if severe), oral antibiotics may help in short bowel syndrome, stop propylene glycol
  - False lactic acidosis
    - Ethylene glycol → glycolate and glyoxylate (may cross-react with L-lactate oxidase used in assays performed with blood gas analyzers)
- Ketoacidosis (acetoacetate, β-hydroxybutyrate)
  - Most commonly due to diabetes (DKA) or alcohol (AKA)
  - Bicarbonate therapy not indicated.
    - β-Hydroxybutyrate to acetoacetate ratio 3:1 in DKA, 7:1 in AKA

- Toxin ingestion
  - Many intoxications are associated with an increased osmolal gap (OG) as well as increased AG
    - $OG = $ Measured $P_{osm} - $ Calculated P_{osm}
    - Normal $OG < 10$ mmol/L
    - Calculated $P_{osm} = 2Na + BUN/2.8 + Glucose/18$ (where BUN or blood urea nitrogen and glucose are expressed as mg/dL)
    - Parent compound causes elevation in OG
    - Metabolites cause increase in the AG
    - Toxicity is due to metabolites
    - Use fomepizole to prevent conversion of parent compound to metabolites
    - If OG has resolved, hemodialysis will be necessary to remove the toxic metabolites
  - Elevated AG and OG: ethanol, ethylene glycol, propylene glycol, methanol
  - Normal AG with elevated OG: isopropanol
  - Elevated AG with normal OG: salicylates

  - Salicylate (mostly lactate)
    - Symptoms: nausea, vomiting, diarrhea, tinnitus, deafness, vertigo, fever, hyperventilation, noncardiogenic pulmonary edema, seizures, coma
    - Arterial blood gases (ABGs): 60% respiratory alkalosis plus metabolic acidosis; 20% respiratory alkalosis alone; rarely, respiratory and metabolic acidosis
    - Treatment:
    - Alkalinization converts salicylate to ionized form
      - Prevents diffusion of salicylate into central nervous system (CNS)
      - Prevents reabsorption of salicylate by nonionic diffusion, thereby causing trapping of salicylate in distal tubule
    - Avoid intubation; if intubation is necessary, hyperventilate
    - Gastric decontamination
    - Correct hypokalemia
    - Hemodialysis to remove salicylate
  - Methanol (formate)
    - Alcoholic fetor
    - Dilated pupils
    - Retinal and optic edema and blindness
    - Undetectable alcohol
    - Can have rhabdomyolysis and pancreatitis
    - Treatment
      - Keep systemic pH > 7.3
      - This converts formic acid to formate, which is less toxic
      - Folate IV 1 mg/kg
      - This converts formic acid in to CO_2 and water
      - Hemodialysis

- Ethylene glycol (glycolate, glyoxylate, oxalate)
    - Toxicity: inebriation, congestive heart failure (CHF), acute respiratory distress syndrome (ARDS), acute tubular necrosis (ATN)
    - No alcoholic fetor or blindness
    - Lab instruments may not distinguish glycolate from lactate
    - Hypocalcemia
    - Calcium oxalate crystals in urine
    - Urine fluoresces under Wood's lamp
    - Treatment
        - Bicarbonate
        - Ethanol or fomepizole
        - Ethylene glycol > 20 mg/dL, or OG > 10 mmol/L, or suspected ingestion + serum bicarbonate < 20 mmol/L + OG > 10 mmol/L + calcium oxalate crystals in urine
        - Thiamine
        - Pyridoxine
        - Hemodialysis
            - Ethylene glycol > 50 mg/dL
            - Acute kidney injury (AKI)
            - pH < 7.3 or decreasing with treatment
            - End-organ damage
- Failure to excrete inorganic anions (phosphate, sulfate) in renal failure
- Normal-AG (hyperchloremic) acidosis
    - Gastrointestinal (GI) loss of bicarbonate (diarrhea)
    - Renal loss of bicarbonate
        - Proximal RTA (type 2) (Morris, 1969) (see also Chapter 2)
        - Carbonic anhydrase (CA) inhibitors (prevent proximal HCO_3^- reabsorption)
    - Failure to excrete acid
        - Distal RTA (type 1, type 4) (Morris, 1969) (see also Chapter 2)
        - Renal failure
    - Administration of acid
        - Infusion of HCl or its congeners (e.g., ammonium chloride)
    - Administration of large amounts of saline (dilutional acidosis)
    - Ureteral diversion (increased chloride–bicarbonate exchange resulting in bicarbonaturia and/or increased ammonium uptake, which is converted to ammonia and H^+ in the liver; generally, only seen if there is partial obstruction of the conduit; increased urine AG; mimics type 1 RTA)

Treatment of Metabolic Acidosis
- Treat underlying cause(s) (see above for specific examples)
- Bicarbonate (especially with normal-AG acidosis)—Na or K bicarbonate (or bicarbonate former) depending on etiology and electrolyte values

METABOLIC ALKALOSIS

Metabolic alkalosis is defined as a primary increase in the bicarbonate concentration, that is, $[HCO_3^-]$ of the plasma. In primary metabolic alkalosis, the pH of the blood will be elevated (alkalemia). An increase in $[HCO_3^-]$ of 1.0 mEq/L should be accompanied by an increase in pCO_2 of 0.7 mm Hg (this is termed "respiratory adaptation"). The rise in pCO_2 will keep the blood pH near normal (although mild alkalemia will be present). Metabolic alkalosis is also associated with a slightly elevated AG (Madias et al., 1979).

Generation of Metabolic Alkalosis
There are three ways to generate metabolic alkalosis:
- Net loss of hydrogen ions (H^+) from extracellular fluid (ECF)
  - Causes of H^+ loss
    - GI—loss of HCl from stomach (vomiting, gastric drainage)
      HCl secretion by parietal cells of stomach does not normally cause metabolic alkalosis because HCl is titrated by pancreatic sodium bicarbonate:

      $$HCl + NaHCO_3 \rightarrow NaCl + CO_2 + H_2O$$

      However, if HCl is lost from the body because of vomiting or gastric drainage, there is a net gain of bicarbonate. Metabolic alkalosis is then maintained by increased renal bicarbonate reabsorption because of depletion of ECF and chloride (see section Maintenance of Metabolic Alkalosis below).
    - Renal—loss of H^+ into urine (mineralocorticoid excess states). Hydrogen ions generated by protein metabolism are normally excreted by the kidneys primarily in the form of ammonium (NH_4^+) ions. In certain conditions, an inappropriate increase in renal H^+ excretion leads to metabolic alkalosis. This is characteristic of primary mineralocorticoid excess states. Aldosterone (the naturally occurring mineralocorticoid hormone) increases sodium reabsorption and potassium and H^+ secretion in the cortical collecting tubule. Sodium retention expands ECF volume and decreases proximal tubule sodium reabsorption. Metabolic alkalosis then results from the combination of excess mineralocorticoid hormone effect and increased distal delivery of sodium (in the presence of aldosterone, sodium in the lumen will enter the cells of the collecting tubule and potassium and H^+ will exit the cells into the tubule lumen). Administration of diuretic drugs that impair ion transport in the loop of Henle or distal convoluted tubule also results in stimulation of aldosterone secretion (secondary to renin release in response to hypovolemia) and increased sodium delivery to the collecting tubule.
      Of note, high levels of aldosterone per se may not result in metabolic alkalosis in the absence of adequate distal sodium delivery. For instance, in CHF and liver cirrhosis, there is secondary hyperaldosteronism (because of decreased renal

perfusion and increased renin secretion); however, distal sodium delivery is decreased and metabolic alkalosis does not normally occur unless diuretics are administered.
- Shift into cells—severe K^+ deficiency
  With very severe potassium deficiency, K^+ will shift out of cells into the ECF in exchange for H^+. Therefore, H^+ is "lost" into the cells, engendering metabolic alkalosis. The increase in intracellular H^+ in renal tubular cells results in increased H^+ secretion and bicarbonate reabsorption, thus also maintaining metabolic alkalosis (see below).

■ Net addition of HCO_3^- to ECF
  ■ Causes of HCO_3^- gain:
    • Exogenous alkali administration (bicarbonate, lactate, citrate, acetate), especially in the presence of impaired renal function.
■ Loss of fluid containing chloride in excess of bicarbonate ("contraction alkalosis")
  ■ Causes of Cl^--rich fluid loss:
    • GI—villous adenoma, congenital chloridorrhea
      • Villous adenomas are tumors that secrete chloride into the stool; K^+ depletion also contributes to the generation of alkalosis. Congenital chloridorrhea is a rare disorder in which there is a failure of gut reabsorption of chloride secreted by the stomach.
    • Renal—diuretics, Bartter and Gitelman syndromes
      • Diuretics are a very common cause of metabolic alkalosis because chloride reabsorption by the kidney is impaired and volume contraction results in stimulation of the renin–angiotensin–aldosterone axis (secondary hyperaldosteronism)
      • Bartter syndrome is a genetic defect of the loop diuretic–sensitive Na–K–2Cl cotransporter in the loop of Henle ("endogenous loop diuretic") (Simon et al., 1996). Gitelman syndrome is a genetic defect of the thiazide-sensitive Na–Cl cotransporter in the distal tubule ("endogenous thiazide") (Monkawa et al., 2000)
          During chronic hypercapnia (seen frequently in chronic obstructive lung disease), there is an appropriate adaptive increase in renal H^+ secretion and thus bicarbonate reabsorption. This is accompanied by loss of chloride in the urine (sodium is reabsorbed preferentially with bicarbonate rather than chloride). Rapid restoration of pCO_2 to normal with mechanical ventilation is not accompanied by a similarly rapid change in bicarbonate handling by the kidney and may result in severe alkalemia. Because of previous chloride depletion, posthypercapnic metabolic alkalosis is typically associated with a low urine chloride concentration and improves with saline administration.
    • Skin—cystic fibrosis
      Metabolic alkalosis has been described in children with cystic fibrosis resulting from loss of chloride in excess of bicarbonate in sweat.

Maintenance of Metabolic Alkalosis

Under normal physiologic conditions, bicarbonate is filtered by the glomerulus (the filtered load is the product of the glomerular filtration rate [GFR] and the plasma bicarbonate concentration). Virtually, all of the filtered bicarbonate is then reabsorbed, primarily at proximal nephron sites. Because normally about 1 mEq/kg of protons are generated by the body each day, this amount of bicarbonate buffer is titrated in the ECF and needs to be regenerated in the distal nephron. Both reabsorption (also termed "reclamation") of filtered bicarbonate and regeneration of bicarbonate occur by tubular secretion of H^+. H^+ is formed in the tubular cell from the splitting of H_2O into H^+ and OH^-. After the H^+ is secreted into the tubular lumen, OH^- then combines with CO_2 to form HCO_3^-, which is reabsorbed into the peritubular capillary. Reabsorption of filtered bicarbonate occurs by titration of filtered bicarbonate by H^+ in the tubular lumen and addition of bicarbonate formed in the tubular cell into the peritubular capillary. In the distal nephron, luminal bicarbonate is usually absent; therefore, H^+ secretion results in urinary H^+ loss (primarily in the form of ammonium ions or NH_4^+) and thus bicarbonate regeneration (Fig. 7.1).

Once metabolic alkalosis has occurred, its maintenance must indicate a failure of the kidneys to excrete the excess bicarbonate. This can occur either because of a decreased filtered load of bicarbonate (because of a decrease in GFR) or an increase in tubular bicarbonate reabsorption (or decrease in bicarbonate secretion). In the absence of renal failure, inability of the kidneys to excrete the excess bicarbonate implies the presence of a factor (or factors) that either increase bicarbonate reabsorption or decrease its secretion, such as ECF chloride depletion, potassium depletion, and hypercapnia. The mechanism(s) by which these factors maintain metabolic alkalosis are given below.

- ECF depletion
  - Decreases GFR
  - Increases proximal tubular Na^+ and HCO_3^- reabsorption (because there is hypochloremia, decreased filtration of chloride leads to bicarbonate reabsorption with sodium in an attempt to maintain ECF volume)
  - Stimulates renin secretion leading to secondary hyperaldosteronism (increases H^+ secretion and HCO_3^- generation in the collecting tubule)
- Chloride depletion (recent data suggest that this is the most important mechanism) (Oh & Carroll, 2002)
  - Increases distal tubular HCO_3^- reabsorption (decreased tubular fluid chloride concentration promotes H^+ secretion and chloride–bicarbonate exchange by type A intercalated cells in the distal tubule) (Fig. 7.2)
  - Decreases distal tubular HCO_3^- secretion (decreased tubular fluid chloride concentration inhibits chloride–bicarbonate exchange by type B intercalated cells in the distal tubule) (Fig. 7.3). Note that type B cells have the opposite configuration

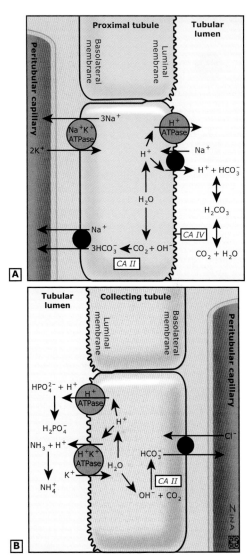

FIGURE 7.1. Mechanism of bicarbonate reabsorption and regeneration by tubular cells. The figure depicts the major cellular and luminal events in bicarbonate reabsorption in the proximal tubule **(A)** and regeneration in the collecting tubules **(B)**. In the proximal tubule, H^+ ions are secreted into the lumen by the Na^+–H^+ exchanger, whereas HCO_3^- ions are returned to the systemic circulation primarily via an Na^+–$3HCO_3^-$ cotransporter. In the collecting tubule, an H^+–ATPase pump and a Cl^-–HCO_3^- exchanger mediate these processes. In the proximal tubule, secreted H^+ combines with filtered HCO_3^- to form CO_2 and H_2O. (This reaction is facilitated by carbonic anhydrase [CA] in the brush border.) Bicarbonate is typically mostly reabsorbed by the time the tubular fluid reaches the collecting duct; H^+ secretion will then result in regeneration of bicarbonate. Note that the collecting tubule cell shown is a type A intercalated cell; there are also type B intercalated cells, which will be discussed below. (Reproduced with permission from Emmett M, Szerlip H. Pathogenesis of metabolic alkalosis. In: Post TW, ed. *UpToDate.* Waltham, MA: UpToDate. Accessed November 29, 2018. Copyright © 2018 UpToDate, Inc. For more information visit www.uptodate.com.)

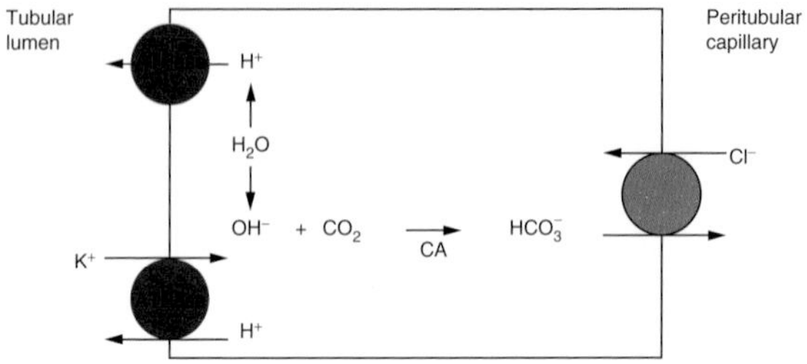

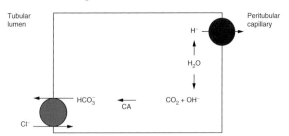

FIGURE 7.2. Transport mechanisms involved in hydrogen secretion and bicarbonate reabsorption by type A intercalated cells in the distal tubule. (Reproduced with permission from Emmett M, Szerlip H. Causes of metabolic alkalosis. In: Post TW, ed. *UpToDate*. Waltham, MA: UpToDate. Accessed August 14, 2012. Copyright © 2018 UpToDate, Inc. For more information visit www.uptodate.com.)

to type A cells, that is, the location of the H^+–ATPase and chloride–bicarbonate exchangers are reversed
- Directly stimulates renin production (leading to secondary hyperaldosteronism and increased H^+ excretion)
- K^+ depletion
  - Increases tubular HCO_3^- reabsorption
- Hypercapnia (increased pCO_2)
  - Increases tubular HCO_3^- reabsorption
    Note that K^+ depletion and hypercapnia will both lead to intracellular acidosis, which increases H^+ secretion (K^+ depletion leads to shift of K^+ out of cells and H^+ into cells; CO_2 movement into cells results in acidosis because CO_2 combines with OH^- [formed from splitting of H_2O into H^+ and OH^-]).

Clinical Features of Metabolic Alkalosis
- History
  - Vomiting
  - Gastric drainage
  - Diuretics
- Symptoms
  - Often none
  - Sometimes cramps

FIGURE 7.3. Transport mechanisms involved in the secretion of bicarbonate into the tubular lumen by type B intercalated cells in the distal tubule. (Reproduced with permission from Emmett M, Szerlip H. Pathogenesis of metabolic alkalosis. In: Post TW, ed. *UpToDate*. Waltham, MA: UpToDate. Accessed August 14, 2012. Copyright © 2018 UpToDate, Inc. For more information visit www.uptodate.com.)

- Signs
  - Hypertension (in primary mineralocorticoid excess states)
  - Hypoventilation (usually not evident on physical examination)
  - Tetany and/or increased deep tendon reflexes (metabolic alkalosis results in increased negative charges on serum albumin, thus increasing binding of calcium to albumin and decreasing the concentration of free or ionized calcium)
  - Cardiac arrhythmias (especially in the presence of digoxin) (Brater & Morelli, 1981)

Laboratory Findings in Metabolic Alkalosis
- ABGs: increased pH, $[HCO_3^-]$, and pCO_2
- Electrolytes: elevated $[HCO_3^-]$, decreased $[Cl^-]$, usually low $[K^+]$, slight increase in AG (increased negative charges on albumin, increased lactate because of increased intracellular pH)
- BUN: frequently increased (because of volume depletion)
- Hematocrit: frequently increased (volume depletion)
- Urine chloride $[Cl^-]$: very helpful in differential diagnosis (value <10 mEq/L indicates volume/chloride depletion)
- Note that urine $[Na^+]$ may not be low despite volume depletion because urinary loss of bicarbonate obligates urinary cation (Na^+ and K^+) excretion.

Differential Diagnosis of Metabolic Alkalosis
- Chloride-responsive type (urine Cl^- low, that is, <10 mEq/L):
    In these conditions, the kidney is avidly reabsorbing chloride because of persistent volume (and chloride) depletion that developed during the generation of metabolic alkalosis.
  - GI—vomiting, gastric drainage, villous adenoma, chloride diarrhea
  - Renal—diuretics (after drug cessation)
  - Skin—cystic fibrosis
- Chloride-resistant type (urine Cl^- high, i.e., >20 mEq/L)
  - Renal—mineralocorticoid excess states—can be either primary (low renin) of secondary (high renin)

Primary	Secondary
Primary hyperaldosteronism	Renal artery stenosis
Cushing syndrome	Accelerated hypertension
Licorice ingestion (stimulates hyperaldosteronism)	Renin-secreting tumor

  - Other—profound potassium depletion

Treatment of Metabolic Alkalosis
- In general, metabolic alkalosis in the presence of ECF excess (as occurs in mineralocorticoid excess states) is mild and does not require treatment. Alkalosis of sufficient severity to require treatment is generally associated with volume depletion and can be corrected with sodium chloride administration. Volume expansion will decrease HCO_3^- reabsorption. Administration of potassium is indicated if hypokalemia is present, because entry of K^+ into cells in exchange for H^+ will buffer excess ECF HCO_3^-.

- Some patients, such as those with severe CHF, may have metabolic alkalosis because of relative plasma volume depletion (because of loop diuretics) but still have increased ECF volume (edema). In this setting, administration of a CA inhibitor such as acetazolamide may be beneficial. CA inhibitors are proximally acting diuretics, which result in decreased bicarbonate reabsorption and bicarbonaturia.
- In the presence of life-threatening alkalosis, intravenous ammonium chloride (providing the patient does not have hepatic or renal failure) can be given. Ammonium chloride administration titrates bicarbonate by the following reaction:

$$NH_4Cl + NaHCO_3 \rightarrow NaCl + NH_3 + CO_2 + H_2O$$

- Finally, prevention of metabolic alkalosis in patients undergoing gastric drainage by drugs that inhibit gastric acid secretion (H_2 blockers, omeprazole) is indicated.

References

Brater DC, Morelli HF. Systemic alkalosis and digitalis related arrhythmias. *Acta Med Scand Suppl.* 647:79–85, 1981.

Gabow PA, Kaehny WD, Fennessey PV, et al. Diagnostic importance of an increased anion gap. *N Engl J Med.* 303(15):854–858, 1980.

Javaheri S, Shore NS, Rose B, et al. Compensatory hypoventilation in metabolic alkalosis. *Chest.* 81:296–301, 1982.

Madias NE. Renal acidification responses to respiratory acid-base disorder. *J Nephrol.* 23(suppl 16):S85–S91, 2010.

Madias NE, Ayus JC, Adrogue HJ. Increased anion gap in metabolic alkalosis: the role of plasma-protein equivalency. *N Engl J Med.* 300(25):1421–1423, 1979.

Monkawa T, Kurihara I, Kobayashi K, et al. Novel mutations in thiazide-sensitive Na-Cl cotransporter gene of patients with Gitelman's syndrome. *J Am Soc Nephrol.* 11:65–70, 2000.

Morris RC Jr. Renal tubular acidosis. Mechanisms, classification, and implications. *N Eng J Med.* 281:1405–1413, 1969.

Oh MS, Carroll HJ. Mechanism of chloride deficit in the maintenance of metabolic alkalosis. *Nephron.* 91(3):379–382, 2002.

Pierce NF, Fedson DS, Brigham KL, et al. The ventilatory response to acute base deficit in humans. Time course during development and correction of metabolic acidosis. *Ann Intern Med.* 72:633–640, 1970.

Simon DB, Karet FE, Rodriguez-Soriano J, et al. Genetic heterogeneity of Bartter's syndrome revealed by mutations in the K^+ channel, ROMK. *Nat Genet.* 14:152–156, 1996.

SUPPLEMENT: ACID–BASE ANALYSIS

The basic steps in acid–base analysis will be outlined here. Then, they will be demonstrated in a series of case examples. One will see that acid–base analysis is actually straightforward when an orderly, logical plan is followed. An ABG is necessary for definitive acid–base analysis.

These are the steps to follow:

1. Look at pH to determine whether there is acidemia (pH < 7.35) or alkalemia (pH > 7.45)
   - If pH is low, there must be a primary acidosis.
   - If pH is high, there must be a primary alkalosis.
2. Look at HCO_3^- and pCO_2 to determine the type of acidosis or alkalosis present
   - HCO_3^- is low in metabolic acidosis and high in metabolic alkalosis.

- pCO_2 is low in respiratory alkalosis and high in respiratory acidosis.

    At this point, the primary acid–base process should be evident, that is, metabolic or respiratory acidosis or alkalosis.

3. Determine whether compensation (adaptation) is appropriate

    Henderson's equation shows the relationship between pH, pCO_2, and HCO_3^-

$$[H^+] = (24 \times pCO_2)/[HCO_3^-]$$

    From this formula, it is evident that to maintain $[H^+]$ near normal, a primary change in either HCO_3^- or pCO_2 should result in a counterbalancing change of the other in the same direction, that is,

- Metabolic acidosis is compensated by respiratory alkalosis (hyperventilation).
- Metabolic alkalosis is compensated by respiratory acidosis (hypoventilation).
- Chronic respiratory acidosis is compensated by metabolic alkalosis.
- Chronic respiratory alkalosis is compensated by metabolic acidosis.
- There is little adaptation to acute respiratory acidosis or alkalosis because it requires 24 to 48 hours for the kidneys to adapt to a primary respiratory disorder.

    The expected compensations (adaptations) to primary acid–base disturbances have been determined empirically and are given in Table 7.2.

    When compensation is less or greater than expected, this suggests the presence of another primary disorder. For instance, in metabolic acidosis, if pCO_2 is higher than expected from Table 7.2, there is evidence for a coexisting primary respiratory acidosis (even though the pCO_2 may still be below the normal range).

4. Calculate AG

    As discussed in the Metabolic Acidosis section above, the AG (Oh & Carroll, 1977) is the difference between the plasma concentration of sodium, the major extracellular cation, and the sum of the concentrations of the anions chloride and bicarbonate, that is, $[Na^+ - (Cl^- + HCO_3^-)]$. Stated differently, the AG occurs as a result of a higher concentration of UA (i.e., not chloride or bicarbonate) than UC (i.e., not sodium). The normal AG is about 10 mEq/L, but will vary slightly depending on the specific electrolyte assays used. Note that $[HCO_3^-]$ (calculated from pH and pCO_2 on an ABG) is very similar to the concentration of total CO_2 (the sum of bicarbonate and dissolved carbon dioxide as measured in the chemistry laboratory). Because an ABG is not always available, total CO_2 is conventionally used to calculate AG, although technically this is not correct because total CO_2 includes a small (and clinically insignificant) amount of uncharged carbon dioxide. (By the way, this is why total CO_2 must be expressed as mmol/L, whereas HCO_3^- and other univalent anions such as Na^+, K^+, and Cl^- can be expressed either as mmol/L or mEq/L.) For simplicity, in the case studies in this chapter, the bicarbonate and total CO_2 concentrations have been set to the same value.

If the AG is ≥ 20 mEq/L, there is an AG metabolic acidosis (Gabow et al., 1980). Lesser elevations are less specific, but it should be kept in mind that albumin is an anion and hypoalbuminemia will lower the AG by ~2.5 mEq/L for each decrement of 1.0 g/dL of serum albumin (Feldman et al., 2005).

Theoretically, one would expect that, in a high-AG acidosis, for every millimole (or milliequivalent) of bicarbonate titrated by H^+, there would be 1 mmol (or milliequivalent) of retained anion. This supposition leads to the "delta-delta" concept (also known as "bicarbonate gap"). If the change in (delta) bicarbonate is greater than the change in (delta) AG, this suggests a combined high-AG/normal-AG acidosis. If delta AG is greater than delta bicarbonate, this suggests the presence of a metabolic alkalosis that is independently increasing bicarbonate levels ("hidden" metabolic alkalosis). (We should point out that this latter supposition may not always be true, as with more severe degrees of AG acidosis, buffers other than bicarbonate are also used to titrate H^+, and thus "delta AG" will be greater than "delta bicarbonate." If the delta AG is < 2-times greater than the delta bicarbonate, this is usually a pure high-AG acidosis.)

Therefore, as discussed above

$$AG = Na^+ - (Cl^- + HCO_3^-) = (UA - UC)$$

UA – UC = 10 to 12 mEq/L (usually 10 in most laboratories)

Since

Delta AG (ΔAG) = (AG – 10), and Delta bicarbonate

$$(\Delta HCO_3^-) = (24 - [HCO_3^-])$$

Bicarbonate gap = $\Delta AG - \Delta HCO_3^-$

Bicarbonate gap $>+6$ suggests concomitant metabolic alkalosis

Bicarbonate gap <-6 indicates concomitant non-AG metabolic acidosis

Bicarbonate gap >-6 but <6 is inconclusive (Wrenn, 1990)

Similarly, the ratio of delta AG and delta bicarbonate (delta-delta) may be used. Delta/delta <1 suggests concomitant non-AG metabolic acidosis and delta/delta >2 suggests concomitant metabolic alkalosis. Lactic acidosis has an average value of 1.6.

As mentioned above, the delta-delta or bicarbonate gap analysis may be misleading in some situations, however. With more severe degrees of AG acidosis, buffers other than bicarbonate are also used to titrate H^+, and thus "delta AG" will be greater than "delta bicarbonate." The 1:1 stoichiometry between delta AG and delta bicarbonate may only be present in the early stages of metabolic acidosis. Its maintenance requires that the rates of exit of protons and anions from the ECF, as well as those of the renal generation of new base and excretion of filtered anions must be roughly equal throughout the subsequent course of the metabolic acidosis (Kraut & Madias, 2007).

7

A 70-year-old man presents with weakness. Serum chemistries reveal (in mmol/L): Na^+, 145; K^+, 3.0; Cl^-, 120; CO_2, 16; ABGs reveal: pH, 7.35; pCO_2, 30 mm Hg; HCO_3^-, 16 mEq/L.

The urine pH is 5.2. Urine chemistries reveal (in mmol/L): Na^+, 40; K^+, 5; Cl^-, 100.

Q1: What is the acid–base disturbance?

A1: On the ABG, blood pH is below normal, indicating mild acidemia. Bicarbonate is low, and the AG [$Na^+ - (Cl^- + HCO_3^-)$] is 145 − (120 + 16) = 9. Hence, this is a non-AG or hyperchloremic metabolic acidosis. (Another way to tell that this is hyperchloremic acidosis is that the serum chloride is elevated relative to the serum sodium level—the normal ratio of sodium to chloride is 138:100 or 1.38 and in this case it is 145:120 or 1.21.) The expected respiratory compensation is a decrease of pCO_2. Since the delta bicarbonate is 24 − 16 = 8, the delta pCO_2 should be 1.2 − 8 = 9.6, which corresponds to the actual delta pCO_2 of 10. Thus, this is a simple metabolic acidosis.

The most common causes of a non-AG metabolic acidosis are as follows:

- Chronic kidney disease (CKD) (because of decreased urine acid excretion)
- RTA (Morris, 1969) (because of either decreased urine acid excretion [distal RTA] or increased urine bicarbonate excretion [proximal RTA])
- Diarrhea (because of increased stool bicarbonate loss)

Less common causes are as follows:

- Ileostomy/pancreatic fistula (loss of bicarbonate-containing fluid)
- Partial obstruction of an ileal conduit (classically was thought to be because of increased chloride–bicarbonate exchange by the conduit leading to bicarbonate loss in the urine, but more recent studies suggest that the principal mechanism is because of increased ammonium absorption by the conduit) (McDougal, 1992)
- Total parenteral nutrition (gain of hydrogen ions through several mechanisms)
- Acetazolamide (causes proximal RTA)

Q2: What is the most likely diagnosis?

1. Distal RTA
2. Proximal RTA
3. Diarrhea due to laxative abuse

A2: In patients with normal or near-normal renal function, the cause of hyperchloremic acidosis will usually be RTA or diarrhea. Classic (distal) RTA and proximal RTA as well as diarrhea typically present with hypokalemic hyperchloremic metabolic acidosis. Making the correct diagnosis may be difficult in some cases. A urine pH > 5.5 in the face of acidosis suggests distal RTA, although it can also be elevated with laxative abuse, leading to diarrhea, volume depletion, and impaired distal sodium delivery. Calculation of the urine AG or "net charge" may be helpful (see Chapter 2). The urine "net charge" ($Na^+ + K^+ - Cl^-$) is positive in classic RTA because of impairment of ammonium (NH_4^+) excretion and thus decreased urine Cl^- (an anion must be excreted with the cation); in diarrhea, renal H^+ excretion is enhanced, and thus there is a large amount of ammonium chloride (NH_4Cl) in the urine, and the net charge is typically negative. The net charge is variable in proximal RTA. In the absence of other proximal tubular transport abnormalities (Fanconi syndrome), the diagnosis of proximal RTA required additional testing. The most direct test is to infuse sodium bicarbonate at a rate of 0.5 to 1 mEq/kg/h and measure urine pH and fractional bicarbonate excretion. Owing to urinary bicarbonate losses when filtered load of bicarbonate is increased, the urine pH will increase above 7.5 and the fractional excretion of bicarbonate will exceed 15% to 20%.

The urine "net charge" here is $40 + 5 - 100 = -55$. Hence, the most likely diagnosis is diarrhea caused by laxatives. The very low urine potassium also supports this diagnosis because potassium is lost in the stool and not in the urine.

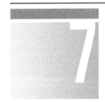

A 30-year-old woman presents with fatigue and weakness. She denies vomiting or diarrhea and takes no medications. Her physical examination is normal except for mild orthostatic hypotension. Serum chemistries reveal (in mmol/L): Na^+, 138; K^+, 2.9; Cl^-, 90; CO_2, 40; ABGs reveal: pH, 7.50; pCO_2, 53 mm Hg; HCO_3^-, 40 mEq/L. The urine pH is 5.5. Urine chemistries reveal (in mmol/L): Na^+, 15; K^+, 15; Cl^-, 5.

Q1: What is the acid–base disorder?

A1: On the ABG, the pH is high, indicating alkalemia, and bicarbonate is high, indicating metabolic alkalosis. Since the delta bicarbonate is $40 - 24 = 16$, the delta pCO_2 should be $0.7 \times 16 = 11.2$, which is close to the actual delta pCO_2 of 13. Therefore, this is a simple metabolic alkalosis.

Q2: What is the likely diagnosis?

1. Diuretic intake
2. Bartter syndrome
3. Gitelman syndrome
4. Vomiting
5. Hypokalemic periodic paralysis

A2: Hypokalemia with low urine K^+ (<20 mmol/L) suggests either extrarenal (such as GI) loss of potassium or previous renal loss that has stopped. Low urine sodium and low urine chloride, coupled with the physical examination, suggest volume depletion. Hence, vomiting would be consistent with these findings. Note that the patient has probably not recently vomited, because in that case, the recent and sudden loss of HCl from the stomach would lead to an abrupt increase in plasma bicarbonate, increasing bicarbonate filtered load and renal bicarbonate excretion. This would result in a high urine pH (often >7) and obligate Na^+ and K^+ loss with the bicarbonate. Diuretic intake would be expected to be associated with an increase in renal electrolyte excretion (however, this might not occur if the diuretic was stopped for 24 hours or more prior to presentation). Bartter and Gitelman syndromes are tubular reabsorptive disorders (Hebert & Gullans, 1996) and would lead to persistently increased renal electrolyte excretion. Hypokalemic periodic paralysis is not associated with metabolic alkalosis. From the data presented, either recent (but not active) surreptitious vomiting or diuretic use is possible, although the very low urine chloride is more suggestive of vomiting.

VIGNETTE **3**

A patient with known CKD presents with uremic symptoms (anorexia, nausea and vomiting, hiccoughs, fatigue). Physical examination reveals pallor and bruising on the skin and 1+ peripheral edema. Serum chemistries reveal (in mmol/L): Na^+, 138; K^+, 6.0; Cl^-, 86; CO_2, 20; ABG: pH, 7.40, pCO_2, 33 mm Hg; HCO_3^-, 20 mEq/L.

Q: What is the acid–base disorder?

1. Metabolic acidosis and metabolic alkalosis
2. Metabolic acidosis and respiratory alkalosis
3. No acid–base abnormality
4. Respiratory acidosis and respiratory alkalosis

A: The pH is normal. Therefore, there is neither no acid–base disorder nor a mixed primary disturbance. The bicarbonate and pCO_2 are low; however, with metabolic acidosis, a delta bicarbonate of

4 would be expected to lead to a delta pCO_2 of $4 \times 1.2 = 4.8$. The actual delta pCO_2 is 7. Thus, there appears to be a mild respiratory alkalosis as well. Remember to always check the AG.

$$AG = Na^+ - (Cl^- + HCO_3^-)$$

$$AG = 138 - (86 + 20) = 32$$

Hence, there is an AG metabolic acidosis, and one must now perform the delta-delta analysis. The delta bicarbonate is only 4, but delta AG is 22. Therefore, there is also a hidden metabolic alkalosis, possibly from uremic vomiting. The final analysis is as follows: high-AG metabolic acidosis, mild respiratory alkalosis, and metabolic alkalosis. The cause of the metabolic acidosis was discovered to be a combination of uremic and lactic acidosis.

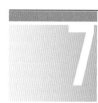

VIGNETTE 4

A 30-year-old male patient presents to the emergency room (ER) with confusion. Serum chemistries reveal (in mmol/L): Na^+, 136; K^+, 3.9; Cl^-, 101; CO_2, 15; ABG: pH, 7.5; pCO_2, 20 mm Hg; HCO_3^-, 15 mEq/L.

Q: What is a probable cause?
1. Acetazolamide ingestion
2. Vomiting
3. Laxative abuse
4. Aspirin poisoning

A: First, the acid–base analysis:

The pH is 7.5, indicating alkalemia, and because pCO_2 is low, there is a respiratory alkalosis. For respiratory alkalosis, the compensation is as follows:

Acute: bicarbonate decreases by 2 mEq/L for each 10 mm Hg decrease in pCO_2

Chronic: bicarbonate decreases by 4 to 5 mEq/L for each 10 mm Hg decrease in pCO_2

Therefore, if this is chronic respiratory alkalosis, the expected bicarbonate would be $24 - 9 = 15$, which is the observed value. Thus far, the data are consistent with a simple chronic respiratory alkalosis.

However, the AG is 20. Alkalemia can cause a mild increase in AG, but this degree of AG suggests the coexistence of an AG acidosis. We are now suspecting an acute respiratory alkalosis with a coexisting high-AG metabolic acidosis.

Acetazolamide causes a non-AG metabolic acidosis. Vomiting causes metabolic alkalosis. Laxatives cause diarrhea, which would cause non-AG metabolic acidosis or sometimes metabolic alkalosis, probably due to hypokalemia. Salicylate toxicity not only causes AG metabolic acidosis but also gives rise to acute respiratory alkalosis and is the likely culprit in this case.

VIGNETTE **5**

A 20-year-old patient has ingested an unknown poison. Serum chemistries (in mmol/L): Na^+, 136; K^+, 4.5; Cl^-, 90; CO_2, 8; ABG: pH, 7.2; pCO_2, 21 mm Hg; HCO_3^-, 8 mEq/L. The urinalysis shows a pH, 5.1 and contains many envelope-shaped crystals.

Q1: What is the acid–base disorder?

A1: The pH is 7.2; therefore, there is an acidemia. HCO_3^- is low, and pCO_2 is also low. This shows that the primary disorder is metabolic acidosis. The expected pCO_2 would be $1.2 \times (24 - 8) = 20$, which is close to the observed value. Thus, this is a simple metabolic acidosis.

The AG is very high at 38. Thus, we must calculate the delta-delta, which would be $(38 - 10) - (24 - 8) = 28 - 16 = 12$. This suggests a hidden metabolic alkalosis.

The full analysis is as follows: AG metabolic acidosis with metabolic alkalosis. However, we should note that metabolic alkalosis may or may not be present, because with very severe metabolic acidosis, buffers other than bicarbonate (e.g., hemoglobin, bone) are also used to titrate the excess acid.

The differential for an AG metabolic acidosis is as follows:

- Lactic acidosis
- Ketoacidosis (DKA, AKA)
- Intoxications (methanol, ethylene glycol, salicylic acid)
- Uremia (due to retention of inorganic anions)

Q2: What type of crystals are they most likely to be?

1. Calcium oxalate
2. Cysteine
3. Struvite
4. Uric acid

A2: Rectangular crystals in the urine represent calcium oxalate crystals, which can be present with ethylene glycol poisoning. The patient's mother arrives and states she gave her son ipecac to induce vomiting. Thus, there is indeed probably a superimposed metabolic alkalosis.

A 55-year-old patient presents to the ER with stomach pain. He denies vomiting. On examination, he is in no distress but is noted to be hyperventilating.

His serum chemistries reveal (in mmol/L): Na, 140; K, 2.6; Cl, 69; CO_2, 40; ABGs: pH, 7.86; pCO_2, 23 mm Hg; HCO_3^-, 40 mEq/L.

Q1: What is the acid–base disorder?

A1: This patient has profound alkalemia, and one suspects the presence of both metabolic and respiratory alkalosis, which are indeed both present. However, remember to always calculate the AG. In this case, the AG is $140 - (69 + 40) = 31$. Therefore, despite a pH of 7.86, the patient has a concomitant high-AG metabolic acidosis.

Q2: What is the etiology?

A2: As it turns out, this realization is key to the correct diagnosis. A salicylate level is in the toxic range. Salicylism causes both high-AG metabolic acidosis (primarily due to lactic acidosis) and primary respiratory alkalosis (because of drug-induced stimulation of the respiratory center).

So far, this sounds like Question 4, but what about the metabolic alkalosis? Upon further questioning, the patient admits to taking high-dose Alka-Seltzer to treat his pain. Alka-Seltzer contains salicylate and bicarbonate.

References

Feldman M, Soni N, Dickson B. Influence of hypoalbuminemia or hyperalbuminemia on the serum anion gap. *J Lab Clin Med*. 146:317–320, 2005.

Gabow PA, Kaehny WD, Fennessey PV, et al. Diagnostic importance of an increased serum anion gap. *N Engl J Med*. 303(15):854–858, 1980.

Hebert SC, Gullans SR. The molecular basis of inherited hypokalemic alkalosis: Bartter's and Gitelman's syndromes. *Am J Physiol Renal Physiol*. 271:F957–F959, 1996.

Kraut JA, Madias NE. Serum anion gap: its uses and limitations in clinical medicine. *Clin J Am Soc Nephrol*. 2(1):162–174, 2007.

McDougal WS. Metabolic complications of urinary intestinal diversion. *J Urol*. 147(5):1199–1208, 1992.

Morris RC Jr. Renal tubular acidosis. Mechanisms, classification and implications. *N Engl J Med*. 281:1405–1413, 1969.

Oh MS, Carroll HJ. The anion gap. *N Engl J Med*. 297:814–817, 1977.

Wrenn K. The delta(delta) gap: an approach to mixed acid-base disorders. *Ann Emerg Med*. 19(11):1310–1313, 1990.

8 Disorders of Calcium/Phosphorus/Magnesium Homeostasis

CALCIUM

Physiology and Measurement

- Normal daily dietary calcium intake in adults is ~1,000 mg; however, net gut absorption is about 100 to 200 mg. In the steady state, the absorbed calcium is excreted in the urine. Vitamin D increases gut absorption. Calcium plays an important role in the strengthening of bones and teeth, muscle contraction, nerve conduction, and blood clotting.

- The vast majority (~99%) of total body calcium is stored in bone. Of the 1% extracellular calcium, ~50% is bound to albumin, with the remainder being free (ionized) calcium or complexed calcium (the latter is a small percentage and can usually be ignored for clinical purposes).

- The normal plasma total calcium (Ca) is 8.5 to 10 mg/dL (2.125–2.5 mmol/L), and ionized calcium (Ca^{2+}) about half of that amount, that is, 4.25 to 5 mg/dL (1.0625–1.25 mmol/L). Because the molecular weight of calcium is 40, 1 mmol of calcium is 40 mg. Thus, to convert mg/dL to mmol/L, divide by 0.1 × molecular weight (i.e., 4). Because calcium is divalent, to convert mmol/L to mEq/L, multiply by 2. Thus, a plasma-ionized calcium level of 5 mg/dL = 1.25 mmol/L = 2.5 mEq/L. All of these units are used in clinical practice.

- Because of calcium–albumin binding, the plasma total calcium decreases by 0.8 mg/dL (0.2 mmol/L) for each 1.0 g/dL (10 g/L) decrease in plasma albumin. Hypoalbuminemia will not affect plasma-ionized calcium. However, ionized (but not total) calcium will fall if there is an increase in pH of the plasma, owing to enhance calcium–albumin binding.

- Plasma calcium is regulated by parathyroid hormone (PTH)/vitamin D. A decrease in plasma-ionized calcium increases PTH secretion, which mobilizes skeletal calcium; stimulates formation of $1\alpha,25$-dihydroxy-vitamin D, thus increasing gut calcium absorption; and decreases urinary calcium excretion. An increase in plasma-ionized calcium will have the opposite effects. These relationships are depicted in Figure 8.1. These effects occur very soon after the calcium level becomes low. The timeline is as follows:
  - Within seconds—PTH is secreted
  - Within hours to days—PTH synthesis is increased
  - Within weeks to months—parathyroid cell proliferation occurs

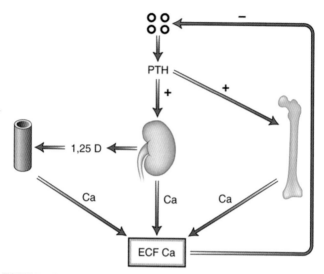

FIGURE 8.1. Effects of PTH on calcium homeostasis. ECF, extracellular fluid; PTH, parathyroid hormone. (From Kronenberg HM, Memed S, Polonsky KS, et al. Hormones and disorders of mineral metabolism. In: Kronenberg H, ed. *Williams Textbook of Endocrinology.* 11th ed. Philadelphia, PA: Saunders; 2007:1024, with permission.)

- After many months—parathyroid glands may become autonomous, that is, tertiary hyperparathyroidism (Silver et al., 1996).
- Hypomagnesemia can cause hypocalcemia by producing PTH resistance or by decreasing PTH secretion (Rude et al., 1976). Hypermagnesemia causes hypocalcemia due in part to the suppressive effects of hypermagnesemia on PTH secretion (Cholst et al., 1984).

CASE STUDY

8.1
A 66-year-old female with pancreatic cancer diagnosed 1 month prior to admission is admitted for evaluation of nausea, vomiting, and diarrhea. She also complains of perioral paresthesias. She is well until 1 month prior to admission when diarrhea started; computed tomography (CT) abdomen with contrast at that time reveals a mass in the pancreatic head; biopsy confirms pancreatic adenocarcinoma. Physical examination reveals the patient to be moderately malnourished. There is no palpable abdominal mass. Inflation of the blood pressure (BP) cuff above systolic pressure leads to carpal spasm (Trousseau's sign). Tapping the facial nerve at the parotid gland leads to a facial twitch (Chvostek's sign). The remainder of the examination is unremarkable.

Blood chemistry:
Sodium: 138 mmol/L
Potassium: 4.0 mmol/L

Chloride: 100 mmol/L

Total CO_2: 24 mmol/L

Urea nitrogen: 30 mg/dL (urea: 10.8 mmol/L)

Creatinine: 1.6 mg/dL (141 mcmol/L)

Lipase: 248 U/L (normal 8–78 U/L)

Total calcium: 7.0 mg/dL (1.75 mmol/L)

Ionized calcium: 0.87 mmol/L (normal 1.16–1.32)

25-Hydroxyvitamin D: 32 ng/mL (80 nmol/L) (normal)

Intact PTH: 150 pg/mL (ng/L) (15.9 pmol/L) (normal 10–65 pg/mL)

Calcitonin: < 2 pg/mL (0.59 pmol/L) (low)

Urine chemistry:

Sodium: 97 mmol/L

Creatinine: 126 mg/dL (11.1 mmol/L)

Fractional excretion of sodium (FENa) : 5.6%

Urine albumin to creatinine ratio (UACR) : 410 mg/g (46 mg/mmol)

Urine protein to creatinine ratio (UPCR) : 1.8 g/g (204 mg/mmol)

Urine calcium to creatinine ratio (Ca:Cr) : < 0.14 mg/mg (low)

Urinalysis:

Specific gravity: 1.010

Protein: 100 mg/dL

Blood: positive

RBC: 50/hpf

WBC: 50/hpf

No bacteria

Urine eosinophils: 5%

Antinuclear antibodies (ANA), antinuclear cytoplasmic antibodies (ANCA), anti-glomerular basement membrane (anti-GBM) antibodies, hepatitis serology, and complements are all normal.

Renal ultrasound shows increased cortical echogenicity and accentuated cortical medullary differentiation.

Question 8.1.1: What are the causes of hypocalcemia?

- Hypoparathyrodism (decreases calcium release from bone)
  - Autoimmune
  - Hungry bone syndrome (Ca shifts into bone for remineralization S/P parathyroidectomy)
- Vitamin D deficiency (decreases gut calcium absorption)
- Gut malabsorption (e.g., intestinal disease)
- Renal failure
  - Deficient $1\alpha,25\text{-}(OH)_2$-vitamin D production, decrease in the number of vitamin D receptors, and resistance to the action of vitamin D (Korkor, 1987). Phosphorus retention leads to an increase in fibroblast growth factor 23 (FGF23) production, which inhibits renal 1α-hydroxylase in the kidney.
  - Hyperphosphatemia per se results in an increase in "calcium–phosphorus product" in blood and favors movement of calcium into tissues, particularly bone.

- Hypocalcemia associated with renal failure results in an increase in PTH secretion (secondary hyperparathyroidism). The typical laboratory constellation in secondary hyperparathyroidism in renal failure is thus low calcium, high phosphorus, and high PTH.
- Acute renal failure associated with rhabdomyolysis can lead to profound hypocalcemia, because of the severity of hyperphosphatemia (muscle breakdown releases phosphorus into the extracellular fluid) and deposition of calcium in damaged muscle.

- Other less common causes of hypocalcemia include acute pancreatitis (calcium–fatty acid precipitation), hypomagnesemia (decreases PTH release and peripheral action), and certain medications (bisphosphonates, cinacalcet, citrate).

CASE STUDY 8.1 CONTINUED

Hypoparathyroidism is ruled out by elevated PTH, and primary hyperparathyroidism excluded by the low plasma calcium. Hence, this is a case of secondary hyperparathyroidism. Although chronic kidney disease (CKD) commonly causes secondary hyperparathyroidism, secondary hyperparathyroidism is not common with acute kidney impairment (AKI). The low urinary Ca:Cr ratio in the presence of normal serum vitamin D makes intestinal malabsorption the most likely cause of hypocalcemia.

Question 8.1.2: What are the signs and symptoms of hypocalcemia?

- Perioral paresthesias
- Tetany
- Carpopedal spasm (Trousseau's sign if occurs after arterial occlusion with BP cuff)
- Chvostek's sign (facial muscle twitching when tapping facial nerve at parotid gland)
- Prolonged QT interval on electrocardiogram (EKG); congestive heart failure (Kazmi & Wall, 2007)

Question 8.1.3: What is the cause of the intestinal malabsorption?

CASE STUDY 8.1 CONTINUED

Upon further history, the patient describes greasy, malodorous stools that float on water, which provides additive support for fat malabsorption. Diarrhea improves with pancreatic enzyme supplementation and with the bile acid sequestrant cholestyramine, which supports the role of pancreatic insufficiency in the etiology of fat malabsorption. Other causes of diarrhea are ruled out by stool studies that are negative for *Campylobacter*, Shiga toxin, ova and parasites, *Clostridium difficile*, and other bacterial pathogens. Pancreatic insufficiency in this patient is due to pancreatic atrophy in the setting of invasive pancreatic adenocarcinoma. Other causes of malabsorption such as inflammatory bowel disease, short bowel syndrome, bariatric surgery (with jejunoileal bypass or Roux-en-Y gastric bypass), celiac disease, recent partial colectomy, and chronic pancreatitis are not present in this patient.

Question 8.1.4: What is the cause of kidney disease in this patient?

CASE STUDY 8.1 CONTINUED

Urinary indices (high FENa) suggest tubular injury, which could be acute and/or chronic. Renal ultrasound does not show hydrone-phrosis but does show increased cortical echogenicity and accentu-ated cortical medullary differentiation suggesting chronic disease.

The presence of hematuria, pyuria, and proteinuria suggests the possibility of a nephritic or vasculitic syndrome. However, subsequent testing for ANA, ANCA, anti-GBM antibodies, hepati-tis serology, and complements was all normal.

A renal biopsy is performed, demonstrating acute and chronic tubulointerstitial nephritis with calcium oxalate crystals in the tubules consistent with oxalosis.

The cause of oxalosis is enteric hyperoxaluria.

Question 8.1.5: What is the cause of renal oxalosis?

- Hyperoxaluria can be primary or secondary. Primary hyper-oxaluria is a rare genetic disorder in which there is deficient liver synthesis of alanine to glyoxylate aminotransferase ratio, glyoxylate reductase, or hydroxypyruvate reductase. Very large amounts of oxalate are produced when the liver is deficient in these enzymes.

- Secondary hyperoxaluria is the result of increased intestinal oxa-late absorption. Causes include a high-oxalate diet, fat malabsorp-tion (enteric hyperoxaluria), alterations of the intestinal oxalate degrading microorganisms, and genetic variations of the intesti-nal oxalate transporter. Hyperoxaluria due to fat malabsorption occurs because of increased intestinal oxalate absorption because excess free fatty acids (FFAs) in the intestinal lumen bind to cal-cium, thus allowing free oxalate to be absorbed in the large bowel. Additionally, bile salts and FFA in the colon may increase perme-ability of the bowel wall and allow increased absorption of oxa-late. Exocrine pancreatic insufficiency is a well-known cause of fat malabsorption and is increasingly being recognized as a cause of acute oxalate nephropathy.

- Compared to healthy patients, those with pancreatic insufficiency and steatorrhea have increased urine oxalate excretion even without renal insufficiency. Decreasing dietary calcium increases urinary oxalate excretion even further. Increasing calcium con-sumption to 3 g/day decreases urinary oxalate excretion to near normal.

Question 8.1.6: What is the treatment of hypocalcemia?

- Treat underlying disease
- Oral or intravenous (IV) (if symptomatic) calcium
- Vitamin D (if indicated)

CASE STUDY 8.1 CONCLUDED

Clinical course: The patient has been placed on pancreatic enzyme supplementation, a low-oxalate diet (oxalate intake < 50 mg/day), and calcium supplementation. Renal function unfortunately has failed to improve.

CASE STUDY 8.2

A 55-year-old previously healthy male presents for evaluation of elevated serum calcium noted on routine laboratory tests. He is asymptomatic. Physical examination is normal.

Blood chemistry:
Sodium: 138 mmol/L
Potassium: 4.0 mmol/L
Chloride: 100 mmol/L
Total CO_2: 24 mmol/L
Urea nitrogen: 30 mg/dL (urea: 10.8 mmol/L)
Creatinine: 1.0 mg/dL (88.4 mcmol/L)
Glucose: 100 mg/dL (11.2 mmol/L)
Uric acid: 6 mg/dL (357 mcmol/L)
Total calcium: 11.0 mg/dL (2.75 mmol/L)
Alkaline phosphatase: 600 U/L (elevated)

Serum and urine protein electrophoresis and serum free light chain kappa:lambda ratio are normal.

Question 8.2.1: What are the causes of hypercalcemia?

- Hyperparathyroidism:
    - Primary hyperparathyroidism—increased calcium release from bone due to parathyroid adenoma
    - Secondary hyperparathyroidism—In early secondary hyperparathyroidism, calcium is low. With prolonged disease, hypercalcemia may develop with adynamic bone disease and markedly reduced bone turnover. In such patients, hypercalcemia that develops with calcium-containing phosphate binders used to treat hyperphosphatemia is due to a marked reduction in the bone uptake of calcium
    - Tertiary hyperparathyroidism—When maximum medical management fails to control secondary hyperparathyroidism, tertiary hyperparathyroidism may result. In this setting, the patient is hypercalcemic, but PTH remains elevated. It may be difficult to distinguish tertiary from primary hyperparathyroidism unless previous history and laboratory values are available. Tertiary hyperparathyroidism is defined as hyperparathyroidism that fails to resolve with maximum medical management or as hyperparathyroidism that persists despite renal transplantation (McIntosh et al., 1966)
- Vitamin D excess (increases gut calcium absorption) (Fetchick et al., 1986)
- Malignancy (multiple mechanisms, including bone resorption, ectopic PTH secretion, secretion of PTH-related peptide)

- Other less common causes of hypercalcemia include granuloma-tous disease (increased activity of renal 25-OH-vitamin D-1a hy-droxylase with increased production of 1a,25-(OH)$_2$-vitamin D), immobilization (increased calcium release from bone) (Stewart et al., 1982), Paget disease (increased bone turnover), thyrotoxi-cosis (increased calcium release from bone) (Mundy et al., 1976), familial hypercalcemic hypocalciuria (inactivating mutation of calcium-sensitive receptor (CaSR) in parathyroid glands and kid-ney tubules, leading to higher set point for plasma calcium to sup-press PTH release and increased renal calcium reabsorption), and certain medications such as thiazides (decreased urinary calcium excretion) (Duarte et al., 1971), lithium (increased PTH release), and calcium plus alkali supplements (Burnett et al., 1949).

Question 8.2.2: What are the symptoms of hypercalcemia?

- Constipation
- Polyuria/polydipsia
- Confusion
- Coma (if severe)
- Shortened QT interval on EKG
- Osteitis fibrosa cystica (Silverberg et al., 1989)

CASE STUDY 8.2 CONTINUED

In our patient, the history is noncontributory and he is asymp-tomatic. Chest X-ray is normal. There is no history of fractures or bone pain, which would have suggested malignancy with bone metastasis. He is not taking any medications, which may cause elevated serum calcium. There is no evidence of paraproteinemia to suggest myeloma.

Question 8.2.3: What additional laboratory tests are indicated?

CASE STUDY 8.2 CONTINUED

Plasma inorganic phosphorus: 1.5 mg/dL (normal 2.5–4.5 mg/dL)
Intact PTH: 100 pg/mL (normal 10–65 pg/mL).

Question 8.2.4: What is the cause of hypercalcemia in this patient?

CASE STUDY 8.2 CONTINUED

The combination of hypercalcemia and hypophosphatemia with elevated PTH is very suggestive of primary hyperparathyroidism. However, one also needs to consider familial hypocalciuric hyper-calcemia (FHH).

Question 8.2.5: How does one distinguish between primary hyperparathyroidism and FHH?

- Primary hyperparathyroidism is due to a parathyroid adenoma. FHH is due to an inactivating mutation of CaSR in the parathyroid glands and kidney tubules. In FHH, hypercalcemia results from a higher set point for plasma calcium to suppress PTH release and increased renal calcium reabsorption.

- In order to distinguish between the two conditions, a 24-hour urine calcium (or urine Ca:Cr ratio) and an ultrasound of the neck are indicated. FHH is characterized by a 24-hour urine calcium of <200 mg (calcium to creatinine clearance ratio < 0.01 or fractional excretion of calcium < 1%), whereas urinary calcium excretion is >200 to 300 mg/day (calcium to creatinine clearance ratio > 0.02 or fractional excretion of calcium > 2%) in primary hyperparathyroidism.

CASE STUDY 8.2 CONTINUED

Clinical Course:
24-hour urine calcium is 350 mg
Ultrasound of the neck: 2 × 2 cm hypoechoic lesion near the left thyroid gland

Question 8.2.6: What is the diagnosis and what is the optimal treatment?

CASE STUDY 8.2 CONTINUED

The diagnosis in this case is primary hyperparathyroidism.

- Indications for parathyroidectomy are as follows:

1. Symptomatic hypercalcemia
2. Asymptomatic hypercalcemia PLUS
   a. Serum calcium elevated by >1 mg/dL or 0.25 mmol/L
   b. Creatinine clearance <60 mL/min/1.73 m^2
   c. Osteoporosis (T score < −2.5)
   d. Age < 50 years
      Options for poor surgical candidates include:
3. Cinacalcet (calcimimetic, which activates CaSR)
4. Bisphosphonates (in the presence of osteoporosis)
5. Vitamin D analogues (if vitamin D deficient; may suppress PTH release but caution advised as worsening hypercalcemia and hypercalciuria can occur)

Question 8.2.7: What urgent measures can be taken to control hypercalcemia?

Treating the underlying condition is the cornerstone of treatment. However, if hypercalcemia is symptomatic and/or severe (even without overt symptoms), prompt treatment to lower the plasma calcium should be undertaken.

- Treatment of hypercalcemia
  - IV fluids (if volume depleted, increases urinary calcium excretion)
  - Furosemide (increases urinary calcium excretion) once volume replete; stop thiazides if being given
  - Bisphosphonates (prevent bone resorption)

- Calcitonin (increases bone uptake of calcium)
- Calcimimetics (activate CaSR in parathyroid glands and kidney tubules, leading to lower set point for plasma calcium to suppress PTH release and decreased renal calcium reabsorption), if appropriate
- Dialysis (removes calcium) (indicated in severe hypercalcemia if coma present)
- Consider urgent parathyroidectomy if appropriate.

CASE STUDY 8.2 CONCLUDED

Since this patient is over 50 years old with mild asymptomatic hypocalcemia, it is elected to follow him in the clinic and obtain a dual-energy X-ray absorptiometry (DEXA) scan to exclude osteoporosis and a 24-hour urine for calcium. If he has a T score < -2.5 or a urine calcium >400 mg/day (>10 mmol/day), he should be considered for parathyroidectomy.

PHOSPHORUS

Physiology and Measurement

- Recommended dietary phosphorus intake in adults is ~700 mg (Institute of Medicine Food and Nutrition Board). Intestinal phosphorus absorption is higher with inorganic phosphate additives (found in processed and "junk" foods) than with organic phosphates naturally found in "whole" foods because the latter are bound to proteins and phytates that limit their absorption. Vitamin D increases phosphorus absorption.
- Most (~80%) of total body phosphorus is stored in bone, with most of the remainder in cells in the form of phospholipids and phosphorylated intermediates.
- The normal plasma inorganic phosphorus level is 2.4 to 4.5 mg/dL (0.76–1.45 mmol/L). Because the molecular weight of phosphorus (P) is 31, 1 mmol P = 31 mg. Thus, to convert mg/dL to mmol/L, divide by $0.1 \times$ molecular weight (i.e., 3.1). At pH 7.4, the valence of phosphates is 1.8. Therefore, to convert mmol/L to mEq/L, multiply by 1.8 (note that this will only be true at physiologic pH). Thus, a plasma phosphorus level of 4 mg/dL = 1.3 mmol/L = 2.3 mEq/L. Owing to the pH-dependent valence of phosphates, it is best to express phosphorus concentrations as mg/dL or mmol/L.
- Classically, plasma phosphorus is regulated by PTH/vitamin D. However, recently, the role of FGF23 has achieved paramount importance in the regulation of phosphorus metabolism. FGF23 is secreted by bone cells, probably in response to local extracellular phosphorus concentration and results in phosphaturia and decreased gut absorption, the latter by inhibition of production of active vitamin D, that is, $1\alpha,25\text{-}(OH)_2$-vitamin D, as shown in Figure 8.2. Phosphorus also stimulates PTH messenger RNA (mRNA) synthesis and increases parathyroid cell proliferation (Silver et al., 1996).

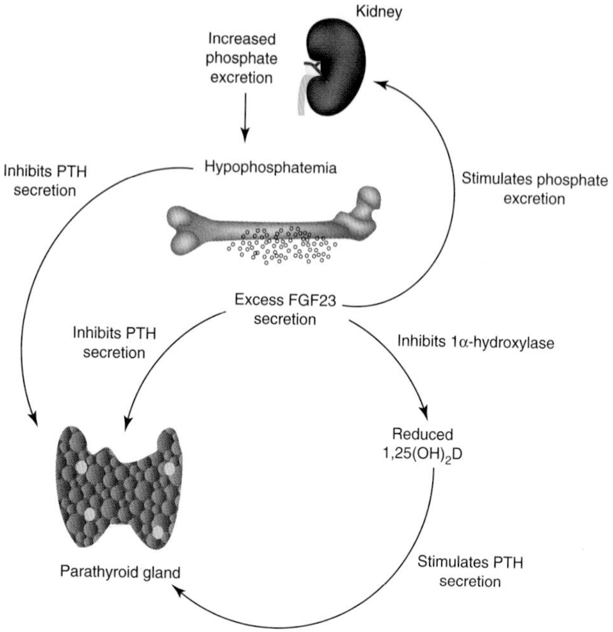

FIGURE 8.2. Effects of FGF23 on phosphate homeostasis. FGF23, fibroblast growth factor 23; PTH, parathyroid hormone. (From Komaba H, Koizumi M, Fukagawa M. Parathyroid resistance to FGF23 in kidney transplant recipients: back to the past or ahead to the future? *Kidney Int.* 78(10):953–955, 2010, with permission.)

CASE STUDY 8.3

A 67-year-old female with diabetes mellitus presents with dysuria, fever, weakness, and hypotension. She has been taking alendronate for osteoporosis. She is admitted to the telemetry unit for BP monitoring and fluid resuscitation. Blood cultures are growing *Escherichia coli* in both bottles. On physical examination, the vitals are as follows: temperature 38°C, pulse 110 beats/min, respirations 30 breaths/min, and blood pressure 80/40 mm Hg. Pulse oximetry 96%. Pertinent physical findings are tachycardia, no murmurs, no rubs, no gallops, clear lung fields, suprapubic tenderness, and no peripheral edema.

Blood chemistry:
Sodium: 135 mmol/L
Potassium: 3.8 mmol/L
Chloride: 110 mmol/L
Total CO_2: 18 mmol/L
Urea nitrogen: 18 mg/dL (urea: 6.4 mmol/L)

Creatinine: 1.0 mg/dL (88.4 mcmol/L)
Glucose: 40 mg/dL (2.2 mmol/L)
Total calcium: 9 mg/dL (2.25 mmol/L)

Magnesium: 2.0 mg/dL (0.82 mmol/L)
Inorganic phosphorus: 1.0 mg/dL (0.32 mmol/L)

Complete blood count:
WBC: 20,000/mm^3
Hemoglobin: 9 g/dL
Hematocrit: 27%
Platelets: 110,000/mm^3

Urinalysis:
Specific gravity: 1.025
Protein: 30 mg/dL
Blood: positive
RBC: 50/hpf
WBC: 50/hpf
Many bacteria

Question 8.3.1: What is the differential diagnosis for hypophosphatemia?

- Shift into cells:
  - Insulin administration (insulin increases P uptake into cells to make adenosine triphosphate [ATP])
  - Refeeding (stimulates insulin release)
  - Respiratory alkalosis (increased intracellular pH stimulates glycolysis and ATP production)
  - Hungry bone syndrome (P shifts into bone for remineralization, S/P parathyroidectomy)
- Renal losses
  - Primary hyperparathyroidism (decreases proximal tubular P reabsorption)
  - FGF23 overproduction (decreases proximal tubular P reabsorption)
  - Vitamin D deficiency (causes secondary hyperparathyroidism)
  - Renal tubular disorders (e.g., Fanconi syndrome) (decreased proximal tubular P reabsorption)
- Decreased gastrointestinal (GI) absorption
  - Malnutrition (low P diet)
  - Vitamin D deficiency (decreased gut P absorption)
  - Malabsorption syndromes (decreased gut P absorption)
  - Phosphorus binders (including over-the-counter [OTC] magnesium- and aluminum-containing antacids)

Question 8.3.2: What is the cause of hypophosphatemia in this patient?

CASE STUDY 8.3 CONCLUDED

In this patient, hypophosphatemia is likely due to shift of phosphorus into cells due to respiratory alkalosis. Although an arterial blood gas (ABG) has not been obtained, the patient is hyperventilating on examination. This patient has sepsis due to urinary tract infection. Not only is sepsis frequently characterized by hypophosphatemia, but hypophosphatemia is a poor prognostic marker in septic patients. Hypoglycemia may indicate a state of insulin excess, which also causes shift of phosphorus into cells.

She is treated with aggressive saline administration and antibiotics that improves the respiratory alkalosis and hypophosphatemia.

Question 8.3.3: Can normal saline contribute to hypophosphatemia?

- Normal saline can cause urinary losses of phosphate and thereby contribute to hypophosphatemia. However, fluid resuscitation should not be stopped if the patient is in a state of shock.

Question 8.3.4: What medications may be playing a role in hypophosphatemia?

- Bisphosphonates such as alendronate can contribute to hypophosphatemia. The enzyme pyrophosphate is an inhibitor of mineralization and can cause bone resorption to occur. However, in most people, alkaline phosphatase destroys the pyrophosphate before it can enter the bone. Bisphosphonates are a chemical modification of pyrophosphate; bisphosphonates cannot be destroyed by alkaline phosphatase, and they prevent bone resorption and strengthen the bony matrix.
- Diuretics can reduce phosphorus by increasing urinary excretion.

Question 8.3.5: What are the symptoms of hypophosphatemia?

Symptoms and Signs of Hypophosphatemia:

- Hypophosphatemia
  - Muscle weakness (including hypoventilation)
  - Rhabdomyolysis
  - Ileus
  - Myocardial depression
  - Cardiac arrhythmias

Question 8.3.6: What is the treatment of hypophosphatemia?

- Treat the underlying cause
- Stop all P binders (if being given)
- Oral or IV phosphorus supplementation. IV P indicated for severe hypophosphatemia (plasma P < 1 mg/dL)
- Add P to dialysate, if appropriate

CASE STUDY

8.4

A 57-year-old male with stage 4 CKD due to diabetes mellitus and hypertension presents for evaluation of paresthesias in his fingers and toes, muscle cramps and weakness. Physical examination is unremarkable.

Blood chemistry:
Sodium: 139 mmol/L
Potassium: 4.1 mmol/L
Chloride: 98 mmol/L
Bicarbonate: 23 mmol/L
Urea nitrogen: 25 mg/dL (urea: 8.9 mmol/L)

Creatinine: 3.0 mg/dL (265 mcmol/L)
Albumin: 3.3 g/dL (33 g/L)
Total calcium: 7.2 mg/dL (1.8 mmol/L)
Magnesium: 1.0 mg/dL (0.4 mmol/L)
Inorganic phosphorus: 8.5 mg/dL (2.7 mmol/L)

Complete blood count:
WBC: 5,000/mm^3
Hemoglobin: 11.8 g/dL
Hematocrit: 35%
Platelets: 200,000/mm^3

Question 8.4.1: What is the differential diagnosis of hyperphosphatemia?

- Shift out of cells
  - Rhabdomyolysis
  - Tumor lysis
- Decreased renal excretion
  - Renal failure
  - Hypoparathyroidism
- Increased gut absorption
  - Vitamin D intoxication
  - Phosphate ingestion (bowel cleansing)

Question 8.4.2: What is the most likely cause of the patient's weakness and paresthesias?

CASE STUDY 8.4 CONTINUED

The clinical picture suggests symptomatic hypocalcemia. Hypocalcemia is primarily caused by phosphorus retention due to CKD. Hypomagnesemia induced hypoparathyroidism resulting in hypocalcemia, and hyperphosphatemia is also likely contributory.

Question 8.4.3: What further labs would support this latter possibility?

CASE STUDY 8.4 CONTINUED

Intact PTH was 10.2 pg/mL (ng/L).
This is abnormally low in the face of hypocalcemia. Even with correction for the mild hypoalbuminemia, the corrected total calcium would still be low (7.9 mg/dL), which should lead to enhanced PTH secretion in an attempt to normalize the blood calcium.

Question 8.4.4: How does hypomagnesemia contribute to hyperphosphatemia?

- Release of calcium from the sarcoplasmic reticulum is inhibited by magnesium. Thus, hypomagnesemia causes decreases in intracellular calcium and decreased PTH release. Hypoparathyroidism leads to decreased renal phosphorus excretion, especially in the setting of stage 4 CKD. Hypoparathyroidism also leads to decreased FGF23 and consequent elevated active vitamin D.

Decreased FGF23 will also cause renal phosphorus retention and elevated vitamin D will increase intestinal phosphorus absorption, both of which will raise serum phosphorus (Fig. 8.2).

Question 8.4.5: What are the symptoms associated with hyperphosphatemia?

- Hyperphosphatemia
  - Usually asymptomatic, unless symptoms of hypocalcemia are present

Question 8.4.6: How should hyperphosphatemia be treated?

- Treat the underlying cause.
- For hypomagnesemia-induced hypoparathyroidism and hyperphosphatemia, magnesium supplementation should increase PTH release, which will normalize serum calcium and phosphorus levels.

CASE STUDY 8.4 CONCLUDED

With magnesium supplementation, follow-up labs were as follows:
Corrected total calcium: 9.5 mg/dL
Inorganic phosphorus: 4.0 mg/dL
Intact PTH: 60 ng/mL

Most cases of hyperphosphatemia are due to decreased renal excretion in the context of AKI or CKD. In these settings, treatment is as follows:

- Diet
  - The normal diet contains 1,000 to 1,500 mg of phosphorus, which is greater than currently recommended amount of ~700 mg. With renal disease, this amount needs to be less (or phosphorus binders need to be taken with meals) to prevent hyperphosphatemia with resulting secondary hyperparathyroidism and vascular calcification.
  - High-phosphorus foods include milk, cheese, cola, and chocolate. Inorganic phosphorus additives are absorbed more than organic phosphorus in foods.
  - Goal: Keep calcium (total) × phosphorus product <55.
- Phosphate binders
  - Calcium-based binders (carbonate or acetate)
    • Inexpensive
    • May cause hypercalcemia
    • Increases vascular calcification
  - Sevelamer
    • Expensive
    • Favorable effect on lipids
    • Lower hospitalization risk
    • Decreases vascular calcification
  - Lanthanum
    • Can have GI side effects
    • Some accumulation in the liver and bone (clinical significance unclear)

- Iron-based binders
  - Sucroferric oxyhydroxide (Velphoro)
    - Does not increase serum iron levels
    - Clinical studies did not include patients with peritonitis (an infection) during peritoneal dialysis, significant gastric or liver disorder, recent major GI surgery, a history of hemochromatosis
  - Ferric citrate (Auryxia)
    - Increases in serum ferritin and transferrin saturation (TSAT) are observed in clinical trials
    - Serum ferritin and TSAT should be checked prior to initiating ferric citrate and during therapy. Reduction in IV or oral iron therapy may be necessary. Contraindicated in iron overload states
    - Aluminum
      - Should not be used chronically
      - Causes encephalopathy, adynamic bone disease, microcytic anemia
  - Dialysis, if appropriate

MAGNESIUM

Physiology and Measurement

- Most magnesium is intracellular (primarily in the bone). Daily dietary intake is about 300 mg, which in the steady state is excreted primarily into the urine.
- The normal plasma total magnesium level (Mg) is 1.8 to 2.4 mg/dL (0.75–1.0 mmol/L). As with calcium, some of the magnesium in the plasma is bound to albumin, though the bound fraction is smaller than it is with calcium. Moreover, ionized magnesium measurements are not generally available in clinical laboratories. Thus, for practical purposes, total magnesium levels are used for the following calculations. Because the molecular weight of magnesium is 24, 1 mmol Mg = 24 mg. To convert mg/dL to mmol/L, divide by 0.1 × molecular weight (i.e., 2.4). Because magnesium is divalent, to convert mmol/L to mEq/L, multiply by 2. Thus, a plasma magnesium level of 2 mg/dL = 0.8 mmol/L = 1.6 mEq/L. In terms of ranges, normal ranges for plasma Mg are 1.8 to 2.4 mg/dL, 0.75 to 1 mmol/L, or 1.5 to 2.0 mEq/L. All of these units are used in clinical practice.
- In contradistinction to calcium and phosphorus, there are no known hormonal regulators of plasma magnesium level. The normal kidney is of paramount importance in preventing loss of magnesium in hypomagnesemic states and increasing urinary excretion of magnesium in response to hypermagnesemia via intrarenal (tubular) mechanisms.
- Hypomagnesemia can cause hypocalcemia by producing PTH resistance or by decreasing PTH secretion (Rude et al., 1976). Hypermagnesemia causes hypocalcemia due in part to the suppressive effects of hypermagnesemia on PTH secretion (Cholst et al., 1984).

CASE STUDY

8.5

A 51-year-old obese male (body mass index [BMI] 40) with **end-stage renal disease** (ESRD) due to diabetes mellitus and hypertension has received a living unrelated kidney transplant from a close friend. He has done well post-transplant. He denies nausea, vomiting, diarrhea, constipation, fever, chills, or abdominal pain. He is referred for evaluation of hypomagnesemia. Medications include prednisone, mycophenolate, and tacrolimus. Physical examination reveals normal vital signs. Other than obesity, there are no abnormal physical findings.

Blood chemistry:
Sodium: 140 mmol/L
Potassium: 4.2 mmol/L
Chloride: 110 mmol/L
Total CO_2: 20 mmol/L
Glucose: 255 mg/dL (14.2 mmol/L)
Urea nitrogen: 20 mg/dL (urea: 7.1 mmol/L)
Creatinine: 4.0 mg/dL (354 mcmol/L)
Total calcium: 9 mg/dL (2.25 mmol/L)
Inorganic phosphorus: 4 mg/dL (1.3 mmol/L)
Magnesium: 1.4 mg/dL (0.58 mmol/L)

Complete blood count:
WBC: 7,800/mm^3
Hemoglobin: 10.6 g/dL
Hematocrit: 34%
Platelets: 160,000/mm^3

Question 8.5.1: What are the causes of hypomagnesemia?

- Shift into cells (thyrotoxicosis, S/P parathyroidectomy)
- Renal losses
  - Diuretics
  - Nephrotoxins (e.g., aminoglycosides, cis-platinum, calcineurin inhibitors, alcohol)
  - Hereditary renal tubular disorders (e.g., Gitelman syndrome)
  - Alcohol
  - Insulin resistance
- GI malabsorption or losses (including decreased absorption owing to proton-pump inhibitors)
- Diarrhea
- Pancreatitis (saponification in fat)

Question 8.5.2: What is the differential diagnosis in this post-transplant patient?

CASE STUDY 8.5 CONTINUED

The etiology is often multifactorial in such patients. Common causes are diuretics, calcineurin inhibitors, insulin resistance, diarrhea, decreased oral intake, and proton-pump inhibitors.

Question 8.5.3: What is the likely cause of hypomagnesemia in this patient?

CASE STUDY 8.5 CONTINUED

Hypomagnesemia is very common in the early post-transplant period for reasons listed above. The cause of hypomagnesemia in this newly transplanted patient is most likely the calcineurin inhibitor tacrolimus.

Question 8.5.4: What are signs and symptoms of hypomagnesemia?

- Symptoms usually due to symptoms of concomitant electrolyte disturbance (hypokalemia, hypocalcemia), if present
- Hypomagnesemia can cause hypoparathyroidism

Question 8.5.5: What is the treatment of hypomagnesemia?

- Oral or IV (if symptoms) Mg. Oral dose often limited by diarrhea.

CASE STUDY 8.6

An 80-year-old woman with severe CKD (estimated glomerular filtration rate [eGFR] 25 mL/min/1.73 m^2) undergoes a colonoscopy to evaluate rectal bleeding. Several hours after completion of the procedure, she is noted to be severely bradycardic. An EKG shows complete heart block. The plasma magnesium level is 5 mg/dL (2.1 mmol/L).

Question 8.6.1: What are the causes of hypermagnesemia?

- IV magnesium administration (e.g., treatment of preeclampsia)
- Decreased renal excretion
- Renal failure, especially with Mg administration (e.g., bowel cleansing)

Question 8.6.2: What are the symptoms and signs of hypermagnesemia?

- Neurologic (paresthesias, hyporeflexia, weakness, respiratory depression)
- Cardiac (bradycardia, hypotension, prolonged PR and QT intervals on EKG, heart block)

Question 8.6.3: What is the treatment of hypermagnesemia?

If asymptomatic, fluids and diuretics (to increase renal excretion) usually sufficient

If symptomatic:

- Magnesium blocks calcium receptors. Emergency antidote is IV calcium. Dosage is 0.5 to 2 mg/kg/h.
- Patients will usually have renal failure. Dialysis is usually needed for removal if severe.

CASE STUDY 8.6 CONCLUDED

This patient is improved with administration of IV calcium. However, urine output is low, so emergency dialysis has been performed.

A 50-year-old man is referred for evaluation of hypercalcemia. His history and physical examination are unremarkable except he admits to stomach pains, which he attributed to "nerves" for which he takes OTC and home remedies. His physical examination is unremarkable. He has rarely seen a doctor before, and there are no previous laboratory studies available.

Blood chemistry:
Sodium: 140 mmol/L
Potassium: 4.0 mmol/L
Chloride: 100 mmol/L
Total CO_2: 24 mmol/L
Urea nitrogen: 55 mg/dL (urea: 19.6 mmol/L)
Creatinine: 2.5 mg/dL (221 mcmol/L)
Total calcium: 12 mg/dL (3 mmol/L)
Inorganic phosphorus: 4.0 mg/dL (1.3 mmol/L)
Magnesium: 2.0 mg/dL (0.8 mmol/L)
Intact PTH: 200 pg/mL (ng/L) (normal: 10–65)
1,25-Dihydroxy-vitamin D: 10 pg/mL (normal: 25–75) (26 pmol/L [normal: 65–195])

Q: What is the most likely diagnosis?

1. Primary hyperparathyroidism
2. Secondary hyperparathyroidism
3. Tertiary hyperparathyroidism
4. None of the above

A: This patient has hypercalcemia associated with elevated PTH. In the face of hypercalcemia, PTH secretion should be suppressed. Therefore, there is clearly hyperparathyroidism. Differentiation between the different types of hyperparathyroidism can be difficult. What type is it? Primary hyperparathyroidism is characterized by the combination of hypercalcemia and hypophosphatemia, the latter caused by impaired renal reabsorption of phosphorus. Plasma phosphorus is normal in this patient. However, there is also kidney disease (which appears to be chronic because dihydroxy-vitamin D level is low), which would be expected to blunt the phosphaturic effect of PTH. Thus, this diagnosis is still possible. Because kidney disease is the most common cause of secondary hyperparathyroidism, one might think this is secondary hyperparathyroidism. However, secondary hyperparathyroidism is typically characterized by the combination of hyperphosphatemia (caused by impaired excretion of phosphorus) and hypocalcemia (due to hyperphosphatemia and low vitamin D). How about tertiary hyperparathyroidism? When patients with secondary hyperparathyroidism ingest large amounts of calcium, they may become hypercalcemic. Predisposing factors are a reduction in bone uptake of calcium in some patients; in other patients, there may be progression from diffuse parathyroid hyperplasia to autonomous overproduction of PTH. Further history revealed that this patient is taking large amounts of Tums (OTC calcium carbonate). A parathyroid scan confirms diffuse parathyroid hyperplasia. Hypercalcemia resolves after Tums are stopped.

VIGNETTE 2

8

A 75-year-old woman is referred to the renal clinic because of CKD and profound hypocalcemia (plasma total calcium, 5 mg/dL). She admits to poor dietary intake for several months, which she thinks is caused by depression. Medications include thyroid hormone and vitamins. She denies circumoral paresthesias, muscle weakness, or cramps. Her physical examination is remarkable for bradycardia (pulse, 50 beats/min), mild hypertension (BP, 135/90 mm Hg), and moderate obesity. Chvostek and Trousseau's signs are negative, and deep tendon reflexes are sluggish. She has a scar in her neck, which she states was the result of an operation many years ago; she does not know what was done at that time.

Blood chemistry:
Sodium: 140 mmol/L
Potassium: 4.0 mmol/L
Chloride: 100 mmol/L
Total CO_2: 24 mmol/L
Urea nitrogen: 55 mg/dL (urea: 19.6 mmol/L)
Creatinine: 2.5 mg/dL (221 mcmol/L)
Total calcium: 4.8 mg/dL (1.2 mmol/L)
Inorganic phosphorus: 5.6 mg/dL (1.8 mmol/L)
Intact PTH: <10 pg/mL (ng/L)
Magnesium: 1.2 mg/dL (0.5 mmol/L)
Thyroid-stimulating hormone: 60 mIU/L (elevated)
Free T4 : 0.5 ng/dL (6.25 pmol/L) (low)

Electrocardiography:
EKG, normal

Q: What is the cause of hypocalcemia?

1. Secondary hyperparathyroidism
2. Hypothyroidism

3. Hypoparathyroidism
4. Hypomagnesemia

A: This patient has hypocalcemia, hyperphosphatemia, and CKD, all characteristic of secondary hyperparathyroidism. However, the low PTH level excludes this diagnosis. She clearly has hypothyroidism (probably she was noncompliant with her thyroid hormone supplement), but this does not cause the abnormalities in divalent mineral metabolism. The correct diagnosis is hypoparathyroidism. After considerable effort, the operative report from 40 years ago was obtained, and it was discovered that the patient had a total thyroidectomy for goiter. Up to 3% of patients undergoing this operation will develop permanent hypoparathyroidism, particularly when the goiter is extensive. Hypomagnesemia can lead to hypocalcemia both by decreasing secretion of PTH and by causing resistance to its effects. However, this severity of hypocalcemia is not seen.

References

Burnett CH, Commons RR, Albright F, et al. Hypercalcemia without hypercalciuria or hypophosphatemia, calcinosis and renal insufficiency: a syndrome following prolonged intake of milk and alkali. *N Engl J Med.* 240:787–794, 1949.

Cholst IN, Steinberg SF, Tropper PJ, et al. The influence of hypermagnesemia on serum calcium and parathyroid hormone levels in human subjects. *N Engl J Med.* 310(19):1221–1225, 1984.

Duarte CG, Winnacker JL, Becker KL, et al. Thiazide-induced hypercalcemia. *N Engl J Med.* 284:828–830, 1971.

Fetchick DA, Bertolini DR, Sarin PS, et al. Production of 1,25-dihydroxyvitamin D3 by human T cell lymphotrophic virus-I-transformed lymphocytes. *J Clin Invest.* 78:592–596, 1986.

Kazmi AS, Wall BM. Reversible congestive heart failure related to profound hypocalcemia secondary to hypoparathyroidism. *Am J Med Sci.* 333:226–229, 2007.

Korkor AB. Reduced binding of [3H]1,25-dihydroxyvitamin D3 in the parathyroid glands of patients with renal failure. *N Engl J Med.* 316(25):1573–1577, 1987.

McIntosh DA, Peterson EW, McRhaul JJ. Autonomy of parathyroid function after renal homotransplantations. *Ann Int Med.* 65:900–907, 1966.

Mundy GR, Shapiro JL, Bandelin JG, et al. Direct stimulation of bone resorption by thyroid hormones. *J Clin Invest.* 58:529–534, 1976.

Rude RK, Oldham SB, Singer FR. Functional hypoparathyroidism and parathyroid hormone end-organ resistance in human magnesium deficiency. *Clin Endocrinol (Oxf).* 5(3):209–224, 1976.

Silver J, Moallem E, Kilav R, et al. New insights into the regulation of parathyroid hormone synthesis and secretion in chronic renal failure. *Nephrol Dial Transplant.* 11(suppl 3):2–5, 1996.

Silverberg SJ, Shane E, de la Cruz L, et al. Skeletal disease in primary hyperparathyroidism. *J Bone Miner Res.* 4:283–291, 1989.

Stewart AF, Adler M, Byers CM, et al. Calcium homeostasis in immobilization: an example of resorptive hypercalciuria. *N Engl J Med.* 306:1136–1140, 1982.

9 Acute Renal Failure

INTRODUCTION

- **Acute renal failure (ARF)** is defined as a sudden (within hours to days) decrease in renal function, leading to retention of nitrogenous waste products (e.g., urea and creatinine [Cr]).

- Classically, ARF is divided into **prerenal failure** (decreased renal blood flow [RBF] leading to decreased glomerular filtration rate [GFR]), **postrenal failure** (urinary obstruction), and **intrinsic renal failure**, due to injury to kidney tissue, most commonly tubules (acute tubular necrosis [ATN]) but also interstitial cells (acute interstitial nephritis [AIN]), and less commonly glomeruli (acute glomerulonephritis [AGN]), or blood vessels (acute vasculitis). An extensive differential diagnosis, organized by anatomic sections of the kidney, should always be developed in the evaluation of ARF (see Fig. 9.1).

- More recently, the term **acute kidney injury** or **AKI** has been used instead of ARF or ATN. However, not all patients with ARF have kidney injury, and there are no biochemical markers of kidney injury in widespread clinical use at this time. Fortunately, "AKI" can also be an acronym for "acute kidney impairment," which will encompass all causes of acute decline in kidney function. The term "ATN" is somewhat problematic because it implies a pathologic change that may or may not be present (however, it is still used by medical coders). Another term that would apply to these conditions would be **acute kidney disease**, although this term is not in widespread use. Further classifications of AKI using the Risk, Injury, Failure, Loss, End-stage (RIFLE) classification (Bellomo et al., 2004) and the Acute Kidney Injury Network (AKIN) classification (Mehta et al., 2007) schema, which use various Cr and urine output criteria, have been recently promulgated. Categorization of ARF as used in this chapter is shown in Figure 9.1.

PRERENAL FAILURE

Definition of Prerenal Failure

- Prerenal failure is a reversible decrease in RBF and GFR. The kidney responds to the decrease in RBF by increasing reabsorption of salt and water (as well as other low–molecular-weight solutes such as urea and uric acid), leading to the characteristic findings of low urine [Na^+] and concentrated urine. Decreased RBF can be either because of an actual decrease in blood volume (hypovolemia) or

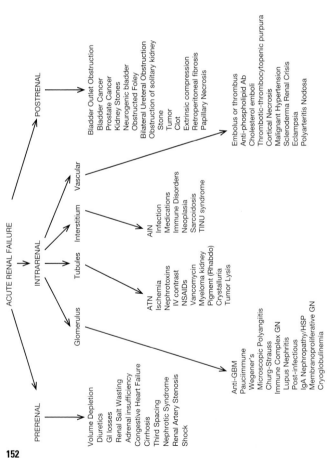

FIGURE 9.1. Categorization of acute renal failure. AIN, acute interstitial nephritis; ATN, acute tubular necrosis; GBM, glomerular basement membrane; GN, glomerulonephritis; HSP, Henoch-Schönlein purpura; IgA, immunoglobulin A; IV, intravenous; NSAIDs, nonsteroidal anti-inflammatory drugs; TINU, tubulointerstitial nephritis and uveitis.

152

blood pressure (BP) (hypotension) or decreased "effective" blood volume. Hypovolemia results in cardiac and arterial underfilling, leading to decreased cardiac output, RBF, and GFR. Decreased effective blood volume (also called decreased effective arterial blood volume [EABV] or arterial underfilling) means that the body senses a decrease in blood volume in the absence of true hypovolemia. Decreased EABV is sensed by high-pressure baroreceptors in the carotid sinus, aortic arch, and the juxtaglomerular apparatus of the kidney; these afferent signals then result in efferent signals (activation of the renin–angiotensin system [RAS], sympathetic system, and vasopressin system) that cause renal vasoconstriction. Decreased EABV caused by decreased cardiac output (as in congestive heart failure [CHF]) or systemic vasodilation (as in liver cirrhosis or sepsis) will decrease RBF and GFR. In CHF, low-pressure volume receptors in the atria and great veins are activated by atrial distension, leading to release of atrial natriuretic peptide (ANP), which somewhat counterbalances the renal vasoconstriction and salt and water retention. From a clinical standpoint, the important thing to remember is that the kidney responds in a similar manner to an actual or "effective" decrease in volume, so the cause of prerenal failure must be deduced clinically (Blantz, 1998).

■ Volume depletion versus dehydration. These are not the same; however, they frequently coexist.
  ■ Volume depletion is characterized by a reduction in the extracellular fluid (ECF) volume and hemodynamic changes, including tachycardia and orthostatic hypotension. Volume depletion indicates sodium and water depletion and is most commonly caused by hemorrhage, vomiting, diarrhea, or third-space sequestration.
  ■ Dehydration, on the other hand, is water depletion; this frequently leads to hypernatremia. Dehydration can lead to confusion, thirst, impaired sensorium, and coma or seizures.

Causes of Prerenal Failure
■ Hypovolemia
  ■ Blood loss
  ■ Gastrointestinal (GI) fluid loss
  ■ Renal fluid loss
    • Diuretics
    • Diuretic phase of recovery from ARF
    • Adrenal insufficiency
    • Hypoaldosteronism (isolated)
    • Renal tubular disorders (e.g., Bartter/Gitelman syndrome)
    • Osmotic diuresis (e.g., hyperglycemia)
    • Salt-wasting nephropathy (e.g., medullary cystic disease)
  ■ Sequestration of ECF that cannot be readily mobilized into the plasma ("third spacing"). Examples include the following:
    • Pancreatitis
    • Intestinal obstruction
    • Peritonitis
    • Crush injuries
    • Bleeding into tissue compartments

- Decreased cardiac output
  - Heart failure
  - Pericardial tamponade (impaired venous inflow into heart)
  - Massive pulmonary embolism (impaired pulmonary blood flow)
- Systemic vasodilation
  - Sepsis (release of vasoactive mediators such as prostacyclin and nitric oxide produced by endothelial cells)
  - Cirrhosis (multifactorial, including endotoxin-induced stimulation of nitric oxide production)
  - Anaphylaxis (release of vasoactive mediators including histamine and bradykinin)
  - Autonomic insufficiency (decreased sympathetic tone)
  - Antihypertensive drugs (several mechanisms, including indirect effects such as decreased sympathetic tone or RAS blockade and direct vasodilator effects)
- Renal vasoconstriction
  - Sepsis (despite systemic vasodilation; complex and not well-understood pathogenesis involving dysregulation of nitric oxide and other factors)
  - Cirrhosis (can lead to marked decrease in RBF and GFR, resulting in hepatorenal syndrome [HRS]; hemodynamically similar to sepsis)
  - Prostaglandin inhibitors (nonsteroidal anti-inflammatory drugs [NSAIDs]) (renal prostaglandins are vasodilatory and attempt to maintain RBF in the setting of renal vasoconstriction)
  - Calcineurin inhibitors (cyclosporine, tacrolimus) (impairment of endothelial cell function, leading to reduced production of vasodilators such as prostaglandins and nitric oxide and enhanced release of vasoconstrictors such as endothelin and thromboxane)
  - Vasoconstrictors (e.g., norepinephrine, phenylephrine)
- Renal vascular disease
  - Macrovascular (see Chapter 15)
  - Microvascular (see Chapter 16)
- Decreased glomerular capillary pressure
  - RAS blockers (dilate efferent > afferent arterioles)

Pathophysiology of Prerenal Failure
- Total body water (TBW) is about 60% of body weight in males and 50% in females. Although water distributes throughout all body compartments, sodium is excluded from the intracellular space. Consequently, total body sodium content determines the size of the ECF compartment (typically about 45% of TBW is extracellular and 55% is intracellular, but is affected by gender and obesity). Normally, 83% (5/6) of the ECF is in the interstitium and 17% (1/6) in the plasma. Thus, in a 70-kg male, TBW = $0.6 \times 70 = 42$ L, ECF is 0.45×42 L = 19 L, and plasma volume is 0.17×19 L = 3.2 L, or about 8% of TBW. Volume depletion occurs when salt loss results in a decrease in ECF.

- With a decrease in either true or EABV (see above), compensatory changes occur to maintain hemodynamic stability. Baroreceptors in the carotid sinus and aortic arch sense volume depletion and cause an increase in sympathetic activity and increased catecholamine release (Kon et al., 1985). Heart rate and contractility increase and peripheral vascular resistance increases to maintain BP. Blood is shunted from nonessential vascular beds such as the skeletal muscle, skin, kidneys, and GI tract toward the coronary and cerebral circulation (Blantz, 1998).
- The juxtaglomerular apparatus in the kidney senses decreased RBF and secretes renin to activate the RAS and increase reabsorption of sodium and water. Stimulation of antidiuretic hormone (ADH), also called arginine vasopressin, also increases water reabsorption. When compensatory mechanisms fail, as with loss of >10% to 20% of blood volume, patients develop orthostatic hypotension, which can progress to supine hypotension and shock (impaired tissue perfusion) (Blantz, 1998).

Symptoms and Signs of Prerenal Failure

- If renal hypoperfusion is due to hypovolemia, tachycardia, postural hypotension, flat neck veins, cool extremities with decreased capillary refill, and poor skin turgor are seen.
- If renal hypoperfusion is due to decreased cardiac output, signs of CHF (distended neck veins, rales, and edema) may be present. Consider cardiac tamponade (check for pulsus paradoxus, which is an accentuated variability in BP with respiration).
- If renal hypoperfusion is due to systemic vasodilation, warm extremities are expected; with liver disease, palmar erythema and spider angiomata are seen.
- If renal hypoperfusion is due to renovascular disease, an abdominal or flank bruit and/or hypertension may be present.
- Decreased urine output is seen in all cases unless prerenal failure is due to renal fluid losses (e.g., diuretics, uncontrolled diabetes).

Laboratory Evaluation in Prerenal Failure

- Plasma sodium is usually normal in volume depletion (because salt and water are both depleted) but will be high in dehydration. Plasma sodium may be low in states of decreased EABV, primarily because of increased ADH release (see Chapter 5).
- Hyperglycemia can cause osmotic diuresis, resulting in both volume depletion and dehydration. (Note: Because hyperglycemia causes water movement from cells to ECF, the extent of dehydration can be underestimated; the "corrected" sodium concentration will be higher than the measured sodium concentration; see Chapter 5.)
- Hypokalemia may exist in patients with diarrhea, taking diuretics, or with renal tubular defects (see Chapter 6).
- Hypercalcemia can cause polyuria and failure of the kidney to respond to ADH (nephrogenic diabetes insipidus), resulting in hypernatremia.

- Acid/base—There can be non–anion gap metabolic acidosis or (rarely) metabolic alkalosis with diarrhea, metabolic alkalosis with vomiting, and lactic acidosis with shock.
- Hemoglobin and hematocrit may be low in patients with blood loss or high with volume depletion or severe dehydration.
- A blood urea nitrogen to creatinine ratio (BUN/Cr) > 20:1 is usually because of increased urea reabsorption and suggests prerenal azotemia. The plasma urea nitrogen is also high in GI bleeding (increased gut nitrogen absorption coupled with prerenal failure), hypercatabolic states, or with glucocorticoid therapy (increased protein breakdown and urea generation).
- A urine sodium or urine chloride <20 mmol/L suggests volume depletion. A fractional excretion of sodium (FENa) < 1% suggests prerenal azotemia. A fractional excretion of urea (FEurea) < 35% also suggests prerenal azotemia and can be used when a patient is on diuretics, because FENa may be elevated if diuretic-induced sodium losses are the causes of prerenal failure. ADH-mediated water retention increases urine osmolality (often to >450 mmol/L). This response to hypertonicity (from either dehydration or dehydration with volume depletion) is incomplete if urinary concentrating ability is impaired.

Treatment of Prerenal Failure

- Treatment is directed at the underlying etiology. Shock or severe intravascular volume depletion requires large volume intravenous (IV) fluid replacement. The choice of resuscitation fluid depends on the cause of the deficit.
  - In hemorrhage, typically both blood transfusion and fluid resuscitation are required. Loss of red blood cells (RBCs) diminishes O_2-carrying capacity, which can only be improved with RBC transfusion.
  - In the absence of hemorrhage, crystalloid solutions (isotonic 0.9% saline or lactated Ringer's solution) are typically used for intravascular volume replenishment. Isotonic fluid remains in the ECF, whereas hypotonic fluid (e.g., 0.45% saline) and free water (e.g., D5W) will also distribute into the intracellular fluid and are not appropriate for initial volume resuscitation. Lactated Ringer's solution will prevent dilutional acidosis from large volume IV fluid replacement because lactate is a bicarbonate former. Alternatively, an isotonic solution containing bicarbonate can be used (e.g., 0.45% saline with 75 mEq/L sodium bicarbonate) if metabolic acidosis is present.
  - Colloid solutions (e.g., hydroxyethyl starch, albumin, dextrans) are also effective for volume replacement and, because they stay at least initially in the plasma space, result in a more rapid increased in blood volume as compared to saline. However, in comparison with isotonic saline, no survival differences have been proven. Albumin may have a negative inotropic effect, and dextrans and hydroxyethyl starch can adversely affect coagulation. However, albumin infusions have been shown to be beneficial in specific circumstances such as after large volume paracentesis or during spontaneous peritonitis of cirrhosis.

■ The best indicator that fluid resuscitation is working is a urine output of 0.5 to 1 mL/kg/h. Heart rate, mental status, and capillary refill are other parameters, but these may not be as useful depending on the underlying illness. Vasoconstriction may make mean arterial pressure less usable, especially if pressors are also used. Central venous pressure (CVP) is the mean pressure in the superior vena cava, reflecting preload. Normal CVP ranges from 2 to 7 mm Hg ($\sim$3–9 cm H_2O). A CVP $<$ 2 mm Hg ($<$2.7 cm H_2O) suggests volume depletion. A CVP 12 to 15 mm Hg indicates that right-sided cardiac filling pressures are adequate and fluid administration may be risky. However, left-sided filling pressures may still be low despite high right-sided pressures in patients with pulmonary hypertension and right ventricular failure, and pulmonary artery catheterization should be considered for diagnosis and treatment/monitoring in such instances.

Hepatorenal Syndrome

■ This is a type of prerenal failure that occurs only in patients with severe liver failure. Patients with HRS typically have jaundice and ascites. The pathogenesis is complex and poorly understood, but is characterized by profound systemic and splanchnic vasodilation leading to relative hypotension, increased cardiac output, but intense renal vasoconstriction. In its classic form, there is no kidney injury, and the syndrome is reversible with improvement of liver function or liver transplantation (Iwatsuki et al., 1973). Because the kidneys may be normal by biopsy, HRS patients are not generally candidates for kidney transplantation. However, HRS can lead to prolonged renal ischemia resulting in ATN; also, administration of aminoglycosides, IV radiocontrast, sepsis, bleeding, and hypotension can also lead to ATN; these patients can be suitable recipients for a kidney allograft if they have required dialysis for many weeks to months.

■ HRS is characterized by activation of the RAS and the sympathetic nervous system (both of which decrease GFR), increased adenosine (which is a systemic vasodilator but a renal vasoconstrictor), and increased systemic but reduced renal nitric oxide and vasodilator prostaglandin generation (Ruiz-del-Arbol et al., 2005). Alternative theories entertain deficiency of a vasodilator factor or an enhanced hepatorenal reflex leading to renal vasoconstriction in HRS.

■ Types of HRS
  ■ Type 1 HRS—characterized by rapid development of renal failure often precipitated by spontaneous bacterial peritonitis or another infection. Without treatment, survival is $<$2 weeks, but selected patients can be supported and undergo successful liver transplantation.
  ■ Type 2 HRS—characterized by moderate, stable, or slowly progressive reduction in GFR. Median survival is 3 to 6 months, but can often undergo successful liver transplantation.

- Diagnosis of HRS
  - Major criteria:
    - Decreased GFR (plasma Cr > 1.5 mg/dL)
    - Absence of shock, sepsis, fluid loss, nephrotoxic drugs
    - No improvement in renal failure after diuretic withdrawal or fluid resuscitation ($\geq$1.5 L)
    - Proteinuria < 500 mg/24 hour; negative renal ultrasound
  - Minor criteria:
    - Urine volume < 500 mL/day
    - Urine sodium < 10 mmol/L
    - Urine osmolality > plasma osmolality
    - Plasma sodium < 130 mmol/L
    - Urine RBCs < 50/hpf
- Treatment of HRS
  - Midodrine or norepinephrine (systemic vasoconstrictor) plus octreotide (splanchnic vasoconstrictor) plus albumin
  - Vasopressin
  - Terlipressin plus albumin—not available in the United States
  - N-acetylcysteine?
  - Liver transplantation is definitive treatment

POSTRENAL FAILURE

Presentation and Pathogenesis

- In postrenal failure, azotemia is caused by reduced RBF resulting from increased pressure within the renal collecting system and is characterized by dilatation of the collecting system on renal imaging (hydronephrosis). The site of obstruction can be intrarenal (pelvicalyceal system) or at the level of the ureters, bladder, or urethra. Upper tract (i.e., intrarenal or ureteral) obstruction can be unilateral or bilateral, whereas lower tract obstruction will affect both the kidneys.
- There may be no symptoms in chronic obstruction, though with lower tract obstruction there will usually be lower urinary tract symptoms, such as hesitancy, urinary dribbling, urgency, and urinary frequency. Acute obstruction of the ureter(s) typically leads to colicky pain starting in the flank(s) and radiating into the groin. In complete obstruction (either bilateral or unilateral in a solitary kidney), there will be anuria, though partial obstruction can be associated with no change in urine output or even polyuria (nephrogenic diabetes insipidus due to tubular damage).
- Normal urine output is thus typical with partial obstruction and does not exclude the diagnosis. Thus, a renal ultrasound is recommended in virtually all cases of ARF.

Causes of Postrenal Failure

- Lower urinary tract
  - Benign prostatic hyperplasia (BPH)
  - Cancer (prostate, bladder)
  - Neurogenic bladder
    - Diabetes mellitus
    - Multiple sclerosis

- Cerebrovascular accident/spinal cord injury
- Alpha-adrenergic blockers
  - Bladder stones/clots
  - Urethral stricture
- Upper urinary tract
  - Cancer (prostate, ovarian, endometrial, cervical, colon, lymphoma)
  - Nephrolithiasis/intratubular crystal deposition (e.g., uric acid, acyclovir, methotrexate)
  - Anatomic abnormalities (e.g., ureteropelvic junction obstruction)
  - Retroperitoneal fibrosis
  - Endometriosis
  - Blood clots
  - Papillary necrosis

Prognosis of Postrenal Failure

- Postrenal azotemia is characterized by hypertension, either because of volume expansion in bilateral obstruction or renin secretion in unilateral obstruction. Two to 8 days following relief of obstruction, postobstructive diuresis may ensue. This is due to an expanded extracellular volume, osmotic diuresis, and a concentrating defect.
- The prognosis for renal functional recovery depends on the duration and extent of obstruction. Based on experimental studies and clinical observations, renal recovery after complete obstruction of the urinary tract in a previously normal kidney is as follows:
  - One week—normal function (Kerr, 1954)
  - Twelve weeks—minimal function (Better et al., 1973)

Laboratory Evaluation in Postrenal Failure

- Urinalysis—hematuria (stone, tumor, clot), pyuria (urinary tract infection [UTI] associated with obstruction), crystals (amorphous—uric acid, tetragon—calcium oxalate, hexagon—cystine, see Chapter 1)
- Abdominal X-ray of the kidneys, ureter, and bladder without contrast (KUB)—most stones are radiopaque, except uric acid
- Renal ultrasound—test of choice for hydronephrosis
  - Although hydronephrosis is the hallmark of urinary obstruction, there are a few settings where it may be absent: (1) recent onset (<3 days) of obstruction, in which there may be inadequate time for dilatation to occur (increased resistive index on duplex Doppler ultrasonography in the affected kidney may be present prior to hydronephrosis in unilateral obstruction); (2) when the collecting systems are encased by retroperitoneal tumor or fibrosis and cannot dilate (this is very rare)
- Computed tomography (CT) abdomen without contrast (this has replaced KUB for acute nephrolithiasis)
- Prostate-specific antigen (PSA) (elevated in prostate cancer)
- Diuretic renogram—increase in urine flow should wash out the radioisotope during a renal scan; if this does not occur, obstruction may be present
- Urodynamics—neurogenic bladder
- Stone evaluation (see Chapter 17).

Treatment of Postrenal Failure

- BPH—alpha blockers, finasteride, transurethral resection of the prostate (TURP) or laser prostatectomy
- Prostate cancer—surgery versus radiation versus watchful waiting (especially in older patients)
- Neurogenic bladder—cholinergic drugs, intermittent self-catheterization, chronic urinary drainage catheter (last resort)
- Nephrolithiasis—for first episode—treat, no need to do extensive diagnostic workup; recurrent episodes require evaluation (see Chapter 17).

ACUTE KIDNEY INJURY

Definition

AKI or intrinsic renal injury is defined as a reversible or irreversible organ failure caused by structural injury to the kidney, generally to the renal tubular epithelial cells. The insult, ischemic or toxic, causes cell death or detachment from the basement membrane causing tubular dysfunction. Although AKI can theoretically be due to acute tubular injury, AIN, AGN, or acute vasculopathy (AV), it is most commonly due to tubular injury (Bellomo et al., 2004).

Causes of AKI (Tubular Injury or ATN)

- Ischemia
  - Hypovolemia or hypotension
  - Renal arterial obstruction (e.g., aortic cross-clamping, thromboembolism)
  - Sepsis (renal vasoconstriction with or without hypotension) (Schrier & Wang, 2004)
- Toxins
  - Exogenous toxins
    - Antibiotics (e.g., aminoglycosides, colistimethate)
    - Radiocontrast (less risk with low- and iso-osmolal contrast)
    - Chemotherapeutic agents (e.g., cis-platinum)
    - Bacterial toxins (especially endotoxin)
  - Endogenous toxins
    - Myoglobin
    - Hemoglobin
    - Uric acid
    - Light chains (myeloma)

Risk Factors for AKI

- Older age
- Preexisting kidney disease
- Cardiac, vascular, or hepatobiliary surgery
- Severe and/or inadequately treated volume depletion
- Severe and/or inadequately treated hypotension
- CHF
- Obstructive jaundice
- Liver cirrhosis
- Multiple myeloma

Pathophysiology of AKI
- Time course
  - Initiation—exposure—may be preventable
  - Maintenance—injury is established
  - Recovery—repair/regeneration
- Mechanisms of ischemic AKI
  - *Failure of autoregulation/renal vasoconstriction.* As BP and renal perfusion decrease, autoregulatory mechanisms initially result in renal vasodilatation to maintain RBF. However, endogenous vasoconstrictor (e.g., angiotensin II, catecholamines, vasopressin) mechanisms are activated to maintain BP. Ultimately, the vasoconstrictor influence is predominant, and there is an increase in afferent arteriolar resistance, leading to a decrease in RBF and a prerenal state. Patients with hypertension and/or chronic kidney disease (CKD) are more susceptible to ischemia because hyalinosis/myointimal hyperplasia causes narrowing of afferent arterioles. Moreover, the renal arterioles in CKD patients tend to be already dilated and, because of impairment of autoregulation, cannot dilate any further in response to low perfusion. Sepsis, liver failure, contrast administration, acute calcineurin inhibitor toxicity, and hypercalcemia are also characterized by renal vasoconstriction. All of these conditions increase the risk of AKI. Severe prerenal failure is thus an important cause of AKI.
  - *Ischemic injury.* With prolonged ischemia, there is adenosine triphosphate (ATP) depletion, leading to apoptosis (Ueda et al., 2000) and necrosis of renal tubular epithelial cells and tubular obstruction (Canfield et al., 1991). Cellular calcium overload (Ye et al., 1999), disruption of the actin cytoskeleton, stimulation of proteases (caspases), inflammation, oxygen radical accumulation, and endothelial injury (Molitoris & Sutton, 2004) are other mechanisms of injury.
- Nephrotoxins can cause intrarenal vasoconstriction, direct tubular toxicity, and/or tubular obstruction. Some toxins (such as contrast) lead to a combination of ischemic and toxic injury, whereas others (aminoglycosides, light chains) are directly toxic to renal cells.

Prognosis of AKI
- Patient survival
  - Many factors determine prognosis of AKI, including patient's age, etiology of AKI, need for dialysis, and comorbid conditions. Older patients in the intensive care unit (ICU) with sepsis, respiratory failure, and dialysis-requiring AKI have an up to 90% mortality rate, whereas young patients with rhabdomyolysis and dialysis-requiring AKI have an excellent prognosis.
  - Patients with multiorgan system failure, including AKI-requiring dialysis, have a very high mortality.
- Renal survival
  - Renal recovery after AKI may be complete or nearly complete in previously healthy patients, but patients with

moderate-to-severe underlying CKD who suffer AKI may not recover renal function.

- Duration of need for dialysis predicts likelihood of renal recovery, with >3-month need for dialysis generally predicting a poor renal prognosis.

Laboratory Evaluation in AKI

- AKI is characterized by the following:
  - Elevated BUN and Cr (BUN/Cr ratio tends to be normal)
  - Electrolyte abnormalities (hyperkalemia, metabolic acidosis most common)
  - Impaired urinary concentration (Uosm < 350 mmol/kg)
  - Impaired sodium reabsorption (Urine Na > 20 and FENa > 1 in AKI; however, in early phases of contrast, sepsis, and rhabdomyolysis, UNa can be <10 and FENa can be <1) (Zarich et al., 1985)
  - Urine sediment—renal tubular epithelial cells, epithelial cell casts, pigmented granular casts ("muddy brown" casts)
  - Normal renal ultrasound
  - Biopsy (not usually done)—loss of cells from tubular epithelium with gaps in denuded basement membrane
- Tests to assess clinical condition—calcium, phosphorus, albumin, liver function, blood gases
- Tests to investigate etiology—depending on the clinical situation, consider collagen-vascular serology (suspected AIN, AGN, or AV), creatine kinase (rhabdomyolysis), uric acid (tumor lysis), blood smear/haptoglobin (thrombotic thrombocytopenic purpura/hemolytic-uremic syndrome [TTP/HUS])
- Distinguishing prerenal failure from tubular injury
  - Classically, they can be distinguished by biochemical and urinary parameters (Fig. 9.2).
  - There is clearly an overlap between these conditions. However, prerenal failure can be improved if renal hemodynamics can be improved (such as with volume resuscitation or improvement in cardiac function), whereas tubular injury does not respond to these measures and portends a worse prognosis.
  - In the future, biomarkers of injury will be used for more accurate diagnosis. In a recent meta-analysis, urine neutrophil gelatinase–associated lipocalin (NGAL) was shown to be an accurate predictor of diagnosis and prognosis (Haase et al., 2009). Measurement of urinary levels of the biomarkers NGAL, kidney injury molecule-1, and interleukin-18 combined with urinary microscopy by trained nephrologists significantly improved upon clinical determination of prognosis (Hall et al., 2011).

Prevention and Treatment of AKI

- Primary prevention:
  - Volume repletion (judicious!)
  - Monitor drug levels and adjust doses. Avoid nephrotoxins (NSAIDs, contrast, aminoglycosides, colistimethate, amphotericin B), if possible
  - Isotonic saline or bicarbonate ± N-acetylcysteine before radiocontrast administration

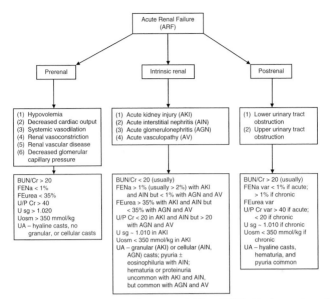

FIGURE 9.2. Laboratory parameters in acute renal failure. BUN/Cr, blood urea nitrogen/creatinine; FENa, fractional excretion of sodium; FEurea, fractional excretion of urea; U/P Cr, urine to plasma creatinine ratio; U sg, urine specific gravity; Uosm, urine osmolality; UA, urinalysis.

- Supportive care in established AKI:
    - Stop nephrotoxins, if possible
    - Avoid further nephrotoxic insults
    - Maintain hemodynamics (prevent hypotensive episodes)
    - Loop diuretics may convert oliguria to nonoliguria and may decrease morbidity associated with fluid overload, although decreased mortality has not been demonstrated in controlled studies
    - Nutrition—25 to 30 kcal/kg/day for anabolism and avoidance of metabolic acidosis (Druml, 2001)
- Dialytic therapy of AKI (Mehta et al., 2001)
    - Indications:
        - Metabolic abnormalities (hyperkalemia, metabolic acidosis; sometimes severe hyponatremia, hypercalcemia, hyperphosphatemia, hypermagnesemia, hyperuricemia)
        - Fluid overload (pulmonary edema)
        - Uremia (anorexia, nausea/vomiting, pericarditis, myoclonus, seizures, unexplained altered mental status)
        - Irreversible oliguria? (some observational studies suggest a benefit of early dialysis, but there are no randomized controlled trials)
    - Methods
        - Continuous renal replacement therapy (hemofiltration or hemodialysis)
        - Intermittent renal replacement therapy (hemodialysis)
        - No controlled studies to support benefit of one modality over the other

Acute Interstitial Nephritis

- AIN is characterized by ARF resulting from immune-mediated tubulointerstitial injury, initiated by medications, infection, and other causes. Patients may present with fever, rash, eosinophilia, arthralgias, malaise, anorexia, nausea/vomiting, and/or oliguria.
- Although some degree of peripheral eosinophilia may be present in AIN, peripheral eosinophilia is not necessary for the diagnosis of AIN. Eosinophiluria may be present, but has poor sensitivity and specificity and is no longer recommended to be used in the diagnosis of AIN. In one study, urine eosinophils are found in a variety of kidney diseases besides AIN, and eosinophiluria performs poorly in distinguishing AIN from other kidney diseases (Muriithi et al., 2013).
- On renal biopsy, most cases of AIN are characterized by patchy edema and focal infiltrates of eosinophils that are globally present. A diffuse interstitial inflammatory process is not a prerequisite for the diagnosis of AIN. The biopsy may also show partially denuded tubules, which is also consistent with AIN because AIN can be characterized by some tubular injury.
  - Causes (based on a review of 128 patients) (Backer & Pusey, 2004)
    - Drugs—71% (usually due to antibiotics)
    - Infection—15%
    - Idiopathic—8%
    - Tubulointerstitial nephritis and uveitis syndrome—5%
    - Sarcoidosis—1%
- Laboratory evaluation
  - Urinalysis—hematuria, proteinuria
  - Urine eosinophils
  - Blood eosinophils
  - Renal ultrasound (echogenic, swollen kidneys, if severe)
  - Renal biopsy—T cells, macrophages, plasma cells, eosinophilic microabscesses (may be necessary to confirm diagnosis)
- Treatment of AIN
  - Discontinue offending agent
  - Supportive care
  - Immunosuppression, if necessary (steroids, mycophenolate, cyclosporine, cyclophosphamide)

Acute Glomerulonephritis

For a detailed treatment, see Chapter 10.

Acute Vasculopathy

For a detailed treatment, see Chapters 15 and 16.

A 61-year-old woman with alcoholic liver cirrhosis presents for evaluation of the new-onset renal failure. She states she has been abstinent from alcohol for the past year. On physical examination, she has stigmata of liver failure, including palmar erythema, icterus, splenomegaly, ascites, and lower extremity edema.

Blood chemistry:
Sodium: 120 mmol/L
Potassium: 5.1 mmol/L
Chloride: 100 mmol/L
Total CO_2: 21 mmol/L
Urea nitrogen: 10 mg/dL (urea: 3.6 mmol/L)
Creatinine: 2.0 mg/dL (177 mcmol/L)
Glucose: 121 mg/dL (6.7 mmol/L)
Total bilirubin: 2.0 mg/dL (34 mcmol/L)
Alkaline phosphatase: 100 U/L
Aspartate transaminase (AST): 15 U/L
Alanine transaminase, 10 U/L
Prothrombin time: 19 s (INR 2.3)
Partial thromboplastin time: 38 s

Complete blood count:
WBCs: 11,000/mm³
Hemoglobin: 13 g/dL (130 g/L)

Hematocrit: 38%
Platelets: 100,000/mm³

Urinalysis:
Color: yellow
pH: 5.0
Specific gravity: 1.015
Protein: negative
Blood: negative
Glucose: negative
Ketones: negative
Bilirubin: moderate
Urobilinogen: moderate
WBCs: 2/hpf
RBCs: 3/hpf
Bacteria: none
Urine sodium: 6 mmol/L
Urine creatinine: 100 mg/dL (8,840 mcmol/L)
Urine osmolality: 450 mmol/kg
Blood cultures × 2: no growth
Renal ultrasound: no hydronephrosis

Renal failure fails to improve after fluid administration (1.5 L of iso-oncotic albumin in 0.9% saline).

Q: Which of the following is not a mechanism of renal vasoconstriction in HRS?

1. Increased prostaglandins
2. Increased adenosine
3. Decreased nitric oxide
4. Increased norepinephrine

A: Deteriorating liver function causes splanchnic vasodilatation and renal vasoconstriction. The renal failure of HRS is thus prerenal in nature and is characterized by the typical findings of prerenal azotemia. In this case, the FENa is very low (0.1%) and the urine is very concentrated, which is typical of the marked sodium and water avidity in this syndrome. The kidneys are normal histologically and will function normally when transplanted into a person with a healthy liver or when the patient with the HRS undergoes a liver transplant. The cause of renal vasoconstriction in liver disease is complex with heightened sympathetic activity, increased adenosine, and decreased renal nitric oxide all appearing to be involved. Downregulation of renal prostaglandins has also been reported. Therapeutic attempts to directly cause renal vasodilation have been unsuccessful, so therapy is directed toward vasoconstriction of the splanchnic and systemic circulations with octreotide and midodrine, respectively. Norepinephrine can be used instead of midodrine in patients in the ICU setting. In Europe, the splanchnic vasoconstrictor terlipressin is also available. Liver transplantation is the definitive therapy.

VIGNETTE 2

A 59-year-old man with hepatitis C cirrhosis with a plasma Cr of 1.2 mg/dL 2 weeks previously develops ARF (plasma Cr 2.4 mg/dL [212 mcmol/L]). Vital signs are normal except for mild stable hypotension (BP 90/60 mm Hg). He appears euvolemic on examination with minimal ascites and no edema. Serum complements (both C3 and C4) are low. Renal ultrasound is normal. 24-hour urine volume is 400 mL. Laboratory tests reveal the following:

Blood chemistry:
Sodium: 124 mmol/L
Potassium: 4.8 mmol/L
Chloride: 100 mmol/L
Total CO_2: 18 mmol/L
Urea nitrogen: 18 mg/dL (urea: 6.4 mmol/L)
Creatinine: 2.4 mg/dL (212 mcmol/L)
Glucose: 100 mg/dL (5.6 mmol/L)

Urine chemistry:
Sodium: 9 mmol/L
Creatinine: 100 mg/dL (8,840 mcmol/L)
Osmolality: 450 mmol/kg
Urine protein to creatinine ratio: 600 mg/g (68 mg/mol)

Urinalysis:
Color: yellow
pH: 5.5
Specific gravity: 1.025

Protein: 2+

Blood: 1+

Glucose: negative

Ketones: 1+

Bilirubin: negative

Urobilinogen: negative

WBCs: 2/hpf

RBCs: 15/hpf

Bacteria: none

A renal biopsy is performed.

Q: The pathology report is unlikely to show which of the following?

1. Normal histology (HRS)
2. Membranoproliferative glomerulonephritis (MPGN)
3. Membranous GN
4. Focal segmental glomerulosclerosis (FSGS)
5. Cryoglobulinemia

A: This patient with hepatitis C cirrhosis has had a doubling of plasma Cr level in 2 weeks and prerenal urinary indices. The FENa is quite low (~0.2%). Although the urine protein to Cr ratio is elevated, it should be noted that 24-hour urine Cr excretion (based on random urine Cr concentration and 24-hour urine volume) is estimated to be only 400 mg (the low value is due to impaired excretion due to ARF coupled with impaired production due to muscle wasting of cirrhosis). The urine protein excretion rate can thus be calculated to be only 240 mg/day. There is absence of shock, sepsis, fluid loss, and nephrotoxic drugs. Proteinuria is <500 mg/24 hours, and urine RBCs are <50/hpf. Therefore, these data are consistent with HRS.

However, remember that HRS is a diagnosis of exclusion. Hepatitis C is known to cause vasculitis and GN, usually MPGN, often associated with cryoglobulinemia. Membranous GN and FSGS have also been reported with hepatitis C. GN can cause a prerenal picture because there is avid tubular sodium and water reabsorption. The renal biopsy in this patient showed MPGN with subendothelial immune deposits, and cryoglobulins in the blood were positive.

VIGNETTE **3**

A 70-year-old man with known BPH presents with dysuria and pyuria and is treated for UTI with ampicillin. Several days later, he develops rash and fever accompanied by nausea and vomiting. Physical examination is significant for hypertension (BP 160/90 mm Hg), low-grade fever (38°C), bibasilar rales in the lungs, bilateral 2+ lower extremity edema, and a diffuse morbilliform rash.

Blood chemistry:
Sodium: 140 mmol/L
Potassium: 5.2 mmol/L
Chloride: 110 mmol/L
Total CO_2: 20 mmol/L
Urea nitrogen: 20 mg/dL (urea: 7.1 mmol/L)
Creatinine: 2.5 mg/dL (221 mcmol/L)
Glucose: 88 mg/dL (4.9 mmol/L)

Complete blood count:
WBCs: 12,000/mm³
Hemoglobin: 14 g/dL
Hematocrit: 42%
Platelets: 200,000/mm³
Neutrophils: 57%
Lymphocytes: 15%
Monocytes: 10%
Eosinophils: 15%
Basophils: 3%

Urinalysis:
Color: yellow
pH: 5.5
Specific gravity: 1.010
Protein: 1+
Blood: negative
Glucose: negative
Ketones: negative
Bilirubin: negative
Urobilinogen: negative
WBCs: 20/hpf
RBCs: 10/hpf
Bacteria: none
Renal ultrasound: no hydronephrosis
Urine chemistry:
Sodium: 70 mmol/L
Osmolality: 300 mmol/kg
Creatinine: 50 mg/dL (4,420 mcmol/L)

Q: What is the next step in the treatment of this patient?

1. Discontinue ampicillin
2. Salt, fluid, and protein restriction
3. Corticosteroids
4. All of the above

A: The working diagnosis in this case is AIN due to ampicillin. The FENa is 2.5% and the urine is isosthenuric, which is consistent with tubulointerstitial injury, and the presence of sterile pyuria and eosinophilia supports this diagnosis. A test for urine eosinophils is sent and is also positive (although the presence of eosinophiluria is not necessary for the diagnosis). AIN is characterized by ARF resulting from immune-mediated tubulointerstitial injury, initiated by medications, infection, and other causes. The most common cause (70%) of AIN is an allergic reaction to a medication, usually a penicillin, cephalosporin, or quinolone. The initial approach to AIN involves avoidance/discontinuation of medications that lead to this condition. Limiting salt and fluid in the diet can improve edema and high BP, and limiting protein in the diet can help control azotemia. Lack of improvement with conservative treatment is the usual indication for use of steroids, though recent studies suggest that moderate doses of corticosteroids at the time of diagnosis may improve renal prognosis (Praga & González, 2010). Some believe that pathologic conformation of interstitial nephritis (plasma cell and lymphocytic infiltrates in the peritubular areas of the interstitium with interstitial edema) is necessary prior to steroid treatment. In patients who do not respond to corticosteroids within 2 to 3 weeks, treatment with cyclophosphamide (Cytoxan) or mycophenolate may be effective.

9

A 56-year-old man in a good state of health except for lumbar spinal stenosis is referred to renal clinic for evaluation of renal failure. He takes 600 mg of ibuprofen three to four times daily for back pain. He has no urinary symptoms. He denies rash or arthralgias. He denies chest pain or shortness of breath. He has mild recurrent sinusitis. He has had recent "flu-like" symptoms and has had poor oral intake for several days. Vital signs are normal; there is no orthostatic hypotension. Physical examination is normal except for a positive straight leg raise that causes severe back pain at 45° elevation. Review of his previous laboratory findings reveals that his serum Cr was 1.0 mg/dL (88.4 mcmol/L) 6 months previously.

Blood chemistry:
Sodium: 141 mmol/L
Potassium: 3.6 mmol/L
Chloride: 115 mmol/L
Total CO_2: 20 mmol/L
Urea nitrogen: 50 mg/dL (urea: 17.8 mmol/L)
Creatinine: 4.2 mg/dL (371 mcmol/L)
Glucose: 95 mg/dL (5.3 mmol/L)

Urinalysis:
Color: yellow
pH: 5.0
Specific gravity: 1.030
Protein: 1+
Blood: negative
Glucose: negative
Ketones: negative
Bili: negative
Urobilinogen: negative
WBCs: 3/hpf
RBCs: 8/hpf
Bacteria: none
Renal ultrasound: normal

The patient is treated with IV fluids. The following labs are ordered: antinuclear antibodies, urine albumin to Cr ratio, urine eosinophils, and urine electrolytes and Cr for calculation of FENa.

Q: Assuming that NSAIDs are the cause of ARF, which of the following is the most likely mechanism of ARF?

1. Renal vasoconstriction (prerenal azotemia)
2. Obstructive uropathy
3. Minimal change disease
4. Interstitial nephritis
5. AKI

A: Renal prostaglandins are vasodilatory and help to maintain renal perfusion in conditions in which there is impaired RBF due to renal vasoconstriction. NSAIDs block prostaglandin production, and in the setting of volume depletion, inability to counteract renal vasoconstriction because of stimulation of the RAS and sympathetic nervous system can result in prerenal ARF. A high urine specific gravity as well as high urine osmolality and low FENa would be expected. Prerenal azotemia can occasionally be severe enough to cause tubular damage (ischemic AKI), but the markedly concentrated urine mitigates against this possibility in this patient.

NSAIDs can rarely cause minimal change disease and resultant nephrotic syndrome. This syndrome is characterized by ARF, and renal biopsy shows fusion of the epithelial cell foot processes and various degrees of interstitial nephritis. Because, in this case, there is minimal dipstick proteinuria even though urine is very concentrated, this diagnosis is very unlikely. Use of NSAIDs has been rarely associated with papillary necrosis, which could cause ureteral obstruction, but the normal renal ultrasound excludes this possibility in this patient.

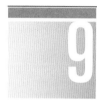

VIGNETTE **5**

A 63-year-old woman with stage 3 CKD is admitted for evaluation of shortness of breath and lethargy. She complains of cough with greenish sputum. She had a fever of 38°C at home. She denies chest pain, abdominal pain, nausea/vomiting, diarrhea, or constipation. One week ago, she was started on a 10-day course of ciprofloxacin for a UTI.

On examination, she is oriented × 3 but is very somnolent. Vital signs are as follows: pulse 115 beats/min, respiratory rate 22 breaths/min, BP 80/60 mm Hg, temperature 38°C. There are rales in the left lower lung area. The neck veins are not distended. Cardiovascular examination reveals tachycardia and a soft ejection murmur. The abdominal examination is unremarkable. There is decreased capillary refill in the toes, but temperature in the feet is normal. There is no edema.

A bolus of 1 L of physiologic saline is given, and antibiotics (azithromycin and ceftriaxone) are initiated. Urine output is initially <20 mL/h.

Blood chemistry:
Sodium: 138 mmol/L
Potassium: 5.2 mmol/L
Chloride: 110 mmol/L
Total CO_2: 20 mmol/L
Urea nitrogen: 40 mg/dL (urea: 14.3 mmol/L)
Creatinine: 2.6 mg/dL (230 mcmol/L)

Glucose: 110 mg/dL (6.1 mmol/L)

Urinalysis:
Color: yellow
pH: 5.5
Specific gravity: 1.010
Protein: 1+
Blood: negative

Glucose: negative
Ketones: negative
Bilirubin: negative
Urobilinogen: negative
WBCs: 3/hpf
RBCs: 3/hpf
Moderate "muddy brown" casts

Urine chemistry:
Sodium: 69 mmol/L
Potassium: 30 mmol/L
Chloride: 75 mmol/L
Osmolality: 310 mmol/kg
Urea nitrogen: 200 mg/dL (urea: 71 mmol/L)
Creatinine: 26 mg/dL (2,298 mcmol/L)

Renal ultrasound: increased echogenicity suggesting medical renal disease, no hydronephrosis. Chest X-ray: L lower lobe consolidation.

Q1: What is the most likely cause of ARF in this patient?

1. Acute tubular injury
2. Prerenal failure from renal hypoperfusion
3. Peri-infectious AGN
4. Drug-induced interstitial nephritis

A1: The FENa is 5% and the FEurea is 50%, the urine specific gravity is 1.010, the urine/plasma osmolality is <1.2, and there are pigmented ("muddy brown") casts in the urine. All of these findings are indicative of acute tubular injury (AKI). Although the patient initially may have had prerenal failure due to hypotension and sepsis leading to renal vasoconstriction, it is clear that this has evolved to tubular injury. There is minimal proteinuria and no hematuria to suggest GN. There is no pyuria to suggest interstitial nephritis.

Q2: Which of the following mechanisms are likely to play a role in the causation of renal tubular injury in this patient?

1. Impaired autoregulation
2. Endotoxemia
3. Endothelial cell injury
4. Tubular obstruction
5. All of the above

A2: The etiology of renal tubular injury in sepsis is complex and poorly understood. In most but not all cases, there is hypoperfusion of the kidneys. Renal autoregulation is impaired, leading to a fall in glomerular and tubular blood flow. Moreover, patients with underlying CKD already have impaired renal autoregulation; such kidneys tend to be maximally vasodilated and do not have the capacity to vasodilate any further in response to a decrease in perfusion pressure. Systemic endotoxemia increases production of nitric oxide that causes systemic vasodilation; however, endothelial injury from endotoxemia will inhibit renal endothelial nitric oxide production, thus furthering impairing renal microperfusion and worsening renal hypoxia and injury. If injury is severe, tubular obstruction may occur because of sloughing of endothelial cells.

9

An 80-year-old man with BPH treated with tamsulosin (Flomax) presents for evaluation of acute urinary retention for 2 days. He has had some hematuria for a few weeks. He has some suprapubic abdominal pain but no nausea, vomiting, diarrhea, constipation, or fever. His urologist has suggested that he might need a TURP. His last PSA 6 months ago was 1.0 ng/mL (normal). Abdominal examination revealed suprapubic dullness to palpation and tenderness, and rectal examination revealed a highly enlarged prostate.

Blood chemistry:
Sodium: 138 mmol/L
Potassium: 4.5 mmol/L
Chloride: 112 mmol/L
Total CO_2: 22 mmol/L
Urea nitrogen: 90 mg/dL (urea: 32 mmol/L)
Creatinine, 5.0 mg/dL (442 mcmol/L)
Total calcium: 9 mg/dL (2.25 mmol/L)
Inorganic phosphorus: 5 mg/dL (1.6 mmol/L)

Compete blood count:
WBCs: 5,000/mm^3
Hemoglobin: 11 g/dL (110 g/L)
Hematocrit: 36% (110 g/L)
Platelets: 200,000/mm^3
Renal ultrasound: bilateral hydronephrosis, no stones, preserved renal cortical thickness.
A Foley catheter was inserted, and 500 mL of urine was drained from the bladder.

Urinalysis:
Color: yellow
pH: 5.5
Specific gravity: 1.012
Protein: 2+
Blood: 1+
Glucose: negative
Ketones: 1+
Bilirubin: negative
Urobilinogen: negative
WBCs: 3/hpf
RBCs: 6/hpf
Bacteria: none
Moderate calcium oxalate crystals: present

The patient is given IV fluids. Two days later, he develops polyuria, producing in excess of 3 L of urine per day.

Q: Which of the following is not the cause of the postobstructive diuresis?

1. Nephrogenic diabetes insipidus
2. Osmotic diuresis
3. Expanded extracellular volume
4. Hypercalciuria

A: This patient has acute urinary retention due to BPH. Acute urinary retention is suggested by the clinical presentation and the presence of 500 mL of urine in the bladder. The plan is for the Foley catheter to be kept in place for 2 weeks while the patient is maintained on the alpha blocker. If a voiding trial 2 weeks later demonstrates a low postvoid residual urine volume, the patient will continue medical management with the alpha blocker. Otherwise, a TURP is planned.

Two to 10 days after bladder decompression, polyuria (defined as >2.5 L of urine per day) may ensue. In this event, urinary retention may have resulted in obstruction of urinary flow and damage to renal parenchyma, leading to impaired urinary concentrating ability with decreased response to ADH (nephrogenic diabetes insipidus). If there is substantial retention of solutes during the period of urinary obstruction, an osmotic diuresis may also be contributing to polyuria. Expansion of the extracellular space with IV fluids is a third reason for the polyuria. The presence of calcium oxalate crystals is a nonspecific finding in this patient and does not necessarily denote hypercalciuria. Hypercalcemia can cause nephrogenic diabetes insipidus and polyuria but was not present in this case.

9

A 55-year-old previously healthy woman presents for evaluation of right-sided flank pain that travels into the right groin. She also has some pain and burning with urination as well as pinkish urine. She denies nausea, vomiting, diarrhea, constipation, fever, or chills. The pain gets better if she is mobile and seems to worsen with rest. She takes only occasional acetaminophen. She has no history of kidney stones. Physical examination reveals her to be in acute distress with difficulty lying in bed. She had low-grade fever, right flank tenderness, suprapubic tenderness, and abdominal guarding without rebound.

Blood chemistry:
Sodium: 140 mmol/L
Potassium: 4.0 mmol/L
Chloride: 110 mmol/L
Total CO_2: 26 mmol/L
Urea nitrogen: 20 mg/dL (urea: 7.1 mmol/L)
Creatinine: 2.0 mg/dL (177 mcmol/L)
Glucose: 120 mg/dL (6.7 mmol/L)

Total calcium: 10 mg/dL (2.5 mmol/L)
Albumin: 4.0 g/dL (40 g/L)
Uric acid: 3 mg/dL (178 mcmol/L)

Complete blood count:
WBCs: 12,000/mm³
Hemoglobin: 14 g/dL (140 g/L)
Hematocrit: 41%
Platelets: 200,000/mm³

Urinalysis:
Color: red
pH: 5.0
Specific gravity: 1.024
Protein: 1+
Blood: 4+
Glucose: negative
Ketones: 1+
Bilirubin: negative

Urobilinogen: negative
Leukocyte esterase: positive
Nitrite: positive
WBCs: 50/hpf
RBCs: 50/hpf
Bacteria: many
Calcium oxalate crystals:
    present

CT abdomen/pelvis without contrast, no hydronephrosis; 4-mm
    stone right midureter

Q: Which of the following is not a necessary intervention in this patient's first episode of renal colic?

1. IV fluids
2. Analgesia
3. Treat UTI
4. 24-hour urine studies

A: The mainstay of treatment for renal colic is analgesia, treatment of infection, and IV fluid administration. If UTI does not
improve promptly, she may require urgent stone removal. Otherwise, a 4-mm stone is likely to spontaneously pass into the bladder. 24-hour urine studies are not needed for the first episode of
kidney stones; this is because only about 50% of patients with a
first episode of kidney stone will have a recurrence. In any event,
they should not be performed during an acute stone episode but
rather in the outpatient setting on the patient's standard diet and
medication regimen.

References

Backer RJ, Pusey CD. The changing profile of acute tubulointerstitial nephritis. *Nephrol Dial Transplant.* 19:8–11, 2004.

Bellomo R, Ronco C, Kellum JA, et al; Acute Dialysis Quality Initiative Workgroup. Acute renal failure—definition, outcome measures, animal models, fluid therapy and information technology needs: the Second International Consensus Conference of the Acute Dialysis Quality Initiative (ADQI) Group. *Crit Care.* 8(4):R204–R212, 2004.

Better OS, Arieff AI, Massry SG, et al. Studies on renal function after relief of complete unilateral ureteral obstruction of three months' duration in man. *Am J Med.* 54(2):234–240, 1973.

Blantz RC. Pathophysiology of pre-renal azotemia. *Kidney Int.* 53:512–523, 1998.

Canfield PE, Geerdes AM, Molitoris BA. Effect of reversible ATP depletion on tight-junction integrity in LLC-PK1 cells. *Am J Physiol.* 261:F1038–F1045, 1991.

Druml W. Nutritional management of acute renal failure. *Am J Kidney Dis.* 37:S89–S94, 2001.

Haase M, Bellomo R, Deverajan P, et al. Accuracy of neutrophil gelatinase-associated lipocalin (NGAL) in diagnosis and prognosis of acute kidney injury: a systematic review and meta-analysis. *Am J Kidney Dis.* 54:1012–1024, 2009.

Hall IE, Coca SG, Perazella MA, et al. Risk of poor outcomes with novel and traditional biomarkers at clinical AKI diagnosis. *Clin J Am Soc Nephrol.* 6:2740–2749, 2011.

Iwatsuki S, Popovtzer MM, Corman JL, et al. Recovery from "hepatorenal syndrome" after orthotopic liver transplantation. *N Engl J Med.* 289:1155–1159, 1973.

Kerr WS Jr. Effect of complete ureteral obstruction for one week on kidney function. *J Appl Physiol.* 6:762–772, 1954.

Kon V, Yared A, Ichikawa I. Role of renal sympathetic nerves in mediating hypoperfusion of renal cortical microcirculation in experimental congestive heart failure and acute extracellular fluid volume depletion. *J Clin Invest.* 76:1913–1920, 1985.

Mehta RL, Kellum JA, Shah SV, et al; Acute Kidney Injury Network. Acute Kidney Injury Network: report of an initiative to improve outcomes in acute kidney injury. *Crit Care.* 11(2):R31, 2007.

Mehta RL, McDonald B, Gabbai FB, et al. A randomized clinical trial of continuous versus intermittent dialysis for acute renal failure. *Kidney Int.* 60:1154–1163, 2001.

Molitoris BA, Sutton TA. Endothelial injury and dysfunction during ischemic acute renal failure. *Kidney Int.* 66:496–499, 2004.

Muriithi AK, Nasr SH, Leung N. Utility of urine eosinophils in the diagnosis of acute interstitial nephritis. *Clin J Am Soc Nephrol.* 8(11):1857–1862, 2013.

Praga M, González E. Acute interstitial nephritis. *Kidney Int.* 77(11):956–961, 2010.

Ruiz-del-Arbol L, Monescillo A, Arocena C, et al. Circulatory function and hepatorenal syndrome in cirrhosis. *Hepatology.* 42:439–447, 2005.

Schrier RW, Wang W. Acute renal failure and sepsis. *N Engl J Med.* 351:159–169, 2004.

Ueda N, Kaushal GP, Shah SV. Apoptotic mechanisms in acute renal failure. *Am J Med.* 108:403–415, 2000.

Ye J, Tsukamoto T, Sun A, et al. A role for intracellular calcium in tight junction reassembly after ATP depletion-repletion. *Am J Physiol.* 277:F524–F532, 1999.

Zarich S, Fang LS, Diamond JR. Fractional excretion of sodium. Exceptions to its diagnostic value. *Arch Intern Med.* 145:108–112, 1985.

10 Glomerulonephritis

DEFINITIONS

- Glomerular diseases can be divided into diseases that, in their more severe forms, are characterized by massive proteinuria without hematuria (nephrotic syndrome) or diseases that are characterized by an "active" urine sediment (hematuria and/or pyuria) with cellular (red and/or white cell) casts and moderate-to-severe proteinuria (nephritic syndrome). Nephrotic syndrome will be discussed in Chapter 11. This chapter discusses about the nephritic syndromes.

- **Acute glomerulonephritis (AGN)** is most commonly postinfectious in etiology. Classically, it occurs most commonly after streptococcal infection (either pharyngitis or cellulitis). Such patients typically present with acute renal failure (rapidly increasing azotemia over a period of days, often with oliguria), hypertension, and edema; the urinalysis shows red blood cell (RBC) casts and proteinuria. In more recent years, AGN of a "peri-infectious" nature associated with staphylococcal infection (especially endocarditis and bone infection) has become more common than classic poststreptococcal glomerulonephritis (GN) (Nadasdy & Hebert, 2011; Nasr & D'Agati, 2011).

- **Rapidly progressive glomerulonephritis (RPGN)** refers to nephritic syndromes in which there is a rapid decline in kidney function over a period of weeks to months. Pathologically, these diseases are characterized by glomerular epithelial cell proliferation ("crescents"), which are caused by leakage of fibrin and inflammatory mediators into Bowman capsule through the injured glomerular basement membrane (GBM). Thus, the term "crescentic glomerulonephritis" is also often used. Any type of nephritis can present as RPGN, although this presentation is more common with some diseases (such as anti-GBM disease). Some patients with RPGN have associated pulmonary involvement, usually presenting as hemoptysis ("renal-pulmonary syndrome").

- **Chronic glomerulonephritis (CGN)** refers to nephritic syndromes in which there is usually a slow decline in kidney function over a period of months to years. In many patients, the initial immune-based injury has resolved, the urine sediment is no longer "active" (no or minimal hematuria, no cellular casts), and only manifestations of chronic kidney disease (CKD) (e.g., hypertension and proteinuria) are evident (see Chapter 12).

CASE STUDY

A 23-year-old female with no past medical history presents for evaluation of oral ulcers and rash that began a month ago. Intermittent fever started 2 weeks ago. She recently has noted ulcers on her lips and lip swelling. A dermatologist gave her a topical corticosteroid, which resulted in some relief. She denies photosensitivity, malar rash, or arthralgias. She also denies neurologic symptoms, chest pain, shortness of breath, or abdominal pain. Menstruation is regular. She is an occasional drinker and smoker. She has been sexually active with one sexual partner. On physical examination, the vital signs are normal. There are oral ulcers, weeping ulcers of the lips, and raised red circular lesions on the forearms and palms without nail involvement. The remainder of the examination is unremarkable.

Blood chemistry:
Sodium: 138 mmol/L
Potassium: 3.3 mmol/L
Chloride: 113 mmol/L
Total CO_2: 18 mmol/L
Urea nitrogen: 26 mg/dL
(urea: 9.3 mmol/L)
Creatinine: 1.6 mg/dL
(142 mcmol/L) (previous creatinine: 0.8 mg/dL)
Liver function tests: normal
Total calcium: 7.6 mg/dL
(1.9 mmol/L)
Inorganic phosphorus:
2.7 mg/dL (0.87 mmol/L)
Magnesium: 2.0 mg/dL
(0.82 mmol/L)
Prothrombin time: 12.1 seconds (international normalized ratio: 0.9)
Partial thromboplastin time: 30.8 seconds

Complete blood count:
WBCs: 3,200/mm^3
Hemoglobin: 11.1 g/dL (111 g/L)
Hematocrit: 32%
Platelets: 55,000/mm^3

Urinalysis:
Specific gravity: 1.017
pH: 6.5
Protein: 300 mg/dL
RBCs : 16/hpf
WBCs: 4/hpf
No bacteria
Dysmorphic RBCs
RBC casts seen

Urine albumin to creatinine ratio (UACR): 1,346 mg/g (152 mg/mmol)
Urine protein to creatinine ratio (UPCR): 1,975 mg/g (223 mg/mmol)

Question 10.1.1: The patient has acute kidney injury (AKI) with nephritic urine, that is, dysmorphic RBCs and RBC casts. The etiology of AKI is thus one of the glomerulonephritides. The first step is to take a detailed but directed history to hone in on the differential diagnosis. What is the differential of GN?

■ In addition to characterizing glomerulonephritides into the three categories of AGN, RPGN, and CGN (see above), they can also be divided into the three types based on etiology. Type I is characterized by the presence of autoantibodies directed against the GBM, type II is characterized by immune complex deposition in the

TABLE 10.1	Causes of Glomerulonephritis	
Anti–glomerular Basement Membrane (Anti-GBM) Disease	**Immune Complex Disease**	**Pauci-immune Disease (ANCA-Associated)**
Goodpasture syndrome Renal-limited anti-GBM nephritis (i.e., no pulmonary symptoms or signs)	Lupus nephritis IgA nephropathy Postinfectious GN Peri-infectious GN Membranoproliferative GN Cryoglobulinemia	Granulomatous polyangiitis (Wegener granulomatosis) Other vasculitides (microscopic polyarteritis, Churg-Strauss disease)

ANCA, antineutrophil cytoplasmic antibody; GN, glomerulonephritis; IgA, immunoglobulin A.

glomerulus, and type III is characterized by a paucity of immune complexes (hence, pauci-immune) (Table 10.1).

Question 10.1.2: What questions should you ask in an effort to get a detailed history?

GN should be evaluated by asking directed questions and a focused examination.

- History—dark (cola-colored) urine, decreased urine output, low-grade fever, malaise, edema (note these findings are most typical of AGN, may or may not be present in RPGN, and are generally absent in CGN).
- Goodpasture—hemoptysis
- Immune complex disease—
  - Lupus—malar rash, discoid lesions, oral ulcers, photosensitivity, confusion, seizures, serositis, arthritis, Raynaud phenomenon
  - IgA nephropathy—gross hematuria; if associated with vasculitis, that is, Henoch-Schönlein: nausea, vomiting, abdominal pain, palpable purpura
  - Infection-associated GN—pharyngitis (*Streptococcus*), visceral abscess or skin/foot infection (typically *Staphylococcus*), hepatitis exposure, travel history, valve replacement, intravenous (IV) drug abuse
  - MPGN—fatigue; pallor; drusen on funduscopic examination and fat atrophy usually affecting the upper limbs, trunk, and face (in dense deposit disease [DDD]); hypertension
  - Cryoglobulinemia—acrocyanosis, retinal hemorrhage, Raynaud syndrome with digital ulceration, livedo reticularis, purpura, joint involvement (usually arthralgias in the proximal interphalangeal [PIP] joints, metacarpophalangeal [MCP]

joints, knees, and ankles), fatigue, myalgias, peripheral neuropathy and rash (cutaneous vasculitis)
■ Pauci-immune GN—sinusitis, hemoptysis, pulmonary infiltrates,
levamisole-contaminated cocaine use

Question 10.1.3: What laboratory studies should you order?

EVALUATION OF GN

■ GN should be suspected in any patient with combined hematuria
and proteinuria.
■ The sine qua non for GN is the presence of RBC casts (often present even when not detected by the clinical laboratory—physician
should perform own urinalysis!).
■ Workup should include measurement of antinuclear antibodies
(ANAs), complements (C3, C4), hepatitis panel (B and C), and antineutrophil cytoplasmic antibodies (ANCAs). If RPGN, especially
if pulmonary hemorrhage, obtain anti-GBM antibodies. Decreased
serum C3 and C4 suggests classic (immune complex) complement
activation (Hebert et al., 1991), whereas decreased serum C3 with
normal C4 suggests alternate pathway activation. Low C4 with
normal C3 should prompt one to exclude cryoglobulinemia (C4 is
cryoprecipitable). Complement pattern can thus sometimes suggest the diagnosis (Table 10.2).

CASE STUDY 10.1 CONTINUED

The following laboratory results are obtained:

C3: 33 mg/dL (low)   ANA: 1:640
C4: 3 mg/dL (low)   Anti-DNA antibodies detected
Rheumatoid factor: negative   Anti-dsDNA antibodies: 1:320
C-ANCA: negative   Anti-Smith antibodies:
P-ANCA: indeterminate   202 AU/mL
Hepatitis panel: negative

TABLE 10.2 Complement Patterns in Glomerulonephritis

Disease	Complement Pattern
Lupus nephritis	Low C3 and C4
Peri-infectious (endocarditis, osteomyelitis, visceral abscess)	Low C3 and C4
Postinfectious (poststreptococcal)	Low C3; low (slight) or normal C4
Membranoproliferative glomerulonephritis	Low C3; normal C4
Cryoglobulinemia	Low or normal C3, low C4 (often very low)

Question 10.1.4: At what dilution is an ANA titer highly suggestive of active lupus?

An ANA titer of at least 1:160 is consistent with active systemic lupus erythematosus.

Question 10.1.5: What is the most likely diagnosis and how should you confirm it?

Lupus nephritis is the most likely diagnosis, but it should be confirmed with a kidney biopsy.

Question 10.1.6: What are the typical findings on kidney biopsy for the nephritic syndromes?

Typical kidney biopsy findings are shown in Table 10.3.

TABLE 10.3 Pathologic Patterns in Glomerulonephritis

Glomerulonephritis	Light Microscopy	Immunofluorescence	Electron Microscopy
Goodpasture (and renal-limited anti-GBM disease)	Crescents	Linear IgG in GBM	Pauci-immune
Systemic lupus erythematosus	Wire loops (subendothelial immune deposits) Hematoxylin bodies (rare but pathognomonic) Endocapillary proliferation	"Full house": IgG 90% IgA 60%–70% IgM 80% C3 C1q	Electron-dense deposits: Subendothelial Subepithelial (mainly in membranous lupus) Endothelial cell tubuloreticular inclusions
Drug-induced lupus May have P-ANCA, anti-lactoferrin, anti-elastase, anti-dsDNA	Necrotizing GN	Little or no immune complex deposits	Little or no immune complex deposits
Infection-related GN	Hypercellular "Exudative" (neutrophils, macrophages, mesangial and endothelial cells) Endocapillary proliferation	Granular IgG, IgM, C3; C1q negative (classic postinfectious GN) Granular IgA, C3 (peri-infectious, e.g., staphylococcal GN)	Subepithelial humps Acute phase (subepithelial, intramembranous, subendothelial and mesangial deposits)

TABLE 10.3	Pathologic Patterns in Glomerulonephritis (*continued*)		
C3 glomerulopathies	Four types possible: Mesangioproliferative MPGN Endocapillary Crescentic	Dense deposit disease—band-like C3 C3 GN—granular C3 (Ig absent or very low)	Dense deposit disease—dense deposits in basement membrane C3 GN—subendothelial, mesangial, sometimes subepithelial deposits
MPGN	Mesangiocapillary Double contours Endocapillary proliferation Lobulation Mesangial interposition	Idiopathic—C3, IgG, IgM—IgA is less frequent C1q deposition may occur Hepatitis C—IgM, C3 Monoclonal gammopathy—light chain restriction (kappa or lambda, not both) Lupus—"full house"	Subendothelial deposits Mesangial deposits Mesangial interposition New basement membrane formation Podocyte effacement
Granulomatous polyangiitis (Wegener granulomatosis) Microscopic polyangiitis Churg-Strauss vasculitis	Necrotizing Granulomas (may not be seen) Crescentic	Pauci-immune	Fibrin
IgA nephropathy	Mesangial proliferative Focal proliferative Can be crescentic Endocapillary proliferation can occur	IgA (also IgG and less commonly IgM mesangial) deposits which may also involve glomerular capillary loops C3 deposits	Paramesangial deposits May have subendothelial, subepithelial, or intramembranous deposits
Thrombotic microangiopathy	Fibrin thrombi Platelet plugs Double contour (split appearance of basement membrane) (if chronic)	No immune complex deposits	Fibrin tactoids Endothelial cell swelling Expansion of lamina rara interna New basement membrane formation

ANCA, antineutrophil cytoplasmic antibody; dsDNA, double-stranded DNA; GBM, glomerular basement membrane; GN, glomerulonephritis; IgG, immunoglobulin G; MPGN, membranoproliferative glomerulonephritis.

CASE STUDY 10.1 CONTINUED

Renal biopsy showed the following:

Light microscopy: Majority of glomeruli demonstrated inflammation, endocapillary proliferation, and prominent immune complexes characterized by wire loops

Immunofluorescence (IF) microscopy: IgA 3+, IgG 3+, IgM 1+, C3 3+, C1q 3+, kappa 2+, lambda 2+ in glomeruli; C1q 1+ in interstitium

Electron microscopy: Electron-dense granular deposits in the subendothelial region in capillary loops with abundant mesangial deposits; tubuloreticular inclusions in endoplasmic reticulum

Question 10.1.7: What is the classification of LN in this patient?

CASE STUDY 10.1 CONCLUDED

Because >50% of glomeruli demonstrate immune complexes and proliferative changes, this patient has Class IV LN (see section on Lupus Nephritis below).

Question 10.1.8: What is the treatment of LN in this patient?

The Aspreva Lupus Management Study (ALMS) is one of the largest trials ever conducted in LN. Therefore, in the United States, the ALMS protocol is currently used.

- ALMS protocol:
  - Induction is for 6 months.
  - Start with prednisone 60 mg and taper.
  - Start mycophenolate mofetil (MMF) 0.5 g BID for 1 week, then 1 g BID for 1 week, then 1.5 g BID thereafter as tolerated.
  - Maintenance is with MMF. If intolerant of MMF, azathioprine and/or calcineurin inhibitors can be used. Rituximab can be used for relapse.

Question 10.1.9: What is the definition of remission?

Remission is defined as urine RBC <5/hpf. Proteinuria can take up to 6 months to normalize; therefore, it is not used to determine whether a patient is in remission.

GOODPASTURE SYNDROME

Goodpasture syndrome is characterized by (1) proliferative crescentic GN, (2) pulmonary hemorrhage, and (3) anti-GBM antibodies. A renal-limited anti-GBM nephritis can also occur.

Pathogenesis

Circulating autoantibodies directed against an antigen (collagen IV epitope) intrinsic to the GBM and alveolar basement membrane result in tissue injury (Wieslander et al., 1984). It is possible that pulmonary manifestations occur in the setting of preexisting lung injury, whereas patients without previous lung injury present with renal-limited disease.

Laboratory Findings

- Hematuria with RBC casts
- Proteinuria
- Anti-GBM antibodies
- Chest X-ray—infiltrates corresponding to hemorrhage
- Hypoxemia if severe

Pathology

- Light microscopy
  - Focal segmental endocapillary and extracapillary (crescents) proliferation (Fig. 10.1)
  - Diffuse crescentic inflammation is the most common.
  - There may be tubulointerstitial nephritis.
- Immunofluorescence
  - Intense, linear stain for IgG and C3 involving the GBM and sometimes also tubular basement membrane (Fig. 10.2)
- Electron microscopy
  - No electron-dense deposits ("pauci-immune")
  - Widening of the subendothelial space with fibrin
  - Gaps in the GBM and Bowman capsule

Treatment

Plasmapheresis removes the circulating anti-GBM antibodies, whereas immunosuppressive therapy prevents new antibody formation and controls the inflammatory process. These treatments are very effective at treating pulmonary hemorrhage, but the kidneys may be less responsive.

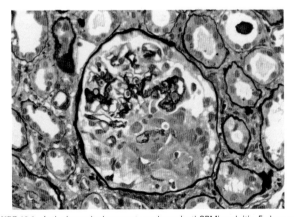

FIGURE 10.1. Anti–glomerular basement membrane (anti-GBM) nephritis. Early segmental fibrinoid necrosis with early cellular crescent formation. This light microscopic finding is that of a pauci-immune necrotizing glomerulonephritis (GN), with a specific diagnosis of anti-GBM antibody-mediated GN made by immunofluorescence (Jones silver stain; original magnification ×400). (Originally published in *Am J Kidney Dis*. 1998;32(3):E1. Copyright by The National Kidney Foundation, with permission.)

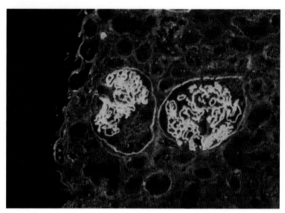

FIGURE 10.2. Anti-glomerular basement membrane (GBM) nephritis. Linear staining of glomerular basement membranes with antibody to immunoglobulin G (IgG) and crescent formation in the glomerulus on the left, diagnostic findings of anti-GBM antibody-mediated glomerulonephritis (immunofluorescence with anti-IgG; original magnification ×200). (Originally published in *Am J Kidney Dis*. 1998;32(3):E1. Copyright by The National Kidney Foundation, with permission.)

LUPUS NEPHRITIS

Systemic lupus erythematosus (SLE) is characterized by skin rash, oral ulcers, photosensitivity, myalgias, neurologic sequelae, arthritis, serositis, and renal involvement, the latter of which may undergo remissions and exacerbations both spontaneously and in response to treatment. Renal prognosis correlates with type and degree of glomerular involvement. Hence, pathologic classification guides treatment and predicts prognosis.

Pathogenesis
Circulating antibodies (including anti-DNA antibodies) formed to an unknown (possibly viral) antigen deposit in the kidney in locations dependent on the size and charge of the antigen and antibody (Hahn, 1998; Isenberg & Collins, 1985). Activation of complement and other inflammatory mechanisms leads to tissue injury.

Laboratory Evaluation
- ANA panel (including anti–double-stranded DNA [dsDNA] and other autoantibodies)
- Complements (C3, C4), CH50 (total hemolytic complement)—These decrease with disease exacerbation and normalize with disease improvement.
- Hence, complements, ANA, anti-dsDNA, and urinalysis (hematuria, proteinuria) can be used to monitor disease progress. In selected cases, rebiopsy is needed.

Pathology

- Light microscopy reveals focal (<50% of glomeruli involved) or diffuse (>50% of glomeruli involved, often associated with crescents) involvement. Karyorrhexis (destructive fragmentation of the nucleus of dying cells) and "wire loop" thickening of basement membranes (due to immune deposits) are seen in severe disease. The World Health Organization classification used for LN classification modified by the International Society of Nephrology/Renal Pathology Society (2003) is currently used.
- Class I—Minimal mesangial involvement
- Class II—Mesangial proliferative LN
  - Classes I and II are associated with a good prognosis and no therapy is generally necessary, although nephrotic syndrome is present, treat like minimal change disease (see below).
- Class III—Focal proliferative LN (<50% of glomeruli involved)
  - There is no consensus as to how class III should be treated. Patients with only mild or moderate proliferative lesions involving a few glomeruli have a good prognosis and may respond to a short course of high-dose corticosteroids. Severe lesions with necrotizing features and crescents will require vigorous therapy (see class IV).
- Class IV—Diffuse proliferative LN (>50% of glomeruli involved, often associated with crescents) (Fig. 10.3)
  - Requires aggressive treatment. Cyclophosphamide and steroids are standard treatment, though in some populations (African Americans, Asians), MMF can be substituted for

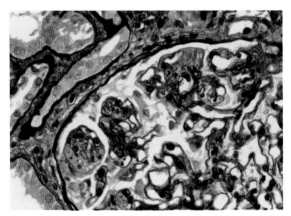

FIGURE 10.3. Lupus nephritis. Diffuse proliferative lupus nephritis (World Health Organization class IV). There is segmental glomerular basement membrane splitting with eosinophilic, large, sausage-shaped subendothelial deposits. In other areas, holes in the basement membrane are seen, representing subepithelial deposits (deposits do not take up the silver stain). Segmental endocapillary proliferation and mesangial proliferation are also present (Jones' silver stain; original magnification ×600). (Originally published in *Am J Kidney Dis*. 1998;31(6):E1. Copyright by The National Kidney Foundation, with permission.)

cyclophosphamide. Many clinicians prefer to use MMF at the outset (see ALMS protocol above). Azathioprine, cyclosporine, and rituximab (anti-CD20) are also used.

- Class V—Membranous nephropathy
  - May be indolent or progressive
  - For patients with a good prognosis (subnephrotic proteinuria, preserved glomerular filtration rate [GFR]), cyclosporine plus corticosteroids may be appropriate. For patients with a poor prognosis (African Americans with nephrotic syndrome), treatment as for class IV is appropriate.
- Class VI—Advanced sclerosing LN
  - Greater than 90% of glomeruli are sclerosed. Immunosuppressive therapy is not indicated.
- Immunofluorescence microscopy—Immune deposits to IgG, IgM, IgA, C3, and C1q in all compartments ("full house").
- Electron microscopy—Electron-dense granular deposits, tubuloreticular inclusions (intracytoplasmic tubular branching structures in cisternae of endoplasmic reticulum). Location of deposits in subendothelial location in classes III and IV (Fig. 10.4) and in subepithelial location in class V; in addition, mesangial deposits are virtually universal.

Treatment

Treatment of LN is based on pathology (see above). In addition to or instead of immune complex disease, some patients with SLE will have renal findings of antiphospholipid syndrome (renal microthrombi)

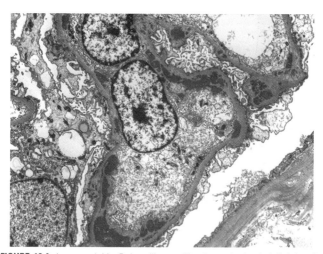

FIGURE 10.4. Lupus nephritis. Endocapillary proliferation and subendothelial deposits characteristic of proliferative lupus nephritis are illustrated in this electron micrograph. Occasional small subepithelial, as well as mesangial, deposits are also present. The capillary loops are segmentally occluded by proliferating endothelial and mesangial cells (transmission electron micrograph; original magnification ×8,000). (Originally published in *Am J Kidney Dis.* 1998;31(6): E1. Copyright by The National Kidney Foundation, with permission.)

and are not treated with immunosuppressives but instead anticoagulation; if severe, plasmapheresis may be indicated.

IGA NEPHROPATHY

IgA nephropathy (nephritis) is characterized by IgA deposition in the mesangium with mesangial proliferation. Clinical features can range from asymptomatic hematuria to RPGN. Prognosis is usually good, but patients with abnormal renal function, severe proteinuria, or hypertension are at risk of renal failure. Though usually an idiopathic disease, it can be secondary to rheumatologic disease (especially ankylosing spondylitis) or liver disease (caused by impaired clearance of IgA immune complexes from the portal circulation).

Pathogenesis

It is postulated that altered mucosal immunity in the setting of exposure to an environmental antigen leads to increased IgA synthesis. If there is abnormal galactosylation of the IgA, there will be decreased clearance by the liver, autoantibody formation to IgA1, and mesangial deposition (Mestecky et al., 1993).

Laboratory Evaluation

- Increased serum IgA in ~50% of cases, but this is not specific
- Normal complements
- Urinalysis with microscopic hematuria ± proteinuria
- Renal biopsy necessary for diagnosis

Pathology

- Light microscopy
  - Nonspecific
  - Mesangioproliferative or proliferative GN (Fig. 10.5)
  - Few have crescents and few may have sclerosed glomeruli.

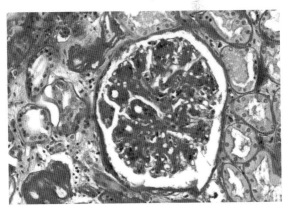

FIGURE 10.5. IgA nephritis. Moderate mesangial expansion with increased matrix and cells are noted (periodic acid-Schiff; original magnification ×200). IgA, immunoglobulin A. (Originally published in *Am J Kidney Dis.* 1998;31(4):E1. Copyright by The National Kidney Foundation, with permission.)

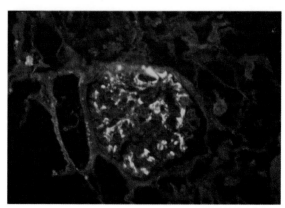

FIGURE 10.6. IgA nephritis. The diagnosis of IgA nephritis depends on the finding of me-sangial IgA deposits on immunofluorescence microscopy. Staining may also be present at lesser intensity for IgG and IgM. C3 is also often present and may be equal in intensity to IgA staining (anti-IgA immunofluorescence, original magnification ×200). IgA, immu-noglobulin A. (Originally published in *Am J Kidney Dis*. 1998;31(4):E1. Copyright by The National Kidney Foundation, with permission.)

- Immunofluorescence
  - IgA and C3 predominantly in the mesangium (Fig. 10.6)
- Electron microscopy
  - Mesangial electron-dense deposits
  - Minority have capillary wall deposits

Treatment

Blood pressure should be treated with angiotensin-converting en-zyme (ACE) inhibitors or angiotensin receptor blockers (ARBs). Immunosuppressives (steroids, cyclophosphamide, azathioprine, mycophenolate) are reserved for progressive active disease and in patients who have persistent proteinuria (>1 g/g creatinine) despite ACE or ARB therapy. There is no evidence for benefit of fish oil, al-though it is frequently used. No treatment is indicated for CKD and extensive fibrosis or glomerulosclerosis.

POST- (AND PERI-) INFECTIOUS GN

Postinfectious GN is usually caused by gram-positive cocci (*Strepto-coccus* and *Staphylococcus*) or other bacteria. It occurs primarily in children aged 2 to 6 years but may occur in adults. Some strains of streptococci are more nephritogenic. Patients present with protein-uria and hematuria and frequently hypertension. There is typically a latency period of a week or so between infection and renal manifesta-tions. Patients may also present with congestive heart failure, edema, or encephalopathy. Resolution usually occurs in 1 to 2 weeks, though the prognosis is more guarded in adults. Recently, a peri-infectious GN predominantly in diabetic patients with staphylococcal infection (usually endocarditis or osteomyelitis) has been described.

Pathogenesis

Bacterial antigens can cross-react with glomerular antigens. Hence, an autoimmune response because of antigen mimicry (Goroncy-Bermes et al., 1987) or an immune complex response is postulated (Michael et al., 1966).

Laboratory Evaluation

- Urinalysis (hematuria, dysmorphic RBCs, RBC casts, proteinuria)
- Decreased GFR
- UPCR: only about 5% are nephrotic
- Low fractional excretion of sodium
- Throat/skin/abscess culture
- Antistreptolysin (ASO) titer usually positive, though if negative, other antibodies (e.g., antihyaluronidase, antistreptokinase, anti-DNase B) should be checked and may be positive.
- Complements: low C3 with normal C4 and low CH50 is typical (these resolve with resolution of disease)

Pathology

- Light microscopy
  - Global hypercellularity, occasional crescents, interstitial edema, and cellular (neutrophil) infiltration
- Immunofluorescence
  - Glomerular immune complex deposits in a subepithelial location ("humps").
  - Classically IgG and C3; predominantly IgA and C3 with "IgA-dominant" glomerulonephritis associated with staphylococcal infection (Fig. 10.7)
- Electron microscopy
  - Subepithelial hump-like dense deposits (Fig. 10.8)

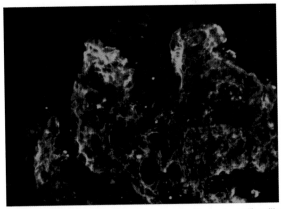

FIGURE 10.7. Postinfectious glomerulonephritis. Irregular ("lumpy-bumpy") capillary loop deposits typically staining for immunoglobulin G (IgG) (seen here) and C3 (immunofluorescence with anti-IgG; original magnification ×400). (Originally published in *Am J Kidney Dis.* 1998;31(5):E1. Copyright by The National Kidney Foundation, with permission.)

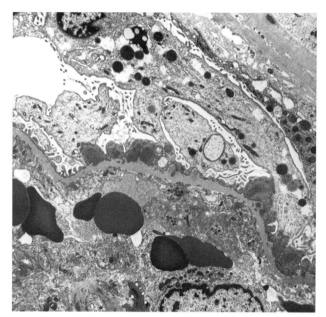

FIGURE 10.8. Postinfectious glomerulonephritis. Large, subepithelial, hump-like scattered deposits are irregularly spaced and sit on top of the basement membrane with little, if any, basement membrane reaction (transmission electron micrograph; original magnification ×6,800). (Originally published in *Am J Kidney Dis.* 1998;31(5):E1. Copyright by The National Kidney Foundation, with permission.)

Treatment

- Treat the infection.
- Supportive (treat volume overload, hypertension, hyperkalemia)
- Steroids are controversial. Some clinicians utilize high-dose steroids if crescents are present.
- Hemodialysis may be necessary.

MEMBRANOPROLIFERATIVE GLOMERULONEPHRITIS

MPGN is also known as mesangiocapillary GN. It is a pathologic description and has multiple causes. It is characterized on pathology by double-contoured GBMs with mesangial interposition and new basement membrane formation. Older classifications based on light and electron microscopic findings have been replaced by a classification based on IF findings.

Idiopathic MPGN is primarily a disease of children. In adults in the United States, many cases are due to hepatitis C. It may present with nephrotic or nephritic syndrome or both. Primary MPGN is idiopathic. Secondary causes include the following (Rennke, 1995):

- Hepatitis B
- Hepatitis C
- Other infections (especially chronic vascular infections including endocarditis, visceral abscess, Lyme disease)

- Rheumatologic causes (lupus, Sjögren syndrome)
- Cancer
- Complement deficiency
- The older MPGN classification based on light and electron micros-copy is being abandoned because it does not provide insight into the cause of MPGN. The older classification based on electron mi-croscopic findings has three histologic types:
  - Type I MPGN—idiopathic (children, no cryoglobulins), hepa-titis C (adults, cryoglobulins usually present). Other causes are hepatitis B, chronic vascular infections (including endocarditis, visceral abscess), cryoglobulinemia (with or without lupus).
    - Pathogenesis: In most cases, it seems to involve complement ac-tivation due to chronic or repeated infection (Varade et al., 1990)
    - Laboratory evaluation
      - Urinalysis (hematuria with RBC casts, proteinuria, may have nephritic or nephrotic syndrome or both)
      - Decreased C3
    - Pathology
      - Light microscopy—global capillary wall thickening with "double contour" (mesangial cell interposition between en-dothelium and GBM), endocapillary hypercellularity, lobu-lar tuft pattern ± crescents (Fig. 10.9)
      - Immunofluorescence—granular to band-like staining of IgG and C3
      - Electron microscopy—mesangial interposition, subendo-thelial immune complex deposits
  - Type II MPGN—DDD—usually due to deficiency of complement factor H
    - Light microscopy—similar to type I, but may only show endo-capillary hypercellularity

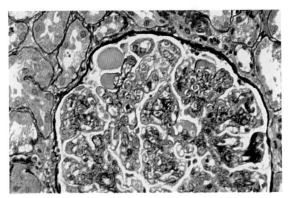

FIGURE 10.9. Membranoproliferative glomerulonephritis. Extensive double contours of the glomerular basement membranes, stained by silver, in membranoproliferative glomeru-lonephritis (MPGN) type I, caused by mesangial interposition and new basement membrane formation in response to subendothelial immune complex deposits (Jones' silver stain; original magnification, ×400). (Originally published in *Am J Kidney Dis.* 1998;31(1):E1. Copyright by The National Kidney Foundation, with permission.)

- Immunofluorescence—band-like staining of C3 (no IgG)
- Electron microscopy—band-like intramembranous electron-dense deposits

■ Type III MPGN—similar to type I, but with additional subepithelial deposits

■ The newer classification is based on immune complex deposition or complement dysregulation. Immune complex–mediated MPGN can be further classified based on two variables: the IF pattern and the presence of monoclonal or polyclonal antibodies in the immune complexes.

■ Immune complex–mediated MPGN:
- Chronic infection. Usually due to hepatitis C. Can be due to hepatitis B, chronic bacterial, fungal, viral, or parasitic infections.
  - Characterized by monoclonal or polyclonal IgM (rheumatoid factor) that binds polyclonal IgG.
  - IF has granular deposition of IgM, C3, and both kappa and lambda light chains.
- Monoclonal gammopathy
  - IF has deposition of kappa or lambda light chains but not both.
  - This is usually due to multiple myeloma but can be due to monoclonal gammopathy of unknown significance (MGUS).
- Autoimmune diseases like lupus, Sjögren, or rheumatoid arthritis
  - IF is typically "full house".

■ Complement dysregulation
- DDD or C3 glomerulonephritis (C3GN)
  - Low C3, normal C4
  - Normal C3 does not exclude DDD or C3GN.
  - IF shows predominantly C3 deposition without significant Ig deposition.
  - DDD can be due to factor H deficiency or autoantibodies to factor H.
  - C3GN can be due to C3 nephritic factor (autoantibody to C3 convertase) or due to deficiency of C3 convertase.

Treatment

■ Treat underlying disease in secondary MPGN (treat chronic infections, multiple myeloma, and autoimmune disease).

■ For DDD or C3GN, treatment is as follows:
- If stable, implement general measures (use ACE inhibitor and control blood pressure).
- If disease is moderately severe and autoantibody present, plasmapheresis combined with rituximab (anti-CD20 antibodies) or eculizumab (anticomplement protein C5).
- If complement deficiency, use fresh-frozen plasma.
- Rapidly progressive disease may require cyclophosphamide and steroids to decrease renal inflammation.

■ In primary MPGN, treatment is as follows:
- MPGN type I—Steroids are first-line therapy. Antiplatelet agents are also commonly used.
- MPGN type II—There is no good form of therapy. Recurs invariably in the transplant.

GRANULOMATOUS POLYANGIITIS (WEGENER GRANULOMATOSIS)

Granulomatous polyangiitis (GPA) is characterized by vasculitis of the respiratory tracts and GN. ANCAs are positive in most patients, usually antiproteinase-3 (anti-PR3) though sometimes antimyeloperoxidase (anti-MPO).

Pathogenesis

Sensitized lymphocytes, exposed to antigen, recruit macrophages that turn into giant cells. ANCA causes exaggerated adhesion, migration, and degranulation of neutrophils (Falk et al., 1990; Savage et al., 1992).

Laboratory Evaluation

- Computed tomography (CT) sinuses—opacification, air fluid levels, masses, erosions
- Chest X-ray or CT chest—nodules, cavitation, infiltrates, interstitial changes
- Normocytic normochromic anemia, leukocytosis, and thrombocytosis are usual.
- Elevated erythrocyte sedimentation rate (ESR), C-reactive protein, and rheumatoid factor
- ANA—normal
- Complements—normal
- ANCA—positive 88% to 96% of the time
    - C-ANCA is anti-PR3.
    - P-ANCA is anti-MPO.
- Urinalysis—hematuria, proteinuria

Pathology

- Light microscopy: Necrotizing granulomas may or may not be seen; fibrous, cellular, or fibrocellular crescents are typical.
- Immunofluorescence: IF is pauci-immune, that is, there is a paucity of immune complexes. Please note that paucity does not mean nonexistent. It is typical to have very small amounts of immune complexes, especially in fulminant lesions. Misinterpretation of these immune complexes should not confuse or delay the diagnosis of GPA.
- Electron microscopy just shows intravascular and subendothelial fibrin and rare immune complexes.

Treatment

The course of the disease may be mild or fulminant. Treatment of choice is cyclophosphamide and steroids with or without plasmapheresis. Protocols used in recent trials are summarized below.

- CYCLOPS protocol:
    - Pulse methylprednisolone (1 g IV × 3) followed by prednisone (1 mg/kg/day)
    - Cyclophosphamide 0.5 g/m^2 IV every 2 weeks or 2 mg/kg orally daily
    - Duration: 3 to 6 months

- RAVE protocol:
  - Rituximab 375 mg/m^2 weekly for 4 weeks
  - Steroids as above
  - Plasmapheresis if:
    - Rising creatinine (>5.7 mg/dL or 500 mcg/L)
    - Pulmonary hemorrhage
    - Coexistent anti-GBM antibodies
  - Maintenance:
    - Azathioprine
    - Second line: mycophenolate
    - Third line: methotrexate

OTHER POLYARTERITIDES

Pathogenesis

There are two forms of polyarteritis. The classic macroscopic form involves medium-sized arteries leading to visceral organ infarction (abdomen, heart, central nervous system) and is quite rare in the United States. The microscopic form involves the lung, skin, and kidney and is associated with ANCA (usually anti-MPO). Wegener granulomatosis is a form of microscopic polyarteritis.

Laboratory Evaluation

- Elevated ESR
- Anemia, leukocytosis, thrombocytosis
- Eosinophilia often present
- Positive ANCA
- Normal complements
- Urinalysis—hematuria with RBC casts, proteinuria

Pathology

- Light microscopy
  - Classic form—glomeruli not primarily affected (secondary ischemic changes may be present). Inflammatory interstitial infiltrates consisting of lymphocytes, neutrophils, monocytes, and eosinophils may be seen.
  - Microscopic form—focal segmental necrotizing GN with crescents. GBM destruction with neutrophils and fibrin in Bowman space. Interstitial inflammatory infiltrate usually seen.
- Immunofluorescence
  - Pauci-immune
  - There are no immune deposits.
- Electron microscopy
  - Epithelial crescents
  - No electron-dense deposits

Treatment

Cyclophosphamide plus corticosteroids (similar to Wegener)

A 50-year-old previously healthy man presents for evaluation of gross hematuria that developed a few days after an upper respiratory infection characterized by sore throat and rhinorrhea. He denies skin rash, oral ulcers, or photosensitivity, myalgias, arthralgias, or neurologic symptoms. The only positive finding on physical examination is trace edema of the hands and feet. The blood pressure is normal.

Blood chemistry:
Sodium: 140 mmol/L
Potassium: 4.5 mmol/L
Chloride: 106 mmol/L
Total CO_2: 26 mmol/L
Urea nitrogen: 10 mg/dL (urea: 3.6 mmol/L)
Creatinine: 1.0 mg/dL (88.4 mcmol/L)
Glucose: 110 mg/dL (6.1 mmol/L)

Urinalysis:
Color: yellow
pH: 5.5

Specific gravity: 1.025
Protein: 2+
Blood: 1+
Glucose: negative
Ketones: negative
Bilirubin: negative
Urobilinogen: negative
WBCs: 2/hpf
RBCs: 10/hpf
Bacteria: none
Urine protein to creatinine ratio (Pr/Cr) : 1.5 g/g (170 mg/mmol)

A renal biopsy is performed. Light microscopy reveals MPGN.

Q: What is the most likely underlying pathophysiology of the disease process in this patient?

1. Mimicry between M-protein on the surface of streptococcal organisms and glomerular antigens causes an autoimmune reaction.
2. Abnormal galactosylation of IgA, decreased clearance by the liver, autoantibody formation to IgA, and mesangial deposition
3. Renal vasculitis with lack of immune deposits
4. Antibody formation to an antigen on type IV collagen that is found in the GBM and the alveolar basement membrane

A: The urinalysis in this patient reveals hematuria and proteinuria and is thus suggestive of GN. The clinical history of this patient (gross hematuria following an upper respiratory infection) suggests IgA nephropathy. In IgA nephropathy, exposure to an allergen or infection causes IgA production and abnormal galactosylation leads to decreased clearance by the liver, autoantibody formation to IgA1, and mesangial deposition. In poststreptococcal GN, M-protein is present on the surface of streptococci and an autoimmune response because of antigen mimicry or an immune complex response causes GN. Although poststreptococcal

GN is in the differential, the lack of latency between infection and hematuria as well as the mesangioproliferative GN argue for IgA nephropathy (in poststreptococcal GN, endocapillary and sometimes epithelial cell proliferation are also expected). A necrotizing GN with lack of immune deposits ("pauci-immune") is typical of renal vasculitis. A necrotizing and frequently crescentic GN caused by antibody formation to an antigen on type IV collagen resulting is typical of anti-GBM disease, which can also be associated with anti–alveolar basement membrane antibodies and pulmonary hemorrhage (Goodpasture syndrome). RPGN (crescentic) is often seen with renal vasculitis or anti-GBM disease and not infrequent with poststreptococcal GN, but is an uncommon mode of presentation for IgA nephropathy.

VIGNETTE 2

10

A 37-year-old woman with a history of chronic sinusitis treated with fluticasone nasal spray and hypertension treated with metoprolol, 25 mg, twice a day; hydralazine, 100 mg, twice a day; and furosemide, 40 mg, daily presents for evaluation of progressive renal failure. Over the past several months, she has developed a facial rash, oral ulcers, photosensitivity, myalgias, and joint pains. She denies urinary symptoms including hematuria. Physical examination is remarkable for a malar rash and a few aphthous ulcers on the tongue and oral palate. The blood pressure is normal.

Blood chemistry:
Sodium: 136 mmol/L
Potassium: 4.5 mmol/L
Chloride: 106 mmol/L
Total CO_2: 26 mmol/L
Urea nitrogen: 40 mg/dL
  (urea: 14.3 mmol/L)
Creatinine: 2.5 mg/dL
  (221 mcmol/L)
Glucose: 110 mg/dL (6.1 mmol/L)

Complete blood count:
WBCs: 13,000/mm^3
Hemoglobin: 10 g/dL
Hematocrit: 30%
Platelets: 400,000/mm^3

ANA: 1:320
ANCA: 1:80 (anti-MPO type)

Urinalysis:
Color: yellow
pH: 5.5
Specific gravity: 1.025
Protein: 2+
Blood: 2+
Glucose: negative
Ketones: 1+
Bilirubin: negative
Urobilinogen: negative
WBCs: 5/hpf
RBCs: 15/hpf
Bacteria: none

Q: What is the most likely diagnosis?

1. LN
2. ANCA-associated vasculitis
3. Drug-induced lupus with immune complex nephritis
4. Drug-induced vasculitis

A: In this woman with symptoms, signs, and laboratory findings suggestive of SLE, LN due to immune complex deposition in the glomeruli is certainly a possibility. However, this patient is taking a relatively high dose of hydralazine, a drug known to cause a dose-related risk of lupus. The renal disease in drug-induced lupus is usually a necrotizing GN with little or no immune complex deposition. Such patients show a P-ANCA pattern on IF microscopy with anti-MPO antibodies.

Hydralazine is discontinued. Several weeks later, renal function has recovered and ANA and ANCA are negative.

References

Falk RJ, Terrell RS, Charles LA, et al. Anti-neutrophil cytoplasmic autoantibodies induce neutrophils to degranulate and produce oxygen radicals in vitro. *Proc Natl Acad Sci U S A*. 1990;87:4115–4119.

Goroncy-Bermes P, Dale JB, Beachey EH, et al. Monoclonal antibody to human renal glomeruli cross-reacts with streptococcal M protein. *Infect Immun*. 1987;55:2416–2419.

Hahn BH. Antibodies to DNA. *N Engl J Med*. 1998;338:1359–1368.

Hebert LA, Cosio FG, Neff JC. Diagnostic significance of hypocomplementemia. *Kidney Int*. 1991;39:811–821.

Isenberg DA, Collins C. Detection of cross-reactive anti-DNA antibody idiotypes on renal tissue bound immunoglobulins from lupus patients. *J Clin Invest*. 1985;76:287–294.

Mestecky J, Tomana M, Crolwey-Nowick PA, et al. Defective galactosylation and clearance of IgA1 molecules as a possible etiopathogenic factor in IgA nephropathy. *Contrib Nephrol*. 1993;104:172–182.

Michael AF Jr, Drummond KN, Good RA, et al. Acute poststreptococcal glomerulonephritis: immune deposit disease. *J Clin Invest*. 1966;45:237–248.

Nadasdy T, Hebert LA. Infection-related glomerulonephritis: understanding mechanisms. *Semin Nephrol*. 2011;31(4):369–375.

Nasr SH, D'Agati VD. IgA-dominant postinfectious glomerulonephritis: a new twist on an old disease. *Nephron Clin Pract*. 2011;119(1):c18–c25.

Rennke HG. Secondary membranoproliferative glomerulonephritis. *Kidney Int*. 1995;47:643–656.

Savage CO, Pottinger BE, Gaskin G, et al. Autoantibodies developing to myeloperoxidase and proteinase 3 in systemic vasculitis stimulate neutrophil cytotoxicity toward cultured endothelial cells. *Am J Pathol*. 1992;141:335–342.

Varade WS, Forristal J, West CD. Patterns of complement activation in idiopathic membranous glomerulonephritis, types I, II, and III. *Am J Kidney Dis*. 1990;16:196–206.

Wieslander J, Barr JF, Butkowski RJ, et al. Goodpasture antigen of the glomerular basement membrane: localization to noncollagenous regions of type IV collagen. *Proc Natl Acad Sci U S A*. 1984;81:3838–3842.

Nephrotic Syndrome

DEFINITION

Nephrotic syndrome is characterized predominantly by massive proteinuria. It is defined by proteinuria of >3.5 g/24 h/1.73 m². Nephrotic syndrome is associated with hypoalbuminemia resulting from urinary loss and renal degradation of albumin. There is edema because of primary retention of sodium by the kidneys and low oncotic pressure; the hypothesis that sodium retention may be due to the renin–angiotensin–aldosterone system (RAAS) has not been supported (Brown et al., 1982). Increased hepatic synthesis of lipoproteins and decreased catabolism leads to hyperlipidemia (Joven et al., 1990). Lipiduria is due to loss of lipoproteins in the urine. Hypercoagulability due to urinary loss of antithrombotic proteins (such as antithrombin III) is also common, especially in severe nephrosis with a serum albumin <2 g/dL (Kauffmann et al., 1978).

CASE STUDY 11.1 A 71-year-old male presents with complaints of weakness, fatigue, and lethargy over the past 8 months. He has been using a motorized wheelchair owing to pain in the right leg. He has also noted bilateral leg swelling for the past 2 months. He denies nonsteroidal anti-inflammatory drug (NSAID) use; he has been taking oxycodone for pain in his right leg. Medications include hydrochlorothiazide 25 mg daily, lisinopril 20 mg daily, metoprolol 75 mg daily, atorvastatin 40 mg daily, and oxycodone 5 mg as needed. Physical examination reveals normal vital signs. He is alert and oriented but appears fatigued. He has an irregular heart rate. There is bilateral lower extremity edema and tenderness over right medial femoral condyle.

Complete blood count:
WBCs: 13,000/mm³
Hemoglobin: 13.2 g/dL
Hematocrit: 40.6%
Platelets: 249,000/mm³

Blood chemistry:
Sodium: 133 mmol/L
Potassium: 4.5 mmol/L
Chloride: 93 mmol/L
Total CO_2: 25 mmol/L

Urea nitrogen: 20 mg/dL (urea: 7.1 mmol/L)
Creatinine: 1.0 mg/dL (88.4 mcmol/L)
Glucose: 125 mg/dL (6.9 mmol/L)
Albumin: 2.5 g/dL (25 g/L)

Urinalysis:
Specific gravity: 1.02
Protein: 3+
RBCs: none
Nitrite: negative
Leukocyte esterase: negative
WBCs: 3/hpf
Few bacteria
Urine protein to creatinine ratio (UPCR): 4.0 g/g (452 mg/mmol)
Knee X-ray: comminuted fracture right medial femoral condyle
Chest X-ray: normal

Question 11.1.1: What are the causes of nephrotic syndrome?

CAUSES OF NEPHROTIC SYNDROME

- Idiopathic or primary (no known cause):
  - Minimal change disease (MCD)
  - Focal segmental glomerulosclerosis (FSGS)
  - Membranous nephropathy (MN)
- Secondary:
  - MCD—Hodgkin disease, NSAIDs
  - FSGS—infections (HIV), drugs (e.g., anabolic steroids, pamidronate, rapamycin), sickle cell disease, reflux nephropathy, renal dysplasia/agenesis, morbid obesity
  - MN—infections (hepatitis B, malaria, syphilis, leprosy, schistosomiasis), malignancy (lung, colon, breast, kidney, lymphoma), collagen disease (especially lupus), drugs (captopril, NSAIDs) (rare)
  - Diabetes mellitus (discussed in Chapter 13)
  - Lupus—especially class V (membranous). Class IV can cause nephritic/nephrotic picture (red blood cell [RBC] casts and massive proteinuria) (discussed in Chapter 10)
  - Amyloidosis (AL or AA type)
  - Light-chain deposition disease (LCDD), immunotactoid glomerulopathy, fibrillary glomerulonephritis (GN)
  - Thrombotic microangiopathy (thrombotic thrombocytopenic purpura/hemolytic-uremic syndrome [TTP/HUS])

Question 11.1.2: What serologic workup is appropriate for this patient with nephrotic syndrome?

The following serologies are useful in honing in on the diagnosis: hepatitis panel, antinuclear antibodies (ANAs), hemoglobin A1c (HbA1c), serum protein electrophoresis (SPEP) and urine protein electrophoresis (UPEP), serum free light chains, complements (C3, C4), and human immunodeficiency virus (HIV).

> ## CASE STUDY 11.1 CONTINUED
>
> Results in this patient are as follows:
>
> Hepatitis panel: negative
> ANA: <1:20
> HbA1c: 6.2%
> C3: 125 (normal 66–185 mg/dL)
> C4: 35 (normal 15–52 mg/dL)
> HIV: test negative
> SPEP/UPEP: no abnormal proteins; no monoclonal bands
> Serum free kappa light chains: 2.7 mg/L
> Serum free lambda light chains: 2.6 mg/L
> Serum kappa:lambda ratio: 1.04 (normal, 0.26–1.65)

Question 11.1.3: What is the differential diagnosis of nephrotic syndrome in this patient?

Idiopathic (primary) nephrotic syndrome is generally caused by MCD, FSGS, or MN. Systemic (secondary) causes of nephrotic syndrome, such as diabetes mellitus and amyloid, should be excluded.

The fact that the serum free kappa:lambda ratio is normal mitigates against monoclonal gammopathies, such as amyloidosis or multiple myeloma. In monoclonal gammopathies, generally either kappa or lambda light chains will be markedly more abundant, and the ratio will be either very high or very low.

Other secondary causes of nephrotic syndrome include infections (such as HIV, syphilis, hepatitis B or C), certain medications, cancer, heroin abuse, and hyperfiltering conditions such as obesity and unilateral renal agenesis.

Question 11.1.4: What are the renal biopsy findings in nephrotic syndrome?

The pathology of nephrotic syndrome is outlined in Table 11.1.

Question 11.1.5: What is the most likely diagnosis in this patient with nephrotic syndrome who is normotensive and has normal renal function with negative serology and absence of paraproteinemia?

MINIMAL CHANGE DISEASE

MCD is the most common cause of nephrotic syndrome in children and can also present in adulthood. Its hallmark is effacement of foot processes on electron microscopy in the absence of changes on light microscopy (Bridges et al., 1982). It does not progress to end-stage kidney disease (ESKD), but nephrosis may be very severe and symptomatic, and episodes of acute renal failure can occur.

Pathogenesis

The cause of MCD is unknown, though a disorder in T lymphocytes is thought to be involved. There is some evidence that a permeability factor produced by T cells with specificity for glomerular epithelial

TABLE 11.1 Pathology of Nephrotic Syndrome

Diagnosis	Light Microscopy	Immunofluorescence	Electron Microscopy
Diabetic nephropathy	Thickening of GBM Diffuse and nodular glomerulosclerosis	Negative	Thickening of GBM. No electron-dense deposits
Membranous nephropathy	Capillary wall thickening with spikes	Capillary wall IgG, C3 In lupus—C1q as well	Subepithelial immune complexes In lupus—mesangial as well
FSGS	Focal and segmental lesions	Sclerosis	Foot process fusion
Minimal change	Normal or minimal mesangial changes	Negative	Foot process fusion
Amyloid	Diffuse amorphous eosinophilic hyaline deposits (PAS negative) Congo red and Thioflavin T positive	AA: typically negative (positive for SAA if done) AL: positive for lambda or kappa light chains	Randomly oriented 10–12 nm fibrils
LCDD	Nodular sclerosing pattern with nodules of eosinophilic material Congo red and Thioflavin T negative	Diffuse linear staining of GBM (usually kappa positive)	Granular deposits (not fibrils)
Fibrillary GN	Mesangial expansion Membranous or MPGN Morphology	IgG, C3, both kappa and lambda light chains	Randomly oriented 16–24 nm fibrils
Immunotactoid GN	Proliferative, membranous or nodular sclerosing pattern	Usually positive for lambda or kappa light chains (light-chain restriction)	Parallel stacks of 30–50 nm fibrils

FSGS, focal segmental glomerulosclerosis; GBM, glomerular basement membrane; GN, glomerulonephritis; IgG, immunoglobulin G; LCDD, light-chain deposition disease; MPGN, membranoproliferative glomerulonephritis; PAS, periodic acid–Schiff; SAA, serum amyloid A.

cells may cause a loss of glomerular negative charge. The glomerular negative charge plays an important role in preventing proteinuria by repelling proteins (such as albumin) that have a negative charge as well. MCD is associated with Hodgkin disease.

Laboratory Evaluation

- Massive albuminuria (selective proteinuria, i.e., most of urinary protein is albumin with little globulin)
- Decreased serum proteins and immunoglobulins (often marked)
- Increased serum lipids (often marked)
- Normal serum complements
- No serologic abnormalities

Pathology

- Light microscopy
  - No glomerular lesions seen (Fig. 11.1)
  - There may be minimal mesangial prominence and flattening of tubular epithelia.
- Immunofluorescence
  - Usually negative
  - Low level of staining for IgM and C3 may be seen.
- Electron microscopy
  - Effacement of visceral epithelial cell foot processes (Fig. 11.2). This is a nonspecific finding that can be found in any proteinuric disease.

Question 11.1.6: What is the treatment of MCD?

Treatment

- Treatment of MCD
  - Low-sodium diet, diuretics, RAAS blockers; avoid calcium channel blockers
  - Corticosteroids are generally effective in MCD and most achieve remission in a few months. Edema improves before serum albumin begins to rise. In children, 60 mg/m^2/d is usually given for 6

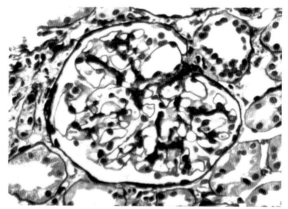

FIGURE 11.1. Minimal change disease. Glomeruli are normal by light microscopy in minimal change disease. Note that the glomerular basement membrane is thin and delicate, and mesangial cellularity and matrix are within normal limits (Jones' silver stain, ×200). (Originally published in Fogo A. Minimal change disease. *Am J Kidney Dis.* 1999;33(3):E1. Copyright by The National Kidney Foundation, with permission.)

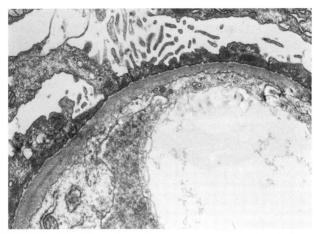

FIGURE 11.2. Minimal change disease. The glomerular basement membrane is of normal thickness without deposits. The visceral epithelial cells show the diffuse effacement of foot processes that occurs in proteinuric states. Foot process effacement is generally quite extensive in minimal change disease (transmission electron microscopy, ×800). (Originally published in Fogo A. Minimal change disease. *Am J Kidney Dis.* 1999;33(3):E1. Copyright by The National Kidney Foundation, with permission.)

weeks. In adults, 1.0 mg/kg/d not to exceed 80 mg/d for a minimum of 8 weeks is recommended even if remission is achieved earlier. Treatment should be tapered 1 to 2 weeks after complete remission is achieved.

- Lack of response by 16 weeks is considered steroid resistance. Most will start a calcineurin inhibitor (such as cyclosporine) along with prednisone (0.15–0.2 mg/kg/d).
- MCD relapse should be treated with a repeat course of prednisone for up to two or three times. For frequent relapses (three or more relapses per year), use continuous low-dose alternate-day prednisone (15 mg every other day or the lowest dose that sustains remission). For steroid toxicity or failure to respond to calcineurin inhibitors, use cyclophosphamide (2 mg/kg/d for 8–12 weeks). For relapse after cyclophosphamide, long-term cyclosporine for 1 to 2 years may be of benefit. For relapse after (or failure to respond to) both cyclophosphamide and cyclosporine, use rituximab (but not in steroid-resistant MCD).
- For steroid-resistant MCD, confirm resistance by documenting failure with pulse methylprednisolone 500 mg × 3. Consider FSGS, IgM nephropathy, idiopathic mesangial proliferation, or C1q nephropathy. Repeat biopsy may be indicated.

CASE STUDY 11.1 CONTINUED

The fracture in the right femur is thought to be pathologic. A magnetic resonance imaging (MRI) of the right lower extremity is performed, which reveals a large tumor. Excisional biopsy reveals diffuse large B-cell lymphoma.

How does the existence of a malignancy change the pretest probability of the differential diagnosis?

Hodgkin lymphoma is associated with MCD. However, this patient has diffuse large B-cell lymphoma. The existence of a non-Hodgkin lymphoma makes secondary membranous or rarely secondary FSGS possible.

FOCAL SEGMENTAL GLOMERULOSCLEROSIS

FSGS is characterized by proteinuria as a result of focal (some glomeruli) and segmental (portions of glomeruli) sclerosis. This form of the nephrotic syndrome has been increasing in incidence and is more frequently found in African Americans and other patients of African descent. Various pathologic types of FSGS (tip lesion, cellular variant, collapsing variant, etc.) have now been described (D'Agati et al., 2004). FSGS often progresses to ESKD.

Pathogenesis

FSGS is a pathologic entity that probably has many etiologies (immune, infectious, hemodynamic, genetic, etc.). It is typically divided up into primary (idiopathic) and secondary FSGS. Primary FSGS may be caused by immune/cytokine dysregulation, similar to MCD. However, podocyte ultrastructural changes (such as loss of mature podocyte markers) have been identified in FSGS but not MCD, which may contribute to focal glomerular basement membrane (GBM) denudation and glomerulosclerosis. In some patients, a circulating glomerular permeability factor seems to be etiologic, and in such cases, rapid recurrence after kidney transplantation is seen. The serum-soluble urokinase receptor is one such putative causative factor (Wei et al., 2011). Many cases of secondary FSGS are thought to be due to low nephron number (as in renal agenesis or in patients born with fewer nephrons) leading to intraglomerular hypertension, which results in endothelial and podocyte injury. Hemodynamic alterations also probably underlie obesity-associated FSGS. The collapsing variant of FSGS is characteristic of HIV-associated nephropathy (HIVAN). Finally, antiserum against transforming growth factor beta ameliorates experimental FSGS (Border et al., 1990).

Laboratory Evaluation

- Massive proteinuria (not only predominantly albuminuria but also globulinuria)
- Decreased serum proteins and immunoglobulins (especially in primary form)
- Increased serum lipids (especially in primary form)
- Normal serum complements
- No serologic abnormalities

Pathology

- Light microscopy
  - Segmental sclerosis in a focal (some glomeruli) and segmental (parts of glomeruli) pattern (Fig. 11.3)

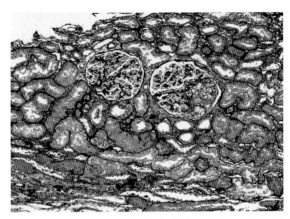

FIGURE 11.3. Focal segmental glomerulosclerosis. The larger of the two glomeruli shown contains two small peripheral foci of segmental sclerosis with intracapillary foam cells and prominence of overlying visceral epithelial cells. This is representative of an early segmental sclerosing lesion in focal segmental glomerulosclerosis. There is also surrounding mild interstitial fibrosis (Jones' silver stain, ×100) (Copyright © 1999 by the National Kidney Foundation). (Originally published in Fogo A. Minimal change disease. *Am J Kidney Dis.* 1999;33(4):E1. Copyright by The National Kidney Foundation, with permission.)

- ■ Immunofluorescence
  - ■ Nonsclerotic glomeruli do not stain for IgG or complement.
  - ■ Sclerotic segments may have irregular staining for IgM, C3, C1q.
- ■ Electron microscopy
  - ■ There is foot process effacement.
  - ■ Electron microscopy is generally used to identify other causes for glomerular scarring.

Treatment

- ■ Exclude secondary causes
  - ■ Test for HIV (if positive, treatment directed at HIV).
  - ■ In massive obesity, weight loss (with or without bariatric surgery) can improve outcomes.
  - ■ Stop medications associated with FSGS (anabolic steroids, pamidronate).
- ■ Primary FSGS may respond to immunosuppressive therapy, though not as well as MCD.
  - ■ Children—Prednisone (same as in MCD) is treatment of choice. Relapse or steroid resistance is also treated as in MCD.
  - ■ Adults—Steroids have been moderately successful. A longer course of therapy with higher doses of prednisone (up to 4 months) will be required. Remission rates have been reported to be as low as 15% to up to 40%. Elderly patients may respond to alternate-day steroid therapy. Other immunosuppressives (calcineurin inhibitors, mycophenolate, cyclophosphamide) have been used.

MEMBRANOUS NEPHROPATHY

MN is the most common form of idiopathic nephrotic syndrome in Caucasian adults (FSGS is more common in African Americans). There are a multitude of secondary causes of MN. In the United States, the most common are lupus, hepatitis B, and malignancy (especially in older patients).

Pathogenesis

MN is characterized by the presence of immune deposits in the GBM in a subepithelial location. Experimental models have suggested that these immune deposits develop in situ, with movement across the GBM of circulating IgG antibodies directed against endogenous podocyte antigens or against circulating antigens that have crossed the GBM. Antigens that have been implicated in MN include the phospholipase A_2 receptor (PLA2R) and neutral endopeptidase. The M-type PLA2R, a transmembrane receptor that is highly expressed in podocytes, has been identified as a major antigen in human idiopathic MN. Circulating autoantibodies to PLA2R have been identified in 70% of patients with idiopathic MN and are associated with disease (Beck et al., 2009). Subsequent studies have confirmed anti-PLA2R antibodies in 60% to 80% of patients with idiopathic MN. Other antigens have been identified in secondary MN, including double-stranded DNA in lupus, thyroglobulin in thyroiditis, hepatitis B antigen, treponemal antigen in syphilis, and carcinoembryonic antigen and prostate-specific antigen in malignancy, though causality has not universally been established. The end result of immune complex formation is complement activation and injury to glomerular epithelial cells (Cybulsky et al., 1986).

Laboratory Evaluation

- Proteinuria (subnephrotic to massive)
- Hypoalbuminemia
- Hyperlipidemia
- Check for hepatitis B, hepatitis C, rapid plasma reagin (RPR) (syphilis), HIV, ANAs, complements (normal complements are seen in idiopathic MN, but may be low in some secondary causes).

Pathology

- Light microscopy
  - Capillary wall thickening
- Immunofluorescence
  - Diffuse granular capillary wall staining for IgG and complement
  - In MN caused by lupus, there is usually high-intensity staining for C1q.
- Electron microscopy
  - Subepithelial immune complex deposits with foot process effacement (Fig. 11.4).
  - Immune complexes may be because of antigens to hepatitis B, tumor antigen, or autoantigen.
  - In secondary MN, the immune complexes may also be in the mesangium.

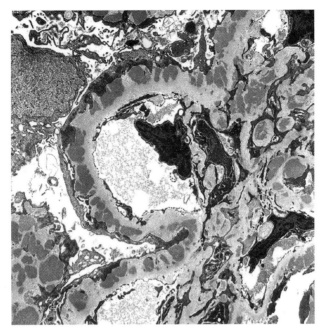

FIGURE 11.4. Membranous nephropathy. Stages II to III membranous glomerulonephritis with thickened capillary wall resulting from numerous medium to large subepithelial dense deposits and basement membrane reaction (transmission electron microscopy, original magnification ×1,650). (Originally published in Fogo A. Membranous glomerulonephritis. *Am J Kidney Dis.* 1998;31(3):E1. Copyright by the National Kidney Foundation, with permission.)

Treatment

- Exclude secondary causes, especially in older patients (malignancy) and patients with risk factors for hepatitis
- Nonimmunosuppressive treatment
  - RAAS blockers
  - Blood pressure control
  - Statins
  - Warfarin for thromboembolic event and possibly with severe hypoalbuminemia
- Idiopathic MN
  - 24-hour urine protein excretion <4 g/d—usually indolent and does not require immunosuppressive treatment
  - 24-hour urine protein excretion 4 to 8 g/d
    - If normal or near-normal renal function, half will undergo spontaneous remission.
    - If persistent, immunosuppression is indicated.
    - Ponticelli protocol:
      Months 1, 3, 5: Methylprednisolone 1 g IV × 3 days followed by prednisone 0.4 mg/kg for 27 days
      Months 2, 4, 6: Cyclophosphamide 2 to 2.5 mg/kg for 30 days orally

- Calcineurin inhibitor regimen:
    Cyclosporine with trough 125 to 225 mcg/L plus prednisone 0.15 mg/kg/d for 26 weeks
    If failure with above, rituximab is an option.
- 24-hour protein excretion >8 g/d for more than 3 months
    Cyclophosphamide plus steroids (if abnormal of decreasing renal function) *or* cyclosporine plus steroids
- Relapsing disease
    - Do not use cyclophosphamide more than twice owing to concerns about bone marrow depression, infection, gonadal toxicity. Can repeat cyclosporine. For resistant disease, consider rituximab.
- Age > 65 years
    - Treat only if proteinuria >8 g/d or declining renal function.

CASE STUDY 11.1 CONCLUDED

The patient is referred to hematology/oncology for treatment of lymphoma. Edema is treated with diuretics. Renal function remains stable. A renal biopsy is deferred as it will not change management.

Most cases of nephrotic syndrome not due to diabetes mellitus will be due to MCD, MGN, or FSGS, though one needs to consider rarer causes.

AMYLOIDOSIS (AL OR AA TYPE)

Amyloidosis refers to diseases caused by extracellular deposition of fibrils within organs. Fibrils are proteins that have an antiparallel beta-pleated sheet configuration that enhances deposition in organs (Husby et al., 1994); these fibrils are resistant to degradation and bind Congo red and Thioflavin T. There are many hereditary amyloidoses, and mutations in diverse proteins may produce amyloid. Only select amyloid fibrils deposit in the kidney. Amyloidoses that affect the kidneys include AL amyloidosis and AA amyloidosis.

Pathogenesis

In **AL amyloidosis**, fibrils are derived from immunoglobulin light chains produced by abnormal clones of plasma cells. These fibrils are derived from the variable region of the light chains (Alim et al., 1999). Multiple myeloma will be present in about 20% of cases. SPEP and UPEP may be negative, but assays for free light chains in the serum are almost always positive (Abraham et al., 2003). Monoclonal lambda light chains are more common than kappa (the opposite is true in multiple myeloma). Typical clinical findings are as follows:

- Symptoms—weight loss, fatigue, dizziness, shortness of breath, edema, peripheral neuropathy, autonomic neuropathy (orthostatic hypotension), carpal tunnel syndrome
- Physical examination—hepatosplenomegaly
- Laboratory—proteinuria (25% nephrotic), urine sediment otherwise bland

In **AA amyloidosis**, there is deposition of serum amyloid A (SAA) (Gilmore et al., 2001). SAA is found mainly in inflammatory processes.

Diagnosis

- Usually biopsy is required (in AL amyloidosis, a bone marrow Bx is usually needed).
- Diagnostic techniques that have been used include the following:
  - Fat pad aspirate
  - Rectal biopsy
  - Bone marrow aspirate
  - Gingival biopsy
  - Skin biopsy
  - Serum amyloid P scintigraphy

Pathology

- Light microscopy
  - Eosinophilic material in the mesangium and capillary walls
  - Spicular projections in GBM
  - Congo red stains orange and apple green birefringence is present under polarized light.
  - Thioflavin T causes fluorescence under ultraviolet light.
- Immunofluorescence
  - AL has positive staining for monoclonal light chains (usually lambda).
  - AA has positive staining for SAA.
- Electron microscopy
  - Fibrils in mesangium. Subepithelial, intramembranous, and subendothelial GBM (Fig. 11.5)

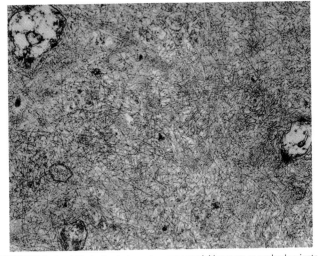

FIGURE 11.5. Amyloidosis. By electron microscopy, amyloid appears as randomly oriented thin fibrils, 10 to 12 nm in diameter, with a loose, flocculent background. The type of amyloid cannot be determined by its appearance on electron microscopy and requires immunofluorescence staining (transmission electron microscopy; original magnification ×51,250). (Originally published in Fogo A. Amyloid. *Am J Kidney Dis*. 1998;32(5):E1. Copyright by The National Kidney Foundation, with permission.)

Treatment

- In general, there is a poor prognosis.
- Treat any inflammatory process and/or infections.
- Chemotherapy (melphalan and prednisone) may be tried for AL amyloidosis.
- Bone marrow transplant has been used for AL amyloidosis.
- Renal transplant is associated with a low survival.

LIGHT-CHAIN DEPOSITION DISEASE

This disease is caused by overproduction and deposition of monoclonal immunoglobulin proteins. However, these proteins are granular and not fibrillar. Congo red and Thioflavin T do not stain these proteins. LCDD protein is derived from the constant region of light chains, whereas amyloid is derived from the variable region of light chains.

LCDD promotes transforming growth factor beta production, which promotes production of collagen, laminin, and fibronectin (Zhu et al., 1995).

The kidney is the most prominent organ to be affected. There is glomerular proteinuria, and half of the patients are nephrotic.

Pathology

- Light microscopy
  - Nodular sclerosing pattern
  - Mesangium has nodules of eosinophilic material.
- Immunofluorescence
  - Diffuse linear staining of GBM due to kappa light chains (as opposed to AL amyloidosis, which are usually lambda)
  - There is staining in nodules, tubular basement membrane, and vessel walls.
- Electron microscopy
  - Fibrils are not seen.
  - Granular deposits in GBM and tubular basement membrane (Fig. 11.6)

Treatment

- Melphalan and prednisone stabilize or improve renal function.
- Marrow or stem cell transplant may be efficacious.
- Suppression of abnormal paraprotein prior to renal transplant is important. Otherwise, there is 70% recurrence.

FIBRILLARY GLOMERULONEPHRITIS

Fibrillary GN usually affects the kidneys in isolation and is associated with deposition of 16- to 24-nm fibrils that are negative for Congo red staining and Thioflavin T staining (Rosenstock et al., 2003).

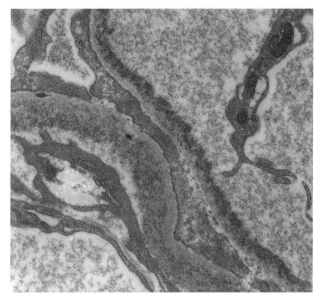

FIGURE 11.6. Light-chain deposition disease. High-power view of the granular, amorphous deposits typical of light-chain deposition disease. These deposits have indistinct borders, are mottled, and are seen on the endothelial aspects of the glomerular basement membrane, the mesangium, and tubular basement membranes (transmission electron microscopy, original magnification ×40,000). (Originally published in Fogo A. Light chain deposition disease. *Am J Kidney Dis.* 1998;32(6):E1. Copyright by The National Kidney Foundation, with permission.)

There is usually proteinuria, hematuria, and hypertension. Progression to end-stage renal disease is common.

Pathology

- Light microscopy
  - Mesangial expansion
  - Membranous
  - Membranoproliferative
  - Crescentic
- Immunofluorescence
  - Stains for IgG, C3, kappa and lambda chains
- Electron microscopy (Fig. 11.7)
  - 16- to 24-nm fibrils
  - Random arrangement of fibrils

Treatment

- No treatment has been shown to be effective.
- Cyclophosphamide and steroids have been tried for crescentic GN.
- Cyclosporine has been tried for membranous GN.

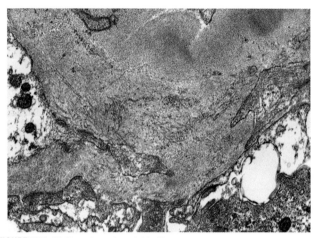

FIGURE 11.7. Fibrillary glomerulonephritis. High-power electron micrograph showing randomly oriented fibrils in the mesangium and glomerular basement membrane in fibrillary glomerulonephritis. These fibrils tend to be slightly larger than those in amyloid, although there is some overlap so that fibril size alone cannot be used to definitively distinguish this from amyloid. A negative Congo red stain should be done to rule out amyloid deposits. (Originally published in Fogo A. Cryoglobulin-related glomerulonephritis. *Am J Kidney Dis.* 1999;33(2):E1. Copyright by The National Kidney Foundation, with permission.)

IMMUNOTACTOID GLOMERULOPATHY

Immunotactoid GN also primarily affects the kidney; there is deposition of fibrils that are 30 to 50 nm (Alpers, 1992). There is usually an association with lymphoproliferative disease. The disease is characterized by proteinuria, hematuria, and hypertension. Progression to end-stage renal disease is common.

Pathology

- Light microscopy
  - Nodular sclerosing
  - Proliferative
  - Membranous
- Immunofluorescence
  - Staining for monoclonal immunoglobulins
- Electron microscopy (Fig. 11.8)
  - 30- to 50-nm fibrils
  - Arrangement in parallel stacks

Treatment

- No treatment has been shown to be effective.

THROMBOTIC MICROANGIOPATHY (TTP/HUS)

See Chapter 16.

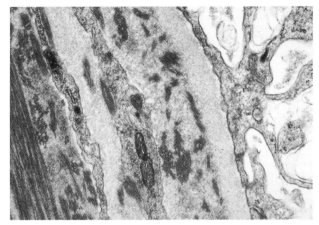

FIGURE 11.8. Immunotactoid glomerulopathy. Deposits show organized structure by electron microscopy, either organized in parallel arrays, and/or with microtubular substructure. Some deposits are cut in cross section, revealing the microtubular substructure, whereas others, stacked in adjacent parallel arrays, are cut longitudinally. These deposits permeate the glomerular basement membrane. (Copyright by The National Kidney Foundation, with permission.)

VIGNETTE 1

A 20-year-old man with no medical history presents for evaluation of an incidental finding of proteinuria on a urinalysis, which has been done because the patient thought his urine is cloudy. He feels well. Physical examination shows bilateral lower extremity edema. The blood pressure is normal.

Blood chemistry:
Sodium: 140 mmol/L
Potassium: 4.0 mmol/L
Chloride: 104 mmol/L
Total CO_2: 26 mmol/L
Urea nitrogen: 20 mg/dL (urea: 7.1 mmol/L)
Creatinine: 1.0 mg/dL (88.4 mcmol/L)
Glucose: 88 mg/dL (4.9 mmol/L)
Albumin: 3.0 g/dL (30 g/L)

Lipid profile:
Total cholesterol: 220 mg/dL (5.7 mmol/L)
Triglycerides: 300 mg/dL (3.4 mmol/L)

Urinalysis:
Color: yellow; slightly turbid
pH: 5.5
Specific gravity: 1.025
Protein: 4+

Blood: negative	WBCs: 2/hpf
Glucose: negative	RBCs: 6/hpf
Ketones: 1+	Bacteria: none
Bilirubin: negative	24-hour urine protein: 4.0 g
Urobilinogen: negative	

Q: In this patient with nephrotic syndrome, match the primary nephrotic syndrome with the expected light microscopic findings:

1. MCD
2. FSGS

3. MN
4. Membranoproliferative

A. Diffuse capillary wall thickening
B. Areas of scarring in some but not all glomeruli
C. Normal findings
D. Capillary wall thickening with glomerulonephritis (MPGN) endocapillary hypercellularity

A: In this young, previously well, patient with nephrotic syndrome, a primary glomerular disease is likely. MCD is the most frequent cause of nephrotic syndrome in children, whereas FSGS or MN becomes more likely in young adulthood. MPGN is usually associated with a chronic infection, most commonly hepatitis C, which can be asymptomatic, so it is still in the differential.

With MCD, the light microscopic findings are usually normal or include minimal mesangial prominence and flattening of tubular epithelia. However, as in all patients with nephrotic syndrome, there will be effacement of podocytes with apparent fusion of foot processes on electron microscopy. There are no immune deposits seen on either electron or immunofluorescence microscopy. In FSGS, the term "focal" refers to the fact that sclerotic lesions are found in some but not all glomeruli; the term "segmental" means that only portions or segments of glomeruli are affected. Again, no immune deposits are seen. MN is characterized by capillary wall thickening because of subepithelial immune complex deposits. In MPGN, there is both capillary wall thickening and endocapillary hypercellularity associated with immune complex deposits, generally in a subendothelial location.

Q: Which of the following is not typical of nephrotic syndrome?

1. Hypercoagulability
2. Hypercholesterolemia
3. Hypoalbuminemia
4. Normal plasma creatinine
5. None of the above

A: Nephrotic syndrome, if severe, can cause profound hypoalbuminemia and hypercoagulability (the pathogenesis of the latter is complex, but a major factor is loss of antithrombin III in the urine). The degree of hypercholesterolemia tends to mirror the severity of hypoalbuminemia because the liver is overproducing lipoproteins (as well as albumin and globulins) in response to low plasma oncotic pressure. Renal function is typically normal at presentation of nephrosis, although progressive renal failure may develop, except in MCD. Hence, the answer is "none of the above."

A 51-year-old white man with a long history of intravenous drug abuse presents for evaluation of abnormal liver enzymes. He has been sharing needles. He has never had a transfusion. He has no symptoms. Vital signs are normal. Physical examination is negative for icterus, caput medusae, or ecchymosis. There is no ascites.

Blood chemistry:
Creatinine: 1.9 mg/dL (168 mcmol/L)
Alanine aminotransferase (ALT): 90 U/L
Aspartate aminotransferase (AST): 88 U/L
Alkaline phosphatase: 90 U/L
Total bilirubin: 2.0 mg/dL (34 mcmol/L)
Albumin: 2.0 g/dL (20 g/L)

Urinalysis:
Color: yellow
pH: 5.5
Specific gravity: 1.025
Protein: 4+

Blood: 1+
Glucose: negative
Ketones: 1+
Bilirubin: negative
Urobilinogen: negative
WBCs: 2/hpf
RBCs: 20/hpf
Blood: negative
Bacteria: none
Cellular and fatty casts seen
24-hour urine protein: 8.7 g

Hepatitis panel:
Hepatitis A antibody: negative
Hepatitis B surface antigen and antibody: negative
Hepatitis C antibody, positive

Q: Which of the following is a likely diagnosis for the nephrotic syndrome in this patient?

1. MCD
2. FSGS
3. MN
4. HIVAN
5. MPGN

A: This patient has nephrotic syndrome with massive proteinuria and fatty casts in the urine. However, there are also hematuria and cellular casts. Thus, this patient has what is sometimes termed the "nephritic-nephrotic syndrome," with features of both glomerular inflammation ("nephritis") and massive protein-uria ("nephrosis"). The differential in such cases includes lupus nephritis, MPGN with or without cryoglobulinemia, and, less commonly, thrombotic microangiopathies such as TTP/HUS. Hepatitis C positivity supports the likelihood of MPGN; additional supportive findings would be hypocomplementemia and cryoglobulinemia. MN has also been described with hepatitis C but is less common. MCD and FSGS are not associated with hepatitis C. HIV is associated with FSGS (HIVAN) and should also be considered in this case, particularly if FSGS is found on biopsy. However, one would not expect the "active" urine sediment (i.e., hematuria, cellular casts) in HIVAN.

References

Abraham RS, Katzmann JA, Clark RJ, et al. Quantitative analysis of serum free light chains. A new marker for the diagnostic evaluation of primary systemic amyloidosis. *Am J Clin Pathol*. 2003;119:274–278.

Alim MA, Yamaki S, Hussein MS, et al. Structural relationship of kappa type light chains with AL amyloid. *Clin Exp Immunol*. 1999;118:334–348.

Alpers CE. Immunotactoid (microtubular) glomerulopathy: an entity distinct from fibrillary glomerulonephritis. *Am J Kidney Dis*. 1992;19:185–191.

Beck LH Jr, Bonegio RG, Lambeau G, et al. M-type phospholipase A2 receptor as target antigen in idiopathic membranous nephropathy. *N Engl J Med*. 2009;361(1):11–21.

Border WA, Okuda S, Languino LR, et al. Suppression of experimental glomerulonephritis by antiserum against transforming growth factor beta I. *Nature*. 1990;346:371–374.

Bridges CR, Myers BD, Brenner BM, et al. Glomerular change alterations in human minimal change nephropathy. *Kidney Int*. 1982;22:677–684.

Brown EA, Markandu ND, Sagnella GA, et al. Evidence that some mechanism other than the renin system causes sodium retention in the nephrotic syndrome. *Lancet*. 1982;2:1237–1240.

Cybulsky AV, Rennke HG, Feintzeig ID, et al. Complement-induced glomerular epithelial cell injury. Role of the membrane attack complex in rat membranous nephrophaty. *J Clin Invest*. 1986;77:1096–1107.

D'Agati VD, Fogo AB, Bruijn JA, et al. Pathologic classification of focal segmental glomerulosclerosis: a working proposal. *Am J Kidney Dis*. 2004;43(2):368–382.

Gilmore JD, Lovat LB, Persey MR, et al. Amyloid load and clinical outcome in AA amyloidosis in relation to circulating concentration of serum amyloid A protein. *Lancet*. 2001;358:24–29.

Husby G, Stenstad T, Magnus JH, et al. Interaction between circulating amyloid fibril protein precursors and extracellular matrix components in the pathogenesis of systemic amyloidosis. *Clin Immunol Immunopathol*. 1994;70:2–9.

Joven J, Villabona C, Vilella E, et al. Abnormalities of lipoprotein metabolism in patients with the nephrotic syndrome. *N Engl J Med*. 1990;323:579–584.

Kauffmann RH, Veltkamp JJ, Van Tilburg NH, et al. Acquired antithrombin III deficiency and thrombosis in the nephrotic syndrome. *Am J Med*. 1978;65(4):607–613.

Rosenstock J, Valeri A, Appel GB, et al. Fibrillary glomerulonephritis. Defining the disease spectrum. *Kidney Int*. 2003;63:1450–1462.

Wei C, El Hindi S, Li J, et al. Circulating urokinase receptor as a cause of focal segmental glomerulosclerosis. *Nat Med*. 2011;17(8):952–960.

Zhu L, Herrera GA, Murphy-Ullrich JE, et al. Pathogenesis of glomerulosclerosis in LCDD: role of TGF-beta. *Am J Pathol*. 1995;147:375–385.

12 Chronic Kidney Disease

DEFINITION

- Chronic kidney disease (CKD) is defined as the presence of clinical and/or pathologic evidence of kidney disease for at least 3 months. CKD is associated with stable renal function over a period of days to months. This distinguishes it from acute renal failure, in which renal function declines over a period of hours to days (see Chapter 9). However, CKD can and often does worsen (progress) with time, i.e., over months to years.
- Kidney disease can be demonstrated by pathologic changes on biopsy, radiologic changes, or laboratory studies such as an abnormal urinalysis or proteinuria.
- Echogenic small kidneys on renal ultrasound confirm CKD (echogenicity alone, especially in association with loss of the corticomedullary junction, is also highly suggestive in normal size kidneys). Large kidneys are characteristic of diabetic kidney disease (DKD), amyloidosis and other infiltrative kidney diseases, and polycystic kidney disease.
- Patients who present with no medical history or records may be inferred to have CKD if the elevated creatinine is stable while in the hospital. However, to confirm the diagnosis of CKD, they should have persistent kidney disease after 3 months (see above). Similarly, albuminuria or total proteinuria (see Chapter 3) should be persistent for 3 months to diagnose CKD based on this parameter, especially if the degree of proteinuria is mild.

CAUSES OF CKD

The causes of CKD and their approximate frequency are given in Table 12.1. It should be recognized that many patients have more than one cause (e.g., diabetes plus hypertension, or hypertension plus ischemia) and that the likelihood of different diseases varies with age, gender, and race. For a discussion of specific types of glomerular disease, see Chapters 10 and 11.

TABLE 12.1 Etiology of CKD

Diabetes mellitus	30%–40%
Hypertensive nephrosclerosis	20%–30%
Chronic glomerulonephritis (primary and secondary)	10%–20%
Chronic tubulointerstitial disease	< 10%
Polycystic kidney disease	~ 5%
Obstructive uropathy	< 5%
Ischemic nephropathy	0%–10%

RISK FACTORS FOR CKD

- Genetic (family history of kidney disease)
- Sociodemographic status (more common in indigent and minority ethnic groups)
- Medical status (e.g., diabetes, hypertension, obesity)

SCREENING FOR CKD

- Screening with urine dipstick for albumin (or complete urinalysis), blood pressure (BP), and serum creatinine (estimated glomerular filtration rate [eGFR]) is indicated in selected populations with the following:
  - Personal or family history of hypertension
  - Diabetes mellitus
  - Edema and/or congestive heart failure (CHF)
  - Atherosclerotic heart or vascular disease
  - Chronic nephrotoxin use (e.g., nonsteroidal anti-inflammatory drugs [NSAIDs], lithium)
  - Personal or family history of kidney disease

CLASSIFICATION OF CKD

- eGFR: The original CKD classification is based on kidney function as assessed by formulae for eGFR (see Chapter 2). Although GFR is a continuum, this classification divides up GFR into stages (Table 12.2). Refinements have been to divide stage 3 CKD into stage 3a (eGFR from 45 to 59) and stage 3b (eGFR from 30 to 44). Some also recommend addition of the suffices p for proteinuria, d for dialysis, and t for transplant.
- eGFR and albuminuria: More recently, the addition of albumin excretion rate (AER), which is associated with progression of CKD, has been included in a revised classification (Table 12.2).

NATURAL HISTORY OF CKD

- Early: Usually asymptomatic in its early stages
- Late: Symptoms and signs (usually related to sodium and water retention, manifesting as hypertension and edema) in association with metabolic and hormonal complications (anemia, vitamin D deficiency, secondary hyperparathyroidism) as well as an increased incidence of cardiovascular disease, infection, and impaired physical function

EVALUATION OF CKD

- Exclude reversible prerenal factors (i.e., renal hypoperfusion): Hypovolemia, hypotension, infection, and administration of drugs that lower the GFR, such as NSAIDs and renin–angiotensin system (RAS) blockers. Unlike the situation in patients with normal kidneys, a low fractional excretion of sodium (FENa) may not be present in CKD because of the decrease in filtered load of sodium (fractional excretion = amount excreted/amount filtered) (see Chapter 9).

TABLE 12.2	Revised CKD Classification Based upon GFR and Albuminuria	
GFR Stages	**GFR (mL/min/1.73 m²)**	**Terms**
G1	>90	Normal or high
G2	60–89	Mildly decreased
G3a	45–59	Mildly to moderately decreased
G3b	30–44	Moderately to severely decreased
G4	15–29	Severely decreased
G5	<15	Kidney failure (add d if treated by dialysis)
Albuminuria Stages	**ACR (mg/g)**	**Terms**
A1	<30 (<3.4 mg/mmol)	Normal to high normal (may be subdivided for risk prediction)
A2	30–300 (3.4–34 mg/mmol)	High
A3	>300 (>34 mg/mmol)	Very high (may be subdivided into nephrotic and non-nephrotic for differential diagnosis, management, and risk prediction)

The cause of CKD is also included in the KDIGO revised classification, but is not included in this table.
Data from National Kidney Foundation. K/DOQI clinical practice guidelines for chronic kidney disease: evaluation, classification, and stratification. *Am J Kidney Dis.* 39(2 suppl 1):S1, 2002.

- Exclude postrenal factors (i.e., obstruction): Usually, this is easily done by ultrasound (bladder scanning and/or renal ultrasound). This is essential in older patients, particularly men. Ultrasound also gives additional helpful information, such as documentation of two kidneys, kidney size, evaluation for renal cysts or masses, exclusion of polycystic disease, identification of nephrocalcinosis or calculi, and, in some centers, evaluation of renal vasculature (see Chapters 9 and 17).

- All patients with CKD should have a basic evaluation, including complete blood count (CBC), urinalysis, electrolytes, renal function (blood urea nitrogen and creatinine), fasting glucose, calcium, phosphorus, magnesium, intact parathyroid hormone (iPTH), 25-(OH)-vitamin D, and urine albumin to creatinine ratio (UACR) and total protein to creatinine ratio. Further evaluations will depend on initial findings and likely diagnostic possibilities. For instance, the presence of hematuria and proteinuria suggests glomerulonephritis (see Chapter 10), and workup should include measurement of antinuclear antibodies, complements (C3, C4), hepatitis panel (B and C), and antineutrophil cytoplasmic antibodies. Nephrotic syndrome should prompt evaluation for diabetes (glycated hemoglobin [Hb]) and consideration of primary AL amyloidosis (serum protein electrophoresis [SPEP], urine protein electrophoresis [UPEP], serum and urine free light chains) and HIV-associated nephropathy (HIVAN) (HIV antibodies, viral load). A high urine total protein without albuminuria suggests paraproteinuria due to myeloma or primary AL (SPEP, UPEP, serum and urine free light chains).

■ Determination of rate of CKD progression: Untreated CKD will typically lead to a progressive decline in GFR at a characteristic rate, depending on the etiology of the disease, the degree of proteinuria, BP control, and other factors. A rate of decline in GFR of >5 mL/min/1.73 m^2/y is considered to be rapid progression; in most patients, GFR will decline at a rate of 2 to 4 mL/min/1.73 m^2/y, though some patients will progress at a very slow rate (<1 mL/min/1.73 m^2/y), a rate not distinguishable from the normal age-related decline in kidney function. In an individual patient, the rate of GFR decline in the past is a very good predictor of the future course of kidney disease and whether to expect end-stage renal disease (ESRD) to develop. For instance, a 55-year-old patient with a GFR of 30 mL/min/1.73 m^2 and a rate of GFR decline of 10 mL/min/1.73 m^2/y despite aggressive management (see below) is almost certain to require dialysis or transplantation in the future (probably in about 2 years), but an 80-year-old patient with a GFR of 20 mL/min/1.73 m^2 and a rate of GFR decline of 1 mL/min/1.73 m^2/y may not live long enough to ever need dialysis.

MANAGEMENT OF CKD

■ **Nutrition:** Before the availability of dialysis, the only therapy for uremia is to reduce protein intake. Although it is clear that protein restriction can decrease uremic symptoms, there is no clear evidence that it can reduce the rate of progression of CKD. However, moderate protein restriction (not <0.8 g/kg/d) may be useful and not detrimental. Phosphate restriction can prevent secondary hyperparathyroidism (see below) and may decrease vascular calcification, although this is still an unproven hypothesis. In the presence of hypertension or edema, sodium restriction is indicated (see below), and potassium restriction is necessary if there is hyperkalemia. The US National Kidney Foundation provides useful dietary guidelines (www.kidney.org).

■ **Salt and water retention:** As GFR declines, the ability of the kidneys to excrete dietary sodium is impaired, leading to a tendency to sodium retention (edema) and development of hypertension. Loop diuretics such as furosemide (Lasix) rather than thiazide diuretics are usually required, in particular when GFR is below 50% of normal. Occasionally, a combination of a loop diuretic and a thiazide-type diuretic (such as hydrochlorothiazide or metolazone) is needed. A brisk diuresis may ensue because of blockade of sodium transport at both the loop and distal tubule (see Chapter 14).

■ **Hypertension:** Edema in a hypertensive patient necessitates dietary salt restriction and institution of or increase in diuretics. Control of BP in patients with CKD almost always requires diuretic therapy in addition to other antihypertensive agents because most patients with CKD and hypertension will be volume overloaded even if edema is absent. RAS inhibitors are preferred in proteinuric

CKD because of their proven renoprotective effects, though it is difficult, if not impossible, to determine whether their beneficial effects are solely owing to lowering of BP or involve mechanisms specific to RAS inhibition. Moreover, hyperkalemia due to decreased aldosterone production or effect is a major problem in many patients. Dihydropyridine calcium blockers can increase proteinuria and glomerular injury and should be avoided in proteinuric CKD if possible. In the absence of proteinuria, there is no specific preferred or nonpreferred agent. Control of hypertension regardless of the drugs used is the most important intervention to slow progression of CKD (indeed, the only proven intervention). Other modalities that may be beneficial include control of blood glucose (in diabetics), lipid (statin therapy), and smoking cessation. Whether or not they affect CKD progression, these interventions are indicated for cardiovascular risk reduction (see Chapter 14).

■ **Cardiovascular disease:** Patients with CKD and especially ESKD have a high rate of cardiovascular disease, which has not been completely explained. Among the traditional risk factors, hypertension, diabetes mellitus, and hyperlipidemia are common in this population. Patients with CKD are also frequently obese with low physical activity. Nontraditional risk factors include proteinuria, oxidative stress, inflammation, hyperphosphatemia (leading to vascular calcification), and, possibly, anemia (although correction of anemia has not been shown to decrease cardiac risk).

CASE STUDY 12.1 A 62-year-old woman with a long history of type 2 diabetes mellitus and hypertension presents for follow-up of CKD. Since her last visit, she missed a few months of her erythropoietin injections and has not been eating well. Her BP has been well controlled. Glycemic control is variable. She denies uremic symptoms including nausea, vomiting, anorexia, dysgeusia, and cognitive changes. She denies changes in voiding habits. She denies chest pain, dyspnea on exertion, orthopnea, lower extremity edema, or symptoms of claudication. However, she does complain of generalized fatigue.

Medications:
Amlodipine: 10 mg daily
Aspirin: 81 mg daily
Calcitriol: 0.25 mcg daily
Carvedilol: 6.25 mg twice daily
Cholecalciferol: 1,000 units daily
Clonidine: 0.3 mg/24 hour patch every 7 days
Ferrous gluconate: 325 mg twice daily
Insulin glargine: 30 units subcutaneously (SC) daily
Insulin lispro: 12 units SC before meals
Losartan: 50 mg daily
Rosuvastatin: 10 mg nightly

Sodium bicarbonate: 1,300 mg twice daily
Epoetin alfa: 10,000 units SC every 30 days

Physical examination:
Vitals: temperature, 36.3°C (97.4°F); pulse, 69 beats/min; respiratory rate, 20 breaths/min; BP, 135/85 mm Hg; height, 5 ft 3 in (160 cm); weight, 77 kg (169 lb 14 oz)
GEN: appears stated age, no apparent distress
HEENT: normocephalic, atraumatic, extraocular muscles intact, anicteric
NECK: no jugular venous distension, no carotid bruits, no lymphadenopathy or thyromegaly
COR: normal S1, S2, no rubs/gallops/murmurs
PULM: clear to auscultation, no rales, no wheezes
ABD: soft, nontender, no bruits
EXT: trace edema, no cyanosis, peripheral pulses symmetrical
SKIN: no lesions, no nail changes, no rash
NEUROPSYCH: mood appropriate, no focal findings

Blood chemistry:
Sodium: 138 mmol/L
Potassium: 4 mmol/L
Chloride: 100 mmol/L
Total CO_2: 18 mmol/L
Urea nitrogen: 28 mg/dL (urea, 10 mmol/L)
Creatinine: 3.3 mg/dL (292 mcmol/L) (eGFR, 18 mL/min)
UACR: 895 mg/g (101 mg/mmol)
Hemoglobin: 9 g/dL
Iron: 80 mcg/dL
Transferrin saturation (TSAT): 25%
Ferritin: 400 ng/mL
Total calcium: 9 mg/dL (2.25 mg/dL)
Inorganic phosphorus: 4.0 mg/dL (1.3 mmol/L)
25-(OH)-vitamin D: 31 ng/mL (77 nmol/L) (normal)
iPTH: 150 pg/mL (15.9 pmol/L) (normal: 10–65 pg/mL)

Question 12.1.1: What is the stage of CKD?

Stage G4 A3 CKD: Clinically, she has DKD based on long-standing diabetes, proteinuria, and retinopathy.

Question 12.1.2: What should be the goals of treatment in this patient?

The patient does not need dialysis at this point, though the likelihood of her needing it in the future is high. Because her eGFR is <20 mL/min/1.73 m^2, she should be evaluated for receipt of a deceased or living donor kidney transplant. Efforts should be aimed at attempting to slow disease progression, including control of BP, proteinuria, glycemic control, avoidance of nephrotoxins, and management of metabolic sequelae associated with CKD.

Question 12.1.3: **What is the significance of the proteinuria?**

Because she has overt proteinuria, the goal should be to maximize losartan as tolerated (avoid hyperkalemia). The BP goal should be <130/80 mm Hg. HbA_{1c} should be <8%. A low-moderate protein diet (0.8 g/kg) may be of benefit. Smoking and NSAIDs should be avoided.

Question 12.1.4: **What is the pathophysiology of anemia?**

- Pathogenesis: As GFR declines, erythropoietin (EPO) production by the kidney is impaired, which typically results in anemia (Hb level <13.0 g/dL in males or <12.0 g/dL in females). Anemia is generally present with moderate CKD, though severe anemia (Hb <9 g/dL) is unusual unless CKD is severe. Other factors, in particular iron deficiency, should be excluded (McGonigle et al., 1984).

- Symptoms: The onset of anemia in CKD is gradual, and patients may not be symptomatic. If present, symptoms may include fatigue, weakness, and lack of energy and enthusiasm. Examination may show pallor. If severe, symptoms of heart failure may occur.

- Laboratory evaluation:
  - CBC—confirms anemia and may suggest an alternative diagnosis other than anemia of CKD (e.g., if there is pancytopenia, schistocytes on the peripheral smear, etc.)
  - Serum iron to total iron-binding capacity (TIBC) ratio (TSAT) and ferritin—iron and ferritin are low, and TIBC is elevated in iron deficiency. Ferritin is an acute-phase reactant and is increased in acute or chronic illness
  - Vitamin B_{12} and folate—may be deficient and should be investigated
  - Reticulocyte count—is a measure of bone marrow response
  - Fecal immunotest for blood—gastrointestinal (GI) bleed is a common confounder
  - Haptoglobin, Coombs—exclude hemolysis
  - EPO levels are generally not necessary unless the degree of anemia is out of proportion to the degree of CKD
  - Reticulocyte Hb content (may be the best marker for functional iron deficiency, but this test is not widely available)
  - Soluble transferrin receptor (sTfR) concentration (directly proportional to EPO rate and inversely proportional to tissue iron availability; thus, iron-deficient patients usually have increased levels of sTfR)

Question 12.1.5: **What are the goals for anemia in a CKD patient?**

Erythropoietin-stimulating agents (ESAs) such as EPO are indicated to treat anemia in CKD not owing to other reversible factors (such as iron deficiency). There is no definitive Hb threshold for starting EPO, though it is agreed that sufficient EPO should be administered to avoid transfusions. We usually start EPO when Hb <9 g/dL and try to keep Hb in the 9 to 11 g/dL range. Hb concentrations >12 g/dL have been associated with increased mortality in CKD and ESRD patients.

In the Normal Hematocrit Study (Besarab et al., 1998), low hematocrit versus normal hematocrit in patients undergoing hemodialysis

(HD) is compared. Achieving a normal hematocrit is associated with an increase in deaths by 30%.

In the Correction of Anemia with Epoetin alfa in Chronic Kidney Disease (CHOIR) study (Singh et al., 2006), the use of epoetin alfa targeting a Hb of 13.5 g/dL is compared to 11.3 g/dL in nondialysis CKD patients. The higher Hb target has a 30% increase in myocardial infarction, stroke, death, and CHF hospitalization.

In a trial of darbepoetin alfa in type 2 diabetes and nondialysis CKD disease (TREAT) (Pfeffer et al., 2009), Hb targets of 13 versus 9 g/dL are compared. Targeting an Hb of 13 g/dL does not have any benefits and is associated with an increased risk of stroke, eightfold higher risk of cancer-related death, and threefold higher risk of recurrent stroke.

This patient's Hb is 9 g/dL. Her TSAT is 25% and ferritin 400 ng/mL, and thus she is not overtly iron deficient. For nondialysis CKD, TSAT should be >20% and ferritin >200 ng/mL.

CKD is a chronic inflammatory state. Inflammatory markers such as C-reactive protein (CRP) are elevated. Hepcidin, synthesized in the liver in response to inflammation, impairs absorption of iron from the gut and prevents iron release from the reticuloendothelial system. In CKD, TSAT is frequently low despite normal ferritin levels. In such patients, oral iron may be poorly absorbed and parenteral iron may more rapidly effective than oral iron, but is associated with increased cost and side effects. Common intravenous (IV) iron preparations include ferric gluconate (Ferrlecit), iron sucrose (Venofer), and ferumoxytol (Feraheme).

> **Question 12.1.6:** How should anemia be treated in CKD?

■ Erythropoietic-stimulating agents (ESAs): epoetin alfa, 50 to 100 units/kg IV/SC, three times a week OR darbepoetin, 0.45 mcg/kg IV/SC, qweek or 0.75 mcg/kg IV/SC, q2weeks OR epoetin beta and methoxy polyethylene glycol, 0.6 mcg/kg IV/SC q2weeks.

■ Iron: oral iron (e.g., ferrous sulfate, 325 mg PO, thrice daily); IV iron (iron sucrose, ferric gluconate, iron dextran, ferumoxytol; various schedules and regimens have been used) may be needed (Moinuddin & Leehey, 2012).

CASE STUDY 12.1 CONTINUED

The iron stores of this patient are replete, so IV iron supplementation is not necessary. However, administration of oral iron is indicated to avoid the later development of iron deficiency associated with iron utilization after EPO administration.

Anemia of CKD is associated with both EPO deficiency and EPO resistance. The role of hypoxia-inducible factor (HIF) has recently been highlighted. HIF alpha and beta subunits dimerize to form HIF alpha/beta that acts on HIF-responsive elements in the *EPO* gene. Prolyl hydroxylase dioxygenase (PHD) hydroxylates HIF and causes its degradation, and its activity is inhibited by hypoxia. Prolyl hydroxylase inhibitors (PHIs) are now being developed with the intent of inhibiting PHD, thereby preventing HIF degradation and decreased

EPO production. Because EPO can be made in both the kidney and the liver, PHIs are effective in both severe CKD and ESRD.

HIF stabilizers may be safer than EPO. They are oral agents and reduce hepcidin, thus increasing GI iron absorption. However, because HIF modulates many genes (including *VEGF*), the role of PHI in angiogenesis and tumor formation is an area of concern. There has been one case of hepatic necrosis leading to death associated with their use.

Question 12.1.7: **What is the pathophysiology of secondary hyperparathyroidism in CKD?**

■ The kidney is the organ primarily responsible for converting 25-(OH)-vitamin D into the active 1,25-(OH)$_2$-vitamin D. With declining GFR, patients will develop active vitamin D deficiency and a resultant fall in serum calcium (albeit not necessarily below the normal range), which then stimulates PTH secretion. PTH serves to release calcium from bone and also stimulates phosphorus excretion and can thereby maintain calcium and phosphorus levels within the normal range well into stage IV CKD. However, owing to declining GFR, the excretion of phosphorus is impaired, leading to a tendency to hyperphosphatemia. Secondary hyperparathyroidism is associated with a classic triad of hypocalcemia, hyperphosphatemia, and elevated PTH levels.

■ As GFR declines, the excretion of phosphorus is impaired, leading to a tendency to hyperphosphatemia. Recently, it has been demonstrated that fibroblast growth factor 23 (FGF23) is stimulated by phosphorus retention; FGF23 causes phosphaturia (via both parathyroid-dependent and parathyroid-independent mechanisms) and maintains serum phosphorus in the normal range until there is a substantial decline in GFR (usually <30 mL/min/1.73 m^2). FGF23 also decreases 1,25-(OH)$_2$-vitamin D (calcitriol) formation, which, in conjunction with hyperphosphatemia, will lead to parathyroid hyperplasia and an increase in PTH secretion. Treatment is dietary phosphorus restriction with or without phosphorus binders (see Chapter 8). Supplementation with vitamin D (patients with CKD are frequently vitamin D deficient) and, possibly, calcitriol are often needed (see Chapter 8).

Question 12.1.8: **What are the goals for bone mineral metabolism?**

It should be noted that guidelines for metabolic bone disease in CKD are often based on a rather low level of evidence. At the present time, it is advised that calcium and phosphorus be maintained in the normal range. Progressive increases in PTH should be treated with calcitriol or vitamin D analogues like doxercalciferol or paricalcitol. Oral cinacalcet or IV etelcalcitide can be used in refractory secondary hyperparathyroidism. These agents are calcium sensing receptor agonists that reduce PTH secretion by reducing the threshold for activation by calcium.

The following goals have been issued, none based on high-quality evidence:

iPTH: stage 3: 35 to 70 pg/mL, stage 4: 70 to 110 pg/mL, stage 5: 150 to 300 pg/mL

Calcium: stages 3 to 4: normal, stage 5: 8.4 to 9.5 mg/dL
Phosphorus: stages 3 to 4: 2.7 to 4.6 mg/dL; stage 5: 3.5 to 5.5 mg/dL
Calcium × phosphorus < 55
25-(OH)-vitamin D (calcidiol) > 30 ng/mL

CASE STUDY 12.1 CONTINUED

In this patient, PTH is at goal for stage 4 CKD (70–110); calcidiol is replete on vitamin D_3 therapy. Phosphorus is at target without binders. Calcitriol may be continued, although recent guidelines now suggest reserving calcitriol for patients in whom iPTH is substantially elevated and progressively increasing or if there are symptoms and/or signs of secondary hyperparathyroidism.

Question 12.1.9: What are the other major electrolyte disturbances in CKD?

As GFR declines, potassium excretion is impaired, which can result in hyperkalemia (see Chapter 6). Metabolic acidosis can be of the hyperchloremic or high–anion gap type or both and should be treated with bicarbonate or other alkali (see Chapter 7); recent data suggest that alkali therapy may slow progression of CKD (de Brito-Ashurst et al., 2009; Mahajan et al., 2010; Phisitkul et al., 2010).

Question 12.1.10: What are the consequences of metabolic acidosis in CKD?

Metabolic acidosis has been associated with bone resorption, systemic inflammation, hypotension, increased mortality, and progression of CKD. It is suggested that a lower limit of 22 mEq/L should be targeted for CKD patients. Sodium bicarbonate or sodium citrate should be administered orally in doses of 0.5 to 1 mEq/kg/d.

Question 12.1.11: What variables are associated with progression of CKD?

Progression of CKD is associated with hypertension, proteinuria, hyperlipidemia, smoking, and metabolic acidosis. Therefore, emphasis should be placed on controlling BP, reducing proteinuria (through moderate protein restriction and angiotensin-converting enzyme inhibitor/angiotensin-receptor blockers [ACE-I/ARBs]), statin therapy, smoking cessation, and alkali therapy.

Question 12.1.12: What long-term strategies should be implemented at this time?

Once eGFR <20, most patients should be referred to an educator(s) knowledgeable in renal replacement therapy (RRT). A major goal is for the patient to choose RRT modality in advance of the need for dialysis. If peritoneal dialysis (PD) is chosen, PD catheter placement can generally be postponed until the patient is expected to need dialysis within a few weeks to months. If HD is chosen, an arteriovenous fistula (AVF) should generally be created at this time (if a graft fistula is required, its placement can be delayed until the patient is near to starting dialysis, similar to PD). Early referral for transplant evaluation is very important. So the patient can be on a waiting list for a deceased donor kidney transplant prior to the need for RRT initiation. In some cases, particularly with living donor transplantation, preemptive transplantation can obviate the need for dialysis.

CASE STUDY 12.1 CONCLUDED

Because this patient does not have any suitable living donors and the wait time for deceased donor transplantation is up to 5 years in many states, it is important to plan for dialysis in this patient, at least as a bridge to transplantation.

Question 12.1.13: What is the role of exercise in CKD?

Aerobic exercise and resistance training have been shown to decrease inflammation, oxidative stress, endothelial dysfunction; reduce BP; improve hyperlipidemia, proteinuria and endurance; decrease insulin resistance; improve obesity; decrease cardiovascular mortality and morbidity; and may decrease the rate of progression of CKD (Castaneda et al., 2004; Heiwe & Jacobson, 2011; Johansen & Painter, 2012; Leehey et al., 2009; Moinuddin & Leehey, 2008, 2010; Tentori, 2008).

Question 12.1.14: When should primary care physicians seek nephrology consultation?

INDICATIONS FOR NEPHROLOGY REFERRAL

- Severely decreased GFR (eGFR <30 mL/min/1.73 m^2, i.e., stage 4CKD), especially in younger patients and/or patients with progressive CKD. This allows for optimization of conservative therapy to delay progression and prevent or treat complications and preparation for RRT (dialysis and/or transplantation)
- Overt proteinuria, i.e., UACR >300 mg/g (34 mg/mmol), especially if the cause is uncertain, as such patients may require kidney biopsy for diagnosis and therapy
- Hematuria not secondary to urologic conditions
- CKD associated with resistant hypertension (uncontrolled BP despite use of three or more drugs at optimal doses)
- Complications such as anemia requiring EPO therapy and abnormalities of bone and mineral metabolism requiring phosphorus binders or vitamin D preparations
- Hyperkalemia (serum potassium > 5.5 mEq/L) resistant to therapy with diet, diuretics, and adjustment of drugs that cause hyperkalemia (see Chapter 6)

12

PROGRESSION OF CKD

A 55-year-old male patient with type 2 diabetes and DKD manifested as proteinuria and hypertension has a GFR of 30 mL/min/1.73 m^2. One year earlier, the GFR was 40, and the year before that, it was 50.

Q1: The patient wants to know whether and when he is likely to require RRT (dialysis and/or transplantation) in the future. What is your answer?

1. Dialysis will likely be necessary in about 1 year
2. Dialysis will likely be necessary in about 2 years
3. Dialysis will probably never be necessary
4. It is impossible to answer this question

A1: At the current rate of decline of kidney function (10 mL/min/1.73 m^2/y), this patient is predicted to have a GFR of 10 mL/min/1.73 m^2 and need RRT in about 2 years.

Q2: What modalities have been proven to slow rate of progression of kidney disease in diabetic patients?

1. Blood glucose control
2. BP control
3. Blood lipid control
4. Treatment of metabolic complications such as hyperphosphatemia
5. Treatment of anemia

A2: The correct answer is BP control. Seminal observations in the late 1970s and early 1980s initially pointed out the importance of BP control in delaying progression of CKD in type 1 diabetic patients with nephropathy. Further support comes from larger studies in type 2 diabetic patients such as UK Prospective Diabetes Study (UKPDS). A number of randomized controlled trials in both type 1 and type 2 diabetes have shown that RAS blockers slow progression more than standard antihypertensive therapy, although BP is usually lower in patients treated with RAS blockers. Although glucose control is important for preventing microvascular complications, it remains uncertain as to whether it can slow progression of established nephropathy. There is no evidence that blood lipid control, control of hyperphosphatemia, or treatment of anemia slows progression.

PROGRESSION OF CKD

An 80-year-old female patient with hypertensive nephrosclerosis and a GFR of 20 mL/min/1.73 m^2 and a rate of GFR decline of 1 mL/min/1.73 m^2/y is referred to you for evaluation. She complains of fatigue and dyspnea on climbing stairs, which were not present 1 year ago. On examination, the BP is 180/70 mm Hg. There is a prominent left ventricular impulse but no signs of fluid overload. There is no proteinuria. An echocardiogram shows left ventricular hypertrophy (LVH) with preserved systolic function. She is severely anemic (Hb 9 g/dL).

Q: Which one of the following are not indicated?

1. Treatment of hypertension
2. Administration of RAS blockers
3. Administration of ESAs such as epoetin alfa
4. Referral for access placement for future HD

A: The most important intervention for prevention of cardiovascular complications is BP control. Although the rate of progression of CKD is very slow in this patient, lowering BP may prevent renal progression as well. RAS blockers are preferred for cardiovascular protection, but the development of hyperkalemia is a concern. Because she is symptomatic with severe anemia, administration of ESAs is indicated for improvement of quality of life and may improve LVH. However, in view of this patient's age and slow rate of progression of CKD, it is unlikely that she will ever require HD, and access placement is not indicated.

ANEMIA

A 71-year-old white female with stage 4 CKD (eGFR 20 mL/min/1.73 m^2) complains of fatigue and dyspnea on exertion. On physical examination, the skin and conjunctivae are pale. Vital signs are normal, and she is not hypoxic.

Blood chemistry:
Sodium: 140 mmol/L
Potassium: 4.0 mmol/L
Chloride: 110 mmol/L
Total CO_2: 26 mmol/L
Urea nitrogen: 40 mg/dL (urea: 14.3 mmol/L)
Creatinine: 2.5 mg/dL (221 mcmol/L)
Glucose: 120 mg/dL (6.7 mmol/L)
Aspartate aminotransferase (AST): 35 U/L
Alanine aminotransferase (ALT): 30 U/L
Alkaline phosphatase: 80 U/L
Total bilirubin: 1.0 mg/dL (17.1 mcmol/L)

Complete blood count:
WBCs: 5,000/mm^3
Hemoglobin: 9.0 g/dL (90 g/L)
Hematocrit: 25%
Mean corpuscular volume: 85 fL
Platelets: 500,000/mm^3

Echocardiogram:
Ejection fraction: 55%
Mitral valve E:A ratio: 1.5
Right ventricular systolic pressure: 25 mm Hg
Persantine thallium stress test, negative for ischemia
Serum ferritin: 50 ng/mL (112 pmol/L)
Serum iron: 25 (4.5 mcmol/L)
TIBC: 250 (4.5 mcmol/L)
TSAT: 10%
Thyroid-stimulating hormone: 2.0 mIU/L (normal)

Q: Which of the following is indicated in this patient?

1. Administration of epoetin alfa to normalize Hb (>13 g/dL)
2. Administration of epoetin alfa to correct Hb to 10 to 11 g/dL
3. Administration of iron to normalize Hb (>13 g/dL)
4. Administration of iron to correct Hb to 10 to 11 g/dL

A: Fatigue in patients with CKD may results from a number of causes, most prominently cardiac disease and anemia. In this case, the echocardiogram is unrevealing, but there is moderately severe anemia. Although EPO deficiency is probably present in a patient with stage 4 CKD, this patient clearly has laboratory findings of iron deficiency (note that in CKD, serum ferritin is usually normal or elevated due to chronic inflammation, so the value of 50 ng/mL, coupled with the low TSAT, is highly suggestive of iron deficiency in this patient). Reticulocyte Hb content and/or sTfR concentration may be useful in some cases, but are not necessary here.

Recent clinical trials such as Correction of Hemoglobin and Outcomes in Renal Insufficiency (CHOIR) and Cardiovascular Reduction Early Anemia Treatment Epoetin beta (CREATE) have provided evidence that normalization of Hb with ESAs such as epoetin alfa (EPO) are not helpful and potentially hazardous owing to a higher rate of cerebrovascular events. Although similar data with iron therapy alone are not available, it would be prudent to only correct Hb to a range of 10 to 11 g/dL, which should be sufficient for relief of symptoms in this patient.

MEDICATION MANAGEMENT

A 55-year-old woman with diabetes mellitus, hypertension, and hyperlipidemia treated with metformin, lisinopril, simvastatin, aspirin, and acetaminophen presents for evaluation of elevated plasma creatinine. She is asymptomatic. She has been checking her blood glucose and has not been hypoglycemic. Her fasting glucose levels at home have been below 140 mg/dL. She does have diabetic retinopathy. She does not complain of chest pain, shortness of breath, or lower extremity rash or ulcers. She is intensely afraid of needles and wants to avoid insulin at all cost. She has been seeing a dietician who monitors her oral intake and her carbohydrate intake. She walks to the local park every day; the round trip takes about 45 minutes.

On physical examination, the BP is 125/80 mm Hg. Cardiopulmonary examination is normal. Kidneys are not palpable. There is no abdominal bruit. Lower extremities are free of onychomycosis, ulcers, rash, and edema.

Blood chemistry:
Sodium: 136 mmol/L
Potassium: 5.0 mmol/L
Chloride: 110 mmol/L
Total CO_2: 20 mmol/L
Urea nitrogen: 30 mg/dL (urea: 10.7 mmol/L)

Creatinine: 2.0 mg/dL (177 mcmol/L)
Glucose: 130 mg/dL (7.2 mmol/L)
eGFR: 32 mL/min/1.73 m^2
UACR: 200 mg/g (22.7 mg/mmol)

Renal ultrasound, kidneys 10 cm long bilaterally; mild increase in echogenicity

Q: Which of the following is usable in diabetic nephropathy stage 3?

1. Metformin 500 mg PO twice daily
2. Glipizide 10 mg PO daily
3. Metformin 500 mg PO daily
4. Sitagliptin (Januvia) 100 mg PO daily
5. Nateglinide 120 mg PO three times daily

A: Metformin can cause lactic acidosis in patients with CKD because it is excreted unchanged in the urine and accumulates with reduction in renal function. Thus, the use of metformin is contraindicated in stages 3 to 5 CKD.

First-generation sulfonylureas are generally contraindicated in CKD. Among second-generation sulfonylureas, glibenclamide undergoes oxidation by the liver to three major metabolites, one of which has 15% potency of glibenclamide and is excreted in the urine. Thus, glibenclamide carries with it the risk of hypoglycemia in CKD. Glimepiride is also metabolized in the liver to two metabolites, one of which is weakly active and excreted in the urine. Thus, glimepiride is also associated with a risk of hypoglycemia in CKD. Glyburide is excreted 50% in the bile and 50% in the urine; its two metabolites have very little, if any, hypoglycemic action. Glyburide is to be avoided in CKD. Glipizide and gliclazide are metabolized by the liver to several inactive metabolites; these are usable in CKD.

The glinides are weak hypoglycemics. Repaglinide and mitiglinide are usable in CKD. A small amount of nateglinide is excreted in the urine, and its active metabolite is also excreted. Thus, in stages 3 to 5 CKD, nateglinide may pose a risk of hypoglycemia. Nateglinide 80 mg PO three times daily may be acceptable.

Exenatide is cleared by the kidney, and its use in advanced CKD (stages 4 and 5) is not recommended. Sitagliptin is excreted in the urine but can be used in reduced doses (50 mg daily in stage 3 CKD and 25 mg daily in stage 4 CKD).

Thiazolidinediones are generally discouraged in all patients because of significant cardiovascular risk, including fluid retention and CHF. These side effects are particularly problematic in CKD.

Acarbose and miglitol are not recommended in CKD. The National Kidney Foundation Disease Outcomes Quality Initiative (KDOQI) guidelines recommend avoidance of these drugs because of lack of data in CKD.

Insulin, in reduced doses, may be used in CKD of any stage. However, insulin is mainly eliminated by the kidney. A 25% decrease in dose is warranted in GFR between 50 and 10 mL/min; a 50% decrease in dose is warranted in GFR <10 mL/min.

References

Besarab A, Bolton WK, Browne JK, et al. The effects of normal as compared with low hematocrit values in patients with cardiac disease who are receiving hemodialysis and epoetin. *N Engl J Med.* 339(9):584–590, 1998.

Castaneda C, Gordon PL, Parker RC, et al. Resistance training to reduce the malnutrition-inflammation complex syndrome of chronic kidney disease. *Am J Kidney Dis.* 43(4):607–616, 2004.

de Brito-Ashurst I, Varagunam M, Raftery MJ, et al. Bicarbonate supplementation slows progression of CKD and improves nutritional status. *J Am Soc Nephrol.* 20(9):2075–2084, 2009.

Heiwe S, Jacobson SH. Exercise training for adults with chronic kidney disease. *Cochrane Database Syst Rev.* (10):CD003236, 2011.

Johansen KL, Painter P. Exercise in individuals with CKD. *Am J Kidney Dis.* 59(1): 126–134, 2012.

Leehey DJ, Moinuddin I, Bast JP, et al. Aerobic exercise in obese diabetic patients with chronic kidney disease: a randomized and controlled pilot study. *Cardiovasc Diabetol.* 8:62, 2009.

Mahajan A, Simoni J, Sheather SJ, et al. Daily oral sodium bicarbonate preserves glomerular filtration rate by slowing its decline in early hypertensive nephropathy. *Kidney Int.* 78(3):303–309, 2010.

McGonigle RJ, Wallin JD, Shadduck RK, et al. Erythropoietin deficiency and inhibition of erythropoiesis in renal insufficiency. *Kidney Int.* 25(2):437–444, 1984.

Moinuddin I, Leehey D. Aerobic exercise in patients with chronic kidney disease. In: Lieberman DC, ed. *Aerobic Exercise and Athletic Performance: Types, Duration, and Health*. New York, NY: Nova Publishers; 2010:323–340.

Moinuddin I, Leehey D. The story of iron: excess, deficiency and therapy. In: Ing TS, Rahman M, Kjellstrand C, eds. *Dialysis: History, Development and Promise*. New Jersey, NJ: World Scientific; 2012.

Moinuddin I, Leehey DJ. A comparison of aerobic exercise and resistance training in patients with and without chronic kidney disease. *Adv Chronic Kidney Dis*. 15(1):83–96, 2008.

Pfeffer MA, Burdmann EA, Chen CY, et al. A trial of darbepoetin alfa in type 2 diabetes and chronic kidney disease. *N Engl J Med*. 361(21):2019–2032, 2009.

Phisitkul S, Khanna A, Simoni J, et al. Amelioration of metabolic acidosis in patients with low GFR reduced kidney endothelin production and kidney injury, and better preserved GFR. *Kidney Int*. 77(7):617–623, 2010.

Singh AK, Szczech L, Tang KL, et al. Correction of anemia with epoetin alfa in chronic kidney disease. *N Engl J Med*. 355(20):2085–2098, 2006.

Tentori F. Focus on: physical exercise in hemodialysis patients. *J Nephrol*. 21(6):808–812, 2008.

13 Diabetic Kidney Disease

DEFINITION

Diabetic kidney disease (DKD), also called diabetic nephropathy and diabetic glomerulosclerosis, is defined as chronic kidney disease (CKD) in a patient with diabetes mellitus (DM) and either macroalbuminuria (>300 mg/24 hours) or microalbuminuria (30–300 mg/24 hours) associated with retinopathy or 10 years duration of type 1 diabetes. This definition assumes absence of other suspected or known causes of CKD (see section on Differential Diagnosis below).

While classically DKD is characterized by proteinuria in the setting of long-standing DM, more recently many patients have been diagnosed with nonproteinuric DKD (Kramer et al., 2003; Robles et al., 2015). Such patients have CKD without significant proteinuria; in those undergoing renal biopsy, some have had typical diabetic glomerulosclerosis. Absence of proteinuria in some patients may be due to control of blood pressure (BP) with antiproteinuric agents such as renin–angiotensin system (RAS) blockers.

BACKGROUND

In 2015, about 9.4% of the US population had DM (American Diabetes Association, 2015) (Centers for Disease Control and Prevention). The current worldwide epidemic of this disease, fueled by rising rates of obesity and inactivity, is responsible for significant morbidity and mortality. In addition to kidney failure, diabetes causes complications such as blindness, myocardial infarctions, cerebrovascular accidents, amputations, and death.

DIAGNOSIS

The diagnosis of DKD requires that the definition criteria are met. Such patients frequently have other diabetic complications such as neuropathy, peripheral vascular disease, stroke, and coronary artery disease. Hypertension is usually present. Nephrotic syndrome (massive proteinuria, edema, hypoalbuminemia, hyperlipidemia, and lipiduria) may be present in severe cases. A kidney biopsy is diagnostic, but is usually not necessary to establish the diagnosis.

PATHOPHYSIOLOGY

- DKD tends to occur in susceptible individuals only; part of this susceptibility involves genetic factors. It has been shown that only up to 40% of diabetic patients will develop kidney disease. Patients destined to develop DKD usually have poorly controlled diabetes and a family history of hypertension and/or kidney disease. They may also have hypertension and, in particular, nocturnal hypertension (nondippers). The pathophysiology involves many factors including sustained hyperglycemia, hypertension, glomerular hyperfiltration, dyslipidemia, proteinuria levels, dietary content of protein and fat, and adverse behaviors (inactivity, smoking).

■ Both hyperglycemia and increased glomerular capillary pressure lead to expansion of the glomerular mesangium. A number of mediators, including platelet-derived growth factor and transforming growth factor-beta (TGF-β), result in fibrosis via collagen and fibronectin accumulation. Elevated glucose leads to increased protein binding and formation of advanced glycosylated end products (AGEs). AGEs also stimulate the release of growth factors such as TGF-β and cause fibrosis. Angiotensin II (AII), elevated in DKD, constricts the efferent arteriole in the glomerulus, causing high glomerular capillary pressures. AII also stimulates fibrosis by upregulating TGF-β (Schena & Gesualdo, 2005).

■ Mesangial expansion is characteristic of early DKD and is followed by fibrosis in the late stages. Kimmelstiel-Wilson nodules, areas of acellular mesangial expansion on biopsy, are the pathologic hallmark of the disease. Increased glomerular basement membrane width, diffuse mesangial sclerosis, hyalinosis, microaneurysms, and hyaline arteriosclerosis are present in addition to tubular and interstitial changes.

SCREENING

■ Because advanced DKD is more resistant to treatment, is associated with greater cardiovascular morbidity and mortality, and is more likely to progress to end-stage kidney disease and dialysis, screening and prevention are recommended.

■ Type 1 diabetic patients should begin annual screening for microalbuminuria 5 years after diagnosis of diabetes, and type 2 diabetic patients should begin annual screening for microalbuminuria at the time of diagnosis of diabetes. Microalbuminuria should be quantified with an albumin to creatinine ratio. An albumin to creatinine ratio between 30 and 300 mg/g (3.4–34 mg/mmol) is classified as microalbuminuria, and an albumin to creatinine ratio >300 mg/g (34 mg/mmol) is consistent with macroalbuminuria. An abnormal albumin to creatinine ratio in the microalbuminuric range should be confirmed with two additional first-void urine specimens over the next 3 to 6 months.

■ Diabetics with CKD may have elevated glomerular filtration rate (eGFR) in the early stages; hence, GFR alone is not useful for screening purposes.

PREVENTION

■ Preventive measures include the use of an angiotensin-converting enzyme inhibitor (ACE-I) or angiotensin-receptor blocker (ARB)

in all diabetic patients with microalbuminuria or macroalbuminuria regardless of BP (most such patients do have hypertension when 24-hour BP readings are obtained).
■ Diet, exercise, and weight loss are preventive of diabetes in all patient populations and are indicated for patients with DKD. Ophthalmologic evaluation, including a comprehensive dilated eye examination, should be performed yearly. Podiatric evaluation should be performed annually, and the feet should be examined at each primary care visit.

DIFFERENTIAL DIAGNOSIS

CKD in diabetes could be caused by a number of disorders other than diabetes. Other considerations include the following:

■ Glomerulonephritis—The urinalysis in DKD typically shows proteinuria and a "bland sediment" (few cells and casts, no cellular casts). A more "active" sediment suggests glomerulonephritis.
■ Obstruction, infection, or stones should be ruled out with renal ultrasound, abdominal X-ray, or computed tomography (CT) scan of the abdomen.
■ Multiple myeloma should be excluded by serum and urine protein electrophoresis and free light-chain determinations if there is clinical suspicion (anemia or pancytopenia, hypercalcemia, lytic bone lesions, proteinuria with minimal albuminuria; see Chapter 3).
■ Hepatitis should be ruled out in patients with intravenous (IV) drug abuse, transfusions, or risky sexual habits.
■ Patients with rash or arthritis should be tested for systemic lupus erythematosus or cryoglobulinemia (antinuclear antibodies, complements, cryoglobulins).
■ Renal artery stenosis should be considered in patients with refractory hypertension and vascular bruits, especially if there is acute renal failure associated with the initiation of a RAS blocker.
■ Consider renal biopsy for an alternate diagnosis if the following are present:
　■ Short duration of diabetes (especially in type 1)
　■ Absence of retinopathy (in type 2)
　■ Rapid decline in renal function
　■ "Active" urine sediment
　■ Evidence of another systemic disease

TREATMENT

■ Treatment of DKD should be comprehensive and should involve simultaneous evaluation and intervention at the level of hyperglycemia, hypertension, dyslipidemia, bone disease, anemia, nutrition, cardiovascular disease, physical fitness (exercise), and behavior (especially smoking) (Gaede et al., 1999).
■ *Hyperglycemia:* Intensive treatment of hyperglycemia can prevent DKD (development of microalbuminuria) as well as progression of microalbuminuria to macroalbuminuria (Reichard

et al., 1993). It is controversial as to whether it can slow progression of CKD in established DKD (The DCCT Group, 1995; Writing Team for the Diabetes Control and Complications Trial/ Epidemiology of Diabetes Intervention and Complications Research Group, 2003). Reversal of lesions of diabetic nephropathy after pancreas transplantation has been observed in type 1 diabetic patients (Fioretto et al., 1998). However, in the Veterans Affairs Diabetes Trial (VADT), intensive glycemic control had no significant overall effect on the progression of renal disease in type 2 diabetes, although it was associated with some protection against increasing albuminuria in patients with more advanced microvascular disease, lower baseline diastolic BP, or higher baseline body mass index (BMI) and on worsening of GFR in patients with high baseline albuminuria (Agrawal et al., 2011). After 11 years of follow-up, there has been a 34% greater odds of maintaining an eGFR of >60 mL/min/1.73 m^2 in individuals with type 2 diabetes who had received intensive glycemic therapy for a median of 5.6 years (Agrawal et al., 2018). Results from the several clinical trials of intensive glucose control in type 2 diabetes, including Action in Diabetes and Vascular Disease (ADVANCE), Action to Control Cardiovascular Risk in Diabetes (ACCORD), and VADT, have raised concern about the benefit versus risk of tight glycemic control in patients with advanced diabetic complications (Terry et al., 2012).

■ *Antidiabetic medications:* Most medications can be used in patients with CKD with appropriate dose adjustment (Leehey et al., 2015). Patients with CKD are at risk for hypoglycemia because of impaired clearance of medications such as insulin or sulfonylureas and because of impaired kidney gluconeogenesis. Metformin is an effective agent but should not be used in patients with eGFR <30 mL/min/1.73 m^2 because of a risk of lactic acidosis. Glipizide is the preferred sulfonylurea because its metabolites have little or no hypoglycemic activity. Glyburide should be avoided owing to accumulation of active metabolites leading to hypoglycemia. Pioglitazone is not cleared by the kidney and will not cause hypoglycemia but may cause edema. The glucagon-like peptide 1 (GLP-1) receptor agonist exenatide is excreted mainly by the kidneys, and its use is not recommended with eGFR <30. However, liraglutide does not require dose adjustment. The dipeptidyl peptidase 4 (DPP-4) inhibitors such as sitagliptin, saxagliptin, and linagliptin can be used (the latter does not require dose adjustment). Sodium-glucose cotransporter 2 (SGLT2) inhibitors such as canagliflozin, dapagliflozin, and empagliflozin, may have renoprotective effects but are ineffective when eGFR <30. The manufacturer recommends not starting empagliflozin if eGFR <45 and discontinuing empagliflozin when GFR falls below 45.

■ *Hypertension:* Treatment of hypertension reduces progression of DKD (Bakris et al., 2003; Lewis et al., 1999). BP should be maintained at 130/80 mm Hg or below, as initially recommended by JNC 7 (Chobanian et al., 2003) and recently recommended by the

American College of Cardiology/American Heart Association (ACC/AHA) (Whelton et al., 2018). First-line treatment should include ACE-Is or ARBs because they have been shown to be beneficial in preventing and slowing progression of DKD (Barnett et al., 2004; Brenner et al., 2001; Lewis et al., 1993, 2001). The beneficial effect of ACE-Is and ARBs may be additive (Jacobsen et al., 2003); however, combined RAS blockade increases the risk of hyperkalemia (Pham et al., 2012). The VA NEPHRON-D trial has been terminated early because of an increased risk of hyperkalemia and acute kidney injury with dual blockade (Fried et al., 2013). Addition of diuretics is usually necessary for BP control and helps to prevent hyperkalemia. Other useful agents are beta-blockers (carvedilol, more than metoprolol, has a beneficial effect on glycemic control as well as insulin resistance) and nondihydropyridine calcium channel blockers (dihydropyridine calcium channel blockers such as amlodipine are not recommended as lone therapy because they worsen proteinuria and have not been shown to improve outcomes; however, they are acceptable if the patient is already on an ACE-I or an ARB).

- *Hyperlipidemia:* Treatment of hyperlipidemia is essential because studies have shown that the lower the low-density lipoprotein (LDL) is, the greater the cardiovascular benefit. The Study of Heart And Renal Protection (SHARP) trial has shown that patients with diabetes and CKD have a very high risk of cardiovascular events and derive substantial benefit from statins (although statins may not be helpful in patients with end-stage kidney disease) (Baigent et al., 2011). LDL should be maintained at least lower than 100 mg/dL and probably lower than 70 mg/dL (Grundy et al., 2004).

- *Other therapies:* There are some data to support the claim that low-protein diets prevent decline in GFR and reduce progression of proteinuria (Hansen et al., 2002). Dietary protein restriction of 0.8 g/kg of ideal body weight is indicated for diabetics with kidney disease. High-protein diets should be avoided. Cessation of smoking, low-dose aspirin, and limited intake of saturated fat, cholesterol, and sodium (2–3 g/d) are also recommended.

- *Prevention:* Nephrotoxic agents, such as nonsteroidal anti-inflammatory drugs (NSAIDs), should be avoided. Radiocontrast media should be minimized; if contrast must be used, use iso-osmolar or nonionic contrast, and minimize the volume of contrast administered. Hydration should be with isotonic saline; there is no role for isotonic bicarbonate or *N*-acetylcysteine. Metformin should be held 48 hours before contrast administration and after exposure until GFR has been demonstrated to be stable.

13

A 57-year-old African American man with a 10-year history of type 2 DM, hypertension, and stage 4 CKD is admitted for a kidney biopsy. He has nephrotic-range proteinuria, but his eye examination in the past month did not reveal retinopathy. His BP is well controlled on ACE-Is lisinopril and furosemide. On physical examination, his vitals are normal. His heart, lungs, and abdominal examinations are normal. He has good distal pulses in his lower extremities, with mild onychomycosis, no foot ulcers, and good sensation.

Blood chemistry:
Sodium: 140 mmol/L
Potassium: 5.0 mmol/L
Chloride: 110 mmol/L
Total CO_2: 26 mmol/L
Urea nitrogen: 30 mg/dL (urea: 10.7 mmol/L)
Creatinine: 3.0 mg/dL (265 mcmol/L)
eGFR: 25 mL/min/1.73 m^2
Urine albumin to creatinine ratio: 3,000 mg/g (340 mg/mmol)
24-hour urine: 5 g of protein
Serum and urine protein electrophoresis: normal
Renal ultrasound: normal

Renal biopsy—most of the glomeruli showed variable mesangial matrix expansion with segmental mesangial cell proliferation. Widespread subintimal hyaline thickening of the arterioles has been detected, suggestive of diabetic glomerulosclerosis.

Q1: Which of the following is not true in diabetic nephropathy?

1. Hyperglycemia causes cross-linking of AGEs
2. Elevated intrarenal AII stimulates fibrotic growth factors
3. Kimmelstiel-Wilson nodules only occur in diabetic nephropathy
4. ACE-Is protect the kidney via lowering BP and via BP-independent effects

A1: Diabetic nephropathy, also known as DKD, is defined as CKD in the presence of macroalbuminuria (>300 mg/24 hours) or CKD with microalbuminuria (30–300 mg/24 hours) associated with retinopathy or 10 years duration of type 1 diabetes. Patients in whom there are atypical findings (such as absence of retinopathy despite nephrotic-range proteinuria) should be considered for kidney biopsy. However, as in this patient, when there is kidney disease in the setting of long-standing diabetes, the biopsy will usually show DKD.

Glucose forms AGEs by binding irreversibly to proteins. Over years, AGEs form cross-links, stimulate the release of growth factors such as TGF-β, and cause fibrosis. AII, which is elevated in diabetic glomeruli, constricts the efferent arteriole in the glomerulus causing high glomerular capillary pressures and also stimulates fibrosis by upregulating growth factors such as TGF-β. By blocking the formation of AII, ACE-Is (and other RAS blockers) are believed to have both BP-dependent and BP-independent renoprotective effects. Mesangial expansion is characteristic of early diabetic glomerulosclerosis and is followed by fibrosis in the late stages. Kimmelstiel-Wilson nodules, areas of mesangial expansion on biopsy, are the hallmark of diabetic glomerulosclerosis and are seen in half the cases of DKD. Kimmelstiel-Wilson nodules can, however, occur in any process characterized by mesangial expansion.

Q2: Which of the following factors have been shown to prevent progression of established DKD?

1. Blood glucose control
2. BP control
3. Blood cholesterol control
4. All of the above

A2: Seminal observations in the 1970s and 1980s first demonstrated the importance of BP control in preventing progression in DKD (as is true for all glomerular disease). Subsequently, large clinical trials have shown benefits of RAS blockers, though in most of these studies, BP control was better in the RAS blocker versus the control group, pointing to the possibility that BP control was an important factor in their added benefit. Without doubt, BP control is the most important intervention to prevent or delay progression of established DKD. The role of blood glucose control remains unclear, with benefits in some subpopulations offset by an increased risk of hypoglycemia. There is also no clear role of lowering blood cholesterol. However, lipid control is important to decrease cardiovascular events independent of its effect on kidney disease.

VIGNETTE 2

A 67-year-old Caucasian man with a 10-year history of type 2 DM and hypertension is seen in clinic complaining of fever and weight loss for the past 2 months. He has a history of microalbuminuria for the past 5 years and persistently normal renal function in the past (plasma creatinine was 1.0 mg/dL [88.4 mcmol/L] when last checked 6 months ago). His most recent eye examination (also 6 months ago) revealed background diabetic retinopathy. Six weeks ago, he saw a urologist for lower urinary tract symptoms (LUTS) and was given ciprofloxacin, which he took for 10 days. His BP has been well controlled on ACE-Is lisinopril and furosemide. He denies other medications including over-the-counter (OTC) meds. On physical examination, his vitals are normal except for low-grade fever (38°C). His HEENT, heart, lung, and abdominal examinations are normal. He has no rash or adenopathy.

Blood chemistry:
Sodium: 140 mmol/L
Potassium: 5.0 mmol/L
Chloride: 110 mmol/L
Total CO_2: 26 mmol/L
Urea nitrogen: 20 mg/dL (urea: 7.1 mmol/L)
Creatinine: 2.0 mg/dL (177 mcmol/L)
eGFR: 36 mL/min/1.73 m^2
Glycated hemoglobin: 9.0%
Urine albumin to creatinine ratio: 300 mg/g (34 mcmol/L)
Urine protein to creatinine ratio: 500 mg/g (57 mg/mmol)

Complete blood count:
WBCs: 15,000/mm^3
Hemoglobin: 9 g/dL (90 g/L)
Hematocrit: 27%
Platelets: 400,000/mm^3
Urobilinogen: negative

WBCs: 5/hpf
RBCs: 50/hpf
Bacteria: none
Granular and few cellular casts seen

Urinalysis:
Color: yellow
pH: 5.5
Specific gravity: 1.012
Protein: 2+
Blood: 2+
Glucose: negative
Ketones: negative
Bilirubin: negative
Renal ultrasound: normal
Urobilinogen: negative
WBCs: 5/hpf
RBCs: 50/hpf
Bacteria: none
Granular and few cellular casts seen

Q: What is the most likely diagnosis in this patient?

1. Diabetic nephropathy
2. Acute glomerulonephritis
3. Drug-induced interstitial nephritis
4. Systemic polyangiitis
5. Multiple myeloma

A: As stated in Vignette 1, diabetic nephropathy, also known as DKD, is defined as CKD in the presence of macroalbuminuria (>300 mg/24 hour) or CKD with microalbuminuria (30–300 mg/24 hour) associated with retinopathy or 10 years duration of diabetes type. The presence of persistent microalbuminuria and retinopathy fits the diagnosis of DKD. However, there are atypical findings for that diagnosis in this case. There are manifestations of a systemic disease (fever, weight loss, anemia, leukocytosis, relative thrombocytosis). More importantly, the renal function has declined at a rate inconsistent with diabetic nephropathy, and he has an "active" urinary sediment with proteinuria, hematuria, and cellular casts. These findings suggest glomerulonephritis, vasculitis, or, possibly, interstitial nephritis. Multiple myeloma is unlikely because he has predominantly albuminuria, and myeloma does not typically cause an active sediment.

Further workup reveals antineutrophil cytoplasmic antibodies to be positive in the perinuclear pattern (P-ANCA). A renal biopsy shows pauci-immune necrotizing glomerulitis consistent with vasculitis, and he is treated with cyclophosphamide and prednisone, leading to improvement in his renal function.

References

Agrawal L, Azad N, Bahn GD, et al; Veterans Affairs Diabetes Trial (VADT) Study Group. Long-term follow-up of intensive glycaemic control on renal outcomes in the Veterans Affairs Diabetes Trial (VADT). *Diabetologia*. 61(2):295–299, 2018.

Agrawal L, Azad N, Emanuele NV, et al; Veterans Affairs Diabetes Trial (VADT) Study Group. Observation on renal outcomes in the Veterans Affairs Diabetes Trial. *Diabetes Care*. 34(9):2090–2094, 2011.

American Diabetes Association. Statistics About Diabetes. 2015. http://www.diabetes.org/diabetes-basics/statistics

Baigent C, Landray MJ, Reith C, et al; SHARP Investigators. The effects of lowering LDL cholesterol with simvastatin plus ezetimibe in patients with CKD (Study of Heart and Renal Protection): a randomised placebo-controlled trial. *Lancet*. 377:2181–2192, 2011.

Bakris GL, Weir MR, Shanifar S, et al. Effects of blood pressure level on progression of diabetic nephropathy: results from the RENAAL Study. *Arch Intern Med*. 163:1555–1565, 2003.

Barnett AH, Bain SC, Bouter P, et al. Angiotensin receptor blockade versus converting enzyme inhibition in type 2 diabetes and nephropathy. *N Engl J Med*. 351:1952–1961, 2004.

Brenner BM, Cooper ME, de Zeeuw D, et al. Effects of losartan on renal and cardiovascular outcomes in patients with type 2 diabetes and nephropathy. *N Engl J Med*. 345:861–869, 2001.

Centers for Disease Control and Prevention. National Diabetes Statistics Report, 2017. https://www.cdc.gov/diabetes/pdfs/data/statistics/national-diabetes-statistics-report.pdf.

Chobanian AV, Bakris GL, Black HR, et al; National Heart Lung and Blood Institute. The Seventh Report of the Joint National Committee on Prevention, Detection, Evaluation, and Treatment of High Blood Pressure: The JNC 7 Report. *Hypertension*. 42(6):1206–1252, 2003.

Fioretto P, Steffes MW, Sutherland DE, et al. Reversal of lesions of diabetic nephropathy after pancreas transplantation. *N Engl J Med*. 339(2):69–75, 1998.

Fried LF, Emanuele N, Zhang JH, et al. Combined angiotensin inhibition for the treatment of diabetic nephropathy. *N Engl J Med*. 369(20):1892–1903, 2013.

Gaede P, Vedel P, Parving HH, et al. Intensified multifactorial intervention in patients with type 2 diabetes and microalbuminuria: the Steno type 2 randomized study. *Lancet*. 353:617–622, 1999.

Grundy SM, Cleeman JI, Merz CN, et al. Implications of recent clinical trials for the National Cholesterol Education Program Adult Treatment Panel III guidelines. *Circulation*. 110:227–239, 2004.

Hansen HP, Tauber-Lassen E, Jensen BR, et al. Effect of dietary protein restriction on prognosis in patients with diabetic nephropathy. *Kidney Int*. 62:220–228, 2002.

Jacobsen P, Andersen S, Jensen BR, et al. Additive effect of ACE inhibition and angiotensin II receptor blockade in type I diabetic patients with diabetic nephropathy. *J Am Soc Nephrol*. 14:992–999, 2003.

Kramer HJ, Nguyen QD, Curhan G, et al. Renal insufficiency in the absence of albuminuria and retinopathy among adults with type 2 diabetes mellitus. *JAMA*. 289(24):3273–3277, 2003.

Leehey DJ, Emanuele MA, Emanuele N. Diabetes. In: Daugirdas JT, Blake P, Ing TS, eds. *Handbook of Dialysis*. 5th ed. Philadelphia, PA: Wolters Kluwer/Lippincott Williams & Wilkins; 2015.

Lewis EJ, Hunsicker LG, Bain RP, et al. The effect of angiotensin-converting-enzyme inhibition on diabetic nephropathy. The Collaborative Study Group. *N Engl J Med*. 329:1456–1462, 1993.

Lewis EJ, Hunsicker LG, Clarke WR, et al. Renoprotective effect of the angiotensin receptor antagonist irbesartan in patients with nephropathy due to type 2 diabetes. *N Engl J Med.* 345:851–860, 2001.

Lewis JB, Berl T, Bain RP, et al. Effect of intensive blood pressure control on the course of type I diabetic nephropathy. Collaborative Study Group. *Am J Kidney Dis.* 34:809–817, 1999.

Pham JT, Schmitt BP, Leehey DJ. Effects of dual blockade of the renin angiotensin system in diabetic kidney disease: a systematic review and meta-analysis. *J Nephrol Therapeutic.* S2:003, 2012. doi:10.4172/2161-0959.S2-003

Reichard P, Nilsson BY, Rosenqvist U. The effect of long term intensified insulin treatment on the development of microvascular complications of diabetes mellitus. *N Engl J Med.* 329:304–309, 1993.

Robles NR, Villa J, Gallego RH. Non-proteinuric diabetic nephropathy. *J Clin Med.* 4(9):1761–1773, 2015.

Schena FP, Gesualdo L. Pathogenetic mechanisms of diabetic nephropathy. *J Am Soc Nephrol.* 16(suppl 1):S30–S33, 2005.

Terry T, Raravikar K, Chokrungvaranon N, et al. Does aggressive glycemic control benefit macrovascular and microvascular disease in type 2 diabetes? Insights from ACCORD, ADVANCE, and VADT. *Curr Cardiol Rep.* 14(1):79–88, 2012.

The Diabetes Control and Complications (DCCT) Research Group. Effect of intensive therapy on the development and progression of diabetic nephropathy in the Diabetes Control and Complications Trial. *Kidney Int.* 47:1703–1720, 1995.

Whelton PK, Carey RM, Aronow WS, et al. 2017 ACC/AHA/AAPA/ABC/ACPM/AGS/APhA/ASH/ASPC/NMA/PCNA guideline for the prevention, detection, evaluation, and management of high blood pressure in adults: a report of the American College of Cardiology/American Heart Association Task Force on Clinical Practice Guidelines. *J Am Coll Cardiol.* 71:e127–e248, 2018.

Writing Team for the Diabetes Control and Complications Trial/Epidemiology of Diabetes Intervention and Complications Research Group. Sustained effect of intensive treatment of type I diabetes mellitus on development and progression of diabetic nephropathy: the Epidemiology of Diabetes Intervention and Complications (EDIC) Study. *JAMA.* 290:2159–2167, 2003.

14 Hypertension and Kidney Disease

DEFINITION

- Elevated blood pressure (BP) may be either the cause or consequence of kidney disease. In virtually all kidney diseases, an increase in BP primarily caused by sodium retention will lead to further worsening of kidney function (progression) (see Chapter 12). In some patients, in particular those of African descent, hypertension per se can cause chronic kidney disease (CKD). The type and severity of renal lesions depend on the degree of BP elevation.

- Classically, chronic hypertension of mild-to-moderate severity leading to slow, insidious scarring of kidneys has been termed "benign nephrosclerosis." On the other end of the spectrum is "malignant nephrosclerosis," in which there can be rapidly progressive impairment of renal function in patients with very elevated BP. Pathologically, benign nephrosclerosis is characterized by hyaline arteriosclerosis, whereas malignant nephrosclerosis is characterized by fibrinoid necrosis and thrombosis in the arterioles and ischemic glomeruli.

PATHOGENESIS

- In patients with essential (primary) hypertension and normal renal function, it has been hypothesized that a primary defect in renal salt excretion results in a compensatory increase in systemic BP to excrete the dietary sodium load ("pressure natriuresis"). The etiology of the defect in renal salt excretion is not usually evident. In some patients, such as those with obesity and/or type 2 diabetes, the mechanism may involve insulin resistance leading to hyperinsulinemia and increased renal sodium reabsorption (Sechi & Bartoli, 1996). Increased angiotensin II, sympathetic tone (Koplin, 1981; Schrier & DeWardener, 1971), and/or aldosterone also increase renal sodium reabsorption.

- According to the hemodynamic formula: BP = cardiac output (CO) × systemic vascular resistance (SVR), either an increase in CO or SVR or both will result in hypertension. It is currently believed that renal sodium retention leads to extracellular fluid (ECF) volume expansion and an increase in CO and BP, which is followed by a compensatory autoregulatory increase in SVR.

■ Hypertension is present in most patients with CKD. Indeed, kidney disease is the most common cause of secondary hypertension. In the face of a diminished number of functioning nephrons, unless dietary salt is restricted, BP will increase because of salt retention. Patients with uncomplicated hypertension usually develop minimal renal damage in response to elevated BP. However, the kidneys of patients with CKD are more vulnerable to elevated BP. The association between hypertension and renal disease is as a result of three factors: (1) the degree of elevated BP, (2) the degree to which this pressure is transmitted to the kidney, and (3) the recruitment of cellular and molecular pathways that mediate tissue injury and fibrosis.

■ Normally, autoregulatory vasoconstriction of the preglomerular vasculature protects the glomeruli from damage due to elevated BP (Imig & Inscho, 2002). However, autoregulation is impaired in patients with CKD, making such patients vulnerable to further glomerular injury. Hypertension per se can cause vascular injury (arteriosclerosis) and also compromise autoregulation. Because autoregulation depends on voltage-gated calcium channels, calcium channel blocking drugs that inhibit these channels (such as dihydropyridines) impair autoregulation (Griffin et al., 1995). In animals, high-protein diets also prevent preglomerular vasoconstriction and cause autoregulatory impairment (Bidani et al., 1987). However, the clinical significance of this phenomenon is unclear.

■ Hypertension causes tissue injury not only by barotrauma but also by induction of oxidative stress and activation of fibrosing factors such as transforming growth factor beta (TGF-β) (August & Suthanthiran, 2006) and plasminogen activator inhibitor 1 (PAI-1). A role of the renin–angiotensin system (RAS) in tissue injury and BP-independent mechanisms in protection from injury by RAS inhibitors such as angiotensin-converting enzyme (ACE) inhibitors and angiotensin-receptor blockers (ARBs) is generally accepted (Scaglione et al., 2005), though it is clear that control of BP per se is of paramount importance in preventing progression of injury to all target organs.

■ Renal nitric oxide production buffers the effects of angiotensin II on renal medullary circulation and reduces BP. Inhibition of nitric oxide increases BP, peripheral vascular resistance, and fractional excretion of sodium (Haynes et al., 1993).

PRIMARY VERSUS SECONDARY HYPERTENSION

Essential (primary) hypertension is a diagnosis of exclusion. Causes of secondary hypertension are given in Table 14.1. Kidney disease is the most common known cause of hypertension and should always be excluded in every hypertensive patient. Evaluation to exclude other secondary disorders depends on the clinical situation (see below).

TABLE 14.1	Causes and Initial Evaluation of Secondary Hypertension
Cause	**Diagnosis and Initial Evaluation**
CKD	Urinalysis ± urine protein to creatinine ratio. eGFR. Renal ultrasound
Insulin resistance (metabolic syndrome)	Obesity, diabetes or impaired glucose tolerance (fasting plasma glucose, glycated hemoglobin), hyperlipidemia
Primary aldosteronism	Hypokalemia with plasma aldosterone to plasma renin activity ratio >20:1 is suggestive of diagnosis
Obstructive sleep apnea	Combination of obesity, daytime sleepiness, and nocturnal snoring should prompt sleep study
Renovascular disease	Resistant hypertension, especially if "flash" pulmonary edema. Vascular (especially femoral and abdominal) bruits. Optimal screening test dependent on center but usually Doppler ultrasound or MRA (providing eGFR >30 mL/min/1.73 m²)
Corticosteroid excess	Chronic steroid use or signs of Cushing syndrome should prompt consideration of diagnosis
Pheochromocytoma	Clinical suspicion (anxiety, tachycardia, palpitations, orthostatic hypotension) should prompt measurement of plasma fractionated metanephrines
Coarctation of aorta	BP in arms > legs with diminished or delayed femoral pulses (brachial–femoral delay)
Thyroid disease (hyperthyroid or hypothyroid)	Thyroid studies
Hyperparathyroidism	Plasma total calcium (ionized calcium and parathyroid hormone if elevated)
Drug-induced hypertension	History (NSAID use, adrenergic agents, illicit drugs, etc.)

BP, blood pressure; CKD, chronic kidney disease; eGFR, elevated glomerular filtration rate; MRA, magnetic resonance angiography; NSAID, nonsteroidal anti-inflammatory drug.

CLINICAL EVALUATION

■ *History:* Duration of hypertension, lifestyle (including dietary salt intake, caloric intake, tobacco use, and exercise), cardiovascular risk factors, history of target organ damage (brain, heart, kidney), drugs that can raise BP (nonsteroidal anti-inflammatory drugs [NSAIDs], adrenergic agents such as nasal sprays and decongestants, illicit drugs [cocaine, methamphetamine, anabolic steroids], oral contraceptives, adrenal steroids), symptoms that suggest secondary hypertension (sudden onset, "flash" pulmonary edema, recent worsening, sympathetic overactivity such as anxiety, tachycardia, palpitations, orthostatic hypotension)

- *Physical examination:* BP in both arms and femoral pulses (exclude coarctation, vascular disease), orthostatic BP (autonomic failure, pheochromocytoma), body mass index (obesity, sleep apnea), funduscopic examination (if malignant hypertension suspected), bruits (carotid, flank, femoral), cardiovascular (prominent left ventricular impulse suggests left ventricular hypertrophy [LVH]), chest (rales due to left ventricular failure), lower extremity edema
  - BP measurement: Proper procedure for measuring BP is of paramount importance
    - Quiet sitting for ≥5 minutes
    - Support arm at heart level
    - Only arm cuffs should be used. Cuff bladder should encircle 80% of arm. Do not use same size cuff on all patients, as too large a cuff will underestimate and too small a cuff will overestimate BP
    - Measurements should be repeated after 1 to 2 minutes
    - Measure in both arms and, if different, use arm with higher value for all subsequent readings
  - Home BP: Hypertensive patients should monitor BP twice daily (12-hour apart) (Pickering et al., 2008). Useful in diagnosis of "white coat" (clinic BP > home BP) and "masked" (home BP > clinic BP) hypertension
  - Ambulatory BP monitoring: May be indicated in specific circumstances
    - Marked clinic and/or home BP variability
    - Severe "white coat" hypertension
    - Diagnosis of hypertension in specific populations (e.g., prospective kidney donors)

LABORATORY EVALUATION

- Electrolytes: Hypokalemia and metabolic alkalosis with mild hypernatremia suggest primary hyperaldosteronism; similar findings but normal serum sodium in secondary hyperaldosteronism (high plasma renin activity) such as in renovascular disease
- Plasma urea nitrogen and creatinine: Elevated in CKD
- Fasting plasma glucose, glycated hemoglobin: Metabolic syndrome, diabetes
- Plasma total calcium: Hyperparathyroidism
- Lipid profile: Metabolic syndrome
- Electrocardiogram (EKG): Exclude LVH
- Urinalysis: Typically shows minimal proteinuria with few cells or casts present ("bland sediment") in essential hypertension. Marked proteinuria or an "active sediment" (the presence of cells and casts) suggests the presence of an underlying glomerular disease with secondary hypertension rather than hypertensive kidney disease. Dipstick proteinuria should lead to measurement of urine protein to creatinine ratio
- Renal ultrasound: Will often show a nonspecific increase in echogenicity. Small kidneys are typical of hypertensive kidney disease, though are also frequently seen in chronic glomerular disease

TREATMENT

- The lowering of BP is of utmost importance in decreasing cardio-vascular risk and preventing further progression of target organ damage, including CKD. Current guidelines from the American College of Cardiology/American Heart Association (ACC/AHA) (Whelton et al., 2018) are that BP should be maintained at or below 130/80 mm Hg. The importance of diuretics to normalize ECF volume and BP in essential hypertension has been solidified by the results of the ALLHAT study (2002). Largely based on this study, the Seventh Report of the Joint National Committee on Prevention, Detection, Evaluation, and Treatment of High Blood Pressure (Chobanian et al., 2003) has recommended thiazide di-uretics as the initial therapy of most patients with hypertension, either alone or in combination with another class of antihyper-tensive agent. Because hypertension in CKD is volume dependent, diuretics should also virtually always be used in this population, though loop rather than thiazide-type diuretics are necessary in patients with substantially decreased glomerular filtration rate (GFR) (see Chapter 12). Diuretics and RAS blockers may cause transient worsening of renal function (elevation in serum cre-atinine), but this is an acceptable and expected consequence of reducing BP. In the long run, controlling BP stabilizes and even improves renal function. The African American Study of Kidney Disease (AASK), whose study population had hypertensive neph-rosclerosis, found that ACE inhibitors are somewhat better than calcium blockers and beta-blockers; however, diuretics per se are not evaluated (Wright et al., 2002). The degree of BP control is far more important than the particular agent(s) used to control BP. RAS blockers are beneficial in proteinuric patients with CKD and hypertension (see Chapter 12). Table 14.2 lists typical drugs used in hypertensive CKD.
- Certain pharmacologic agents such as NSAIDs and calcineurin in-hibitors (CNIs) block the transmission of BP to glomeruli via pre-glomerular vasoconstriction. However, these agents actually cause worsening of BP and renal function (Frishman, 2002). Therefore, avoidance of NSAIDs in all patients with hypertension and CKD is prudent, and doses of CNIs in recipients of organ transplants with CKD should be minimized if possible.
- Nonpharmacologic (lifestyle) management is often overlooked but is of great importance in BP control. Achieving a normal weight, eating a low-sodium, Mediterranean-style diet, and exercise are all beneficial. Aerobic exercise (30 minutes, 5–7 days weekly) has been shown to decrease BP and will aid in weight reduction (Ben-jamin, 2010).

RESISTANT HYPERTENSION

- Definition: BP not controlled despite ≥3 drugs at appropriate doses
- Poor compliance is the most common cause

TABLE 14.2 Commonly Used Antihypertensives

Diuretics
  Thiazides (e.g., hydrochlorothiazide)
  Indapamide
  Metolazone
ACE inhibitors
  Captopril
  Enalapril
  Lisinopril
  Ramipril
Beta-blockers
  Metoprolol
  Carvedilol
  Labetalol
ARBs
  Losartan
  Valsartan
Dihydropyridine calcium channel blockers
  Nifedipine
  Felodipine
  Amlodipine
Nondihydropyridine calcium channel blockers
  Diltiazem
  Verapamil
Vasodilators
  Hydralazine
  Minoxidil
  Nitroprusside (parenteral only)
α_1 Blockers
  Terazosin
  Doxazosin
  Phentolamine/phenoxybenzamine (in pheochromocytoma)
α_2 agonists
  Clonidine
  Methyldopa
Aldosterone antagonists
  Spironolactone
  Eplerenone

ACE, angiotensin-converting enzyme; ARB, angiotensin-receptor blockers.

- Failure to use diuretics or inadequate diuretic doses is also a common cause (patients with CKD require loop diuretics)
- Consider dietary salt excess, "white coat" hypertension, secondary hypertension

HYPERTENSIVE EMERGENCIES

- Hypertension is an emergency if it is associated with acute neurologic damage (e.g., encephalopathy, papilledema, seizures, hemorrhagic stroke), cardiovascular compromise (e.g., angina or myocardial infarction, pulmonary edema, aortic dissection), or worsening of another life-threatening event (e.g., head trauma, arterial bleeding). The term "urgency" has been applied to hypertension without acute end-organ damage but deemed to require prompt lowering of BP to prevent such an event (this is a rather vague concept).

- Normally, an elevation in BP will cause vasoconstriction in organ beds, limiting the amount of pressure transmitted to the arterioles and capillaries. Hypertensive emergencies are often due to a breakdown in autoregulation, leading to acute endothelial damage and fibrin deposition in the microvasculature, with resultant organ ischemia. Microangiopathic hemolytic anemia is characteristically seen because of fragmentation of red blood cells as they traverse the damaged arterioles.

- The degree of BP elevation may be misleading. In a previously normotensive patient, a BP of 150/100 mm Hg may lead to acute neurologic symptoms (as in eclampsia during pregnancy), but a chronic hypertensive patient may have a BP of 260/130 mm Hg without any symptoms. It is known that cerebral and other vital organ beds undergo a shift in autoregulatory threshold in chronic hypertension, which protects against microvascular damage even at very high BP levels (Strandgaard, 1976).

- Clinical evaluation should focus on detecting evidence of acute organ damage (flame hemorrhages or papilledema on funduscopic examination, myocardial ischemia, acute renal failure, neurologic symptoms and signs, microangiopathic hemolytic anemia).

- BP needs to be promptly lowered to safe levels, but not to a normal range, especially in patients with chronic hypertension. Parenteral agents are needed with hypertensive encephalopathy or acute cardiovascular compromise (see Vignette 1).

- When stable, secondary causes of hypertension should generally be excluded.

VIGNETTE 1

14

A 67-year-old woman with hypertension presents for evaluation of chest pain radiating to her left jaw and left shoulder. She also complains of weakness, anxiety, palpitations, diaphoresis, and dizziness. She denies abdominal pain but does have nausea and has vomited several times. Medications include hydrochlorothiazide 25 mg orally daily, extended-release metoprolol 100 mg daily, and lisinopril 40 mg once daily. She smokes one pack per day and admits to excessive alcohol consumption. Vital signs are BP, 210/130 mm Hg; pulse, 100 beats/min; respiratory rate, 22 breaths/min; temperature, 37°C; weight, 100 kg. Funduscopic examination shows flame hemorrhages, but no papilledema is noted. Cardiac examination reveals tachycardia but no murmurs. The lungs are clear. There is no abdominal bruit and no edema. There is an ataxic gait and positive Romberg sign, but no focal neurologic findings.

Blood chemistry:
Sodium: 136 mmol/L
Potassium: 4.0 mmol/L
Chloride: 106 mmol/L
Total CO_2: 24 mmol/L
Urea nitrogen: 44 mg/dL (urea: 15.7 mmol/L)
Creatinine: 2.0 mg/dL (177 mcmol/L)
Glucose: 130 mg/dL (7.2 mmol/L)
Alkaline phosphatase: 100 U/L
Aspartate aminotransferase (AST): 60 U/L
Alanine aminotransferase (ALT): 120 U/L
Albumin: 3.0 g/dL (30 g/L)
Total bilirubin: 2.4 mg/dL (41 mcmol/L)

Complete blood count:
WBCs: 11,000/mm^3
Hemoglobin: 10 g/dL (100 g/L)
Hematocrit: 30%
Platelets: 100,000/mm^3

Peripheral smear: moderate schistocytes seen

Urinalysis:
Color: yellow
pH: 5.5
Specific gravity: 1.028
Protein: 2+
Blood: 1+
Glucose: negative
Ketones: 1+
Bilirubin: 2+
Urobilinogen: 2+
WBCs: 2/hpf
RBCs: 10/hpf
Bacteria: none
EKG—sinus tachycardia, no ST depression or elevation, diffuse T-wave inversions
Troponin: 0.05 ng/mL (mcg/L) (normal)
Creatine kinase: 400 U/L (normal < 200)

Q: What is the first step in the treatment of this patient?

1. Cardiac catheterization
2. Plasma exchange
3. Computed tomography (CT) of the head
4. Intravenous (IV) nitroprusside

A: The gastrointestinal symptoms may be related to alcoholism, a viral syndrome, or severe hypertension per se. Most likely vomiting has resulted in inability to take her medications. Accelerated/malignant hypertension is often accompanied by microangiopathic hemolytic anemia due to fragmentation of RBCs as they traverse damaged arterioles; the presence of schistocytes on peripheral smear combined with moderate thrombocytopenia is typical of this condition. The elevated ALT and mild hyperbilirubinemia with bilirubin and urobilinogen in the urine may be seen with hemolysis, but in this case could also reflect alcoholic hepatitis. There are flame hemorrhages seen on funduscopic examination, indicating acute arteriolar damage. The azotemia, proteinuria, and hematuria probably reflect acute hypertensive damage to renal arterioles and glomeruli.

Acute end-organ damage due to arteriolar injury indicates a hypertensive emergency; the presence of angina-type chest pain also qualifies as a hypertensive emergency. Other hypertensive emergencies include acute aortic dissection and acute cerebral hemorrhage. This patient needs admission to the intensive care unit to promptly lower the BP. However, normalization of the BP is not recommended because this patient has chronic hypertension and likely has a reset in cerebral autoregulation. A reduction in diastolic BP to ~100 to 110 mm Hg over the next 2 to 6 hours is indicated, with further gradual reductions toward a normal BP over the next 24 to 48 hours. The BP must be reduced with parenteral antihypertensives. IV nitroprusside or nitroglycerin or other IV medications such as nicardipine (Cardene) and fenoldopam (Corlopam); ACE inhibitors such as enalaprilat (Vasotec); and beta-blockers such as labetalol (Normodyne, Trandate) and esmolol (Brevibloc) can be used. Hydralazine has less predictable effects and could worsen angina in this patient. If pheochromocytoma is suspected, phentolamine is a reasonable choice (though there is little to suggest this rare diagnosis in this patient).

Cardiac catheterization can be contemplated when the BP has been stabilized. The microangiopathic hemolytic anemia is due to accelerated hypertension and not due to thrombotic thrombocytopenic purpura or hemolytic uremic syndrome, and thus plasma exchange is not indicated. A CT of the head is not essential owing to the absence of focal neurologic findings; in any event, control of BP is the first priority.

VIGNETTE 2

14

A 67-year-old African American man with chronic poorly controlled hypertension is referred to nephrology clinic for resistant hypertension. He denies smoking or alcohol intake. He also denies chest pain, dizziness, headaches, visual abnormalities, hematuria, abdominal pain, nausea, vomiting, diarrhea, constipation, shortness of breath, or heat or cold intolerance. He denies anxiety, depression, or other psychiatric abnormalities. He does lead a stressful lifestyle with his job as store manager and is going through a divorce. He is obese and uses continuous positive airway pressure for obstructive sleep apnea. Both of his parents and three of four siblings are hypertensive. Medications include hydrochlorothiazide 25 mg orally daily, extended-release metoprolol 100 mg daily, and lisinopril 40 mg once daily. Vital signs are BP, 210/130 mm Hg; pulse, 90 beats/min; respiratory rate, 20 breaths/min; temperature, 38°C; weight, 240 lb. There was a midline abdominal systolic bruit, no abdominal striae, and 1+ edema in the lower extremities.

Blood chemistry:
Sodium: 148 mmol/L
Potassium: 3.0 mmol/L
Chloride: 104 mmol/L
Total CO_2: 30 mmol/L
Urea nitrogen: 20 mg/dL (urea: 7.1 mmol/L)
Creatinine: 1.6 mg/dL (141 mcmol/L)
Glucose: 120 mg/dL (6.7 mmol/L)

Complete blood count:
WBCs: 6,000/mm^3
Hemoglobin: 14 g/dL (140 g/L)
Hematocrit: 41%

Platelets: 200,000/mm^3

Urinalysis:
Color: yellow
pH: 5.5
Specific gravity: 1.025
Protein: negative
Blood: negative
Glucose: negative
Ketones: 1+
Bilirubin: negative
Urobilinogen: negative
WBCs: 3/hpf
RBCs: 0/hpf
Bacteria: none

Q: Which of the following are appropriate in this patient?

1. Plasma aldosterone to renin ratio
2. 24-Hour urine cortisol
3. Plasma metanephrines
4. Magnetic resonance angiography (MRA) renal arteries
5. Thyroid-stimulating hormone
6. CT of the adrenals
7. All of the above

A: This patient has resistant hypertension because he is on three medications at appropriate doses. Note that his BP is the same as in the patient in Vignette 1; however, he is asymptomatic and without acute end-organ damage so does not have a hypertensive emergency. Although he has mild azotemia, his elevated GFR calculates to be 56 mL/min/1.73 m^2, and thus a thiazide-type diuretic is acceptable. Moreover, he has no edema. Although it is likely in view of the strong family history that he has essential hypertension, exclusion of secondary causes of hypertension is indicated. In this patient with hypernatremia, hypokalemia, and mild metabolic alkalosis, one should suspect primary hyperaldosteronism. Note that despite renal sodium retention, the absence of edema is typical of this condition. Cushing syndrome should also be considered, but the absence of the characteristic physical findings makes this rare disease even less likely. Likewise, there are no clinical findings to suggest pheochromocytoma or thyroid disease. The abdominal bruit on auscultation of the abdomen raises the possibility of renovascular hypertension. However, the plasma aldosterone is elevated (20 pg/mL) with a plasma aldosterone-to-plasma renin activity ratio of >30:1, which together with the clinical data is highly suggestive of an aldosteronoma. Because high-dose lisinopril would normally be expected to inhibit aldosterone production and increase renin, an elevated ratio in a patient taking ACE inhibitors adds further support to this diagnosis. Renovascular hypertension (as well as sleep apnea) would not be associated with a high aldosterone–renin ratio nor with hypernatremia. After BP is controlled, a 24-hour urine for aldosterone on a high-sodium diet (to document hypersecretion of aldosterone) is elevated (>14 mcg/24 h), and a CT of the adrenals reveals a 3-cm right adrenal adenoma. Laparoscopic right adrenalectomy has resulted in marked improvement of BP and correction of electrolyte abnormalities.

References

ALLHAT Officers and Coordinators for the ALLHAT Collaborative Research Group. Major outcomes in high-risk hypertensive patients randomized to angiotensin-converting enzyme inhibitor or calcium channel blocker vs diuretic: the Antihypertensive and Lipid-Lowering Treatment to Prevent Heart Attack Trial (ALLHAT). *JAMA.* 288(23):2981–2997, 2002.

August P, Suthanthiran M. Transforming growth factor beta signaling, vascular remodeling, and hypertension. *N Engl J Med.* 354(25):2721–2723, 2006.

Benjamin R. *The Surgeon General's Vision for a Healthy and Fit Nation.* Rockville, MD: U.S. Department of Health and Human Services, Public Health Service, Office of the Surgeon General; 2010.

Bidani AK, Schwartz MM, Lewis EJ. Renal autoregulation and vulnerability to hypertensive injury in remnant kidney. *Am J Physiol.* 252(6, pt 2):F1003–F1010, 1987.

Chobanian AV, Bakris GL, Black HR, et al; National Heart Lung and Blood Institute. The Seventh Report of the Joint National Committee on prevention, detection, evaluation, and treatment of high blood pressure. *Hypertension.* 42(6):1206–1252, 2003.

Frishman WH. Effects of non-steroidal anti-inflammatory drug therapy on blood pressure and peripheral edema. *Am J Cardiol.* 89(6A):18D–25D, 2002.

Griffin KA, Picken MM, Bidani AK. Deleterious effects of calcium channel blockade on pressure transmission and glomerular injury in rat remnant kidneys. *J Clin Invest.* 96(2):793–800, 1995.

Haynes WG, Noon JP, Walker BR, et al. Inhibition of nitric oxide synthesis increases blood pressure in healthy humans. *J Hypertens.* 11:1375–1380, 1993.

Imig JD, Inscho EW. Adaptations of the renal microcirculation to hypertension. *Microcirculation.* 9(4):315–328, 2002.

Koplin I, ed. *The Sympathetic Nervous System and Hypertension.* New York, NY: Springer-Verlag; 1981:283–289.

Pickering TG, Miller NH, Ogedegbe G, et al. Call to action on use and reimbursement for home blood pressure monitoring: executive summary: a joint scientific statement from the American Heart Association, American Society of Hypertension, and Preventive Cardiovascular Nurses Association. *Hypertension.* 52(1):1–9, 2008.

Scaglione R, Argano C, Corrao S, et al. Transforming growth factor beta 1 and additional renoprotective effect of combination ACE-I and Ang II receptor blocker in hypertensive subjects with minor renal abnormalities: a 24-week randomized controlled trial. *J Hypertens.* 23(3):657–664, 2005.

Schrier RW, DeWardener HE. Tubular reabsorption of sodium ion: influence of factors other than aldosterone and glomerular filtration rate. *N Engl J Med.* 285(23):1292–1303, 1971.

Sechi LA, Bartoli E. Molecular mechanisms of insulin resistance in arterial hypertension. *Blood Press Suppl.* 1:47–54, 1996.

Strandgaard S. Autoregulation of cerebral blood flow in hypertensive patients. The modifying influence of prolonged antihypertensive treatment on the tolerance to acute, drug-induced hypotension. *Circulation.* 53(4):720–727, 1976.

Whelton PK, Carey RM, Aronow WS, et al. 2017 ACC/AHA/AAPA/ABC/ACPM/AGS/APhA/ASH/ASPC/NMA/PCNA guideline for the prevention, detection, evaluation, and management of high blood pressure in adults: a report of the American College of Cardiology/American Heart Association Task Force on Clinical Practice Guidelines. *J Am Coll Cardiol.* 71:e127–e248, 2018.

Wright JT Jr, Bakris G, Greene T, et al. Effect of blood pressure lowering and antihypertensive drug class on progression of hypertensive kidney disease: results from the AASK trial. *JAMA.* 288(19):2421–2431, 2002.

15 Macrovascular Diseases of the Kidney

RENAL ARTERY STENOSIS

- Definitions:
    - Renal artery stenosis: symptomatic narrowing (>50%–70% stenosis) of one or both renal arteries, either from atherosclerosis or fibromuscular dysplasia
    - Renovascular hypertension: hypertension due to renal artery stenosis
    - Ischemic nephropathy: chronic kidney disease (CKD) due to renal artery stenosis
- Clinical features of renovascular hypertension:
    - Hypertension beginning before the age of 30 or after the age of 55
    - Accelerated hypertension (often in a previously hypertensive patient)
    - Resistant hypertension (i.e., refractory to three or more drugs in combination)
    - Episodes of flash pulmonary edema (acute left ventricular failure)
    - Unexplained progressive renal insufficiency
    - Epigastric bruit (or femoral bruits)
    - Acute renal failure after institution of renin–angiotensin system (RAS) blockers (especially with bilateral renal artery stenosis or unilateral stenosis in a solitary kidney)
    - Diffuse atherosclerosis (i.e., signs and symptoms of peripheral vascular disease)
    - Asymmetric kidney size
    - History of smoking
- Types of renovascular disease:
    - Fibromuscular dysplasia
        - Rare
        - Unknown cause
        - Generally affects young women
        - Renal dysfunction uncommon
        - Can affect proximal or distal arteries
        - Often occurs postpregnancy or post-trauma
    - Atherosclerotic
        - Common
        - Traditional risk factors (diabetes, hypertension, smoking, family history, age, male gender)

- Generally affects older patients
- Patients often have concomitant essential hypertension, CKD, congestive heart failure, stroke, or myocardial infarction (MI)
- Typically proximal or ostial (at origin from aorta)

- Pathophysiology:
  - Renal artery stenosis is an anatomic finding that can lead to renovascular hypertension or ischemic nephropathy or both. In unilateral renal artery stenosis, the affected kidney secretes renin leading to hypertension, which causes pressure natriuresis in the contralateral kidney and consequent hypovolemia. In bilateral renal artery stenosis, patients are hypervolemic because there is no contralateral natriuresis; although plasma renin levels are usually normal, these levels can be considered higher than expected given that hypertension and hypervolemia are present (Fig. 15.1 A and B) (Pickering, 1989).
  - In ischemic nephropathy, CKD develops because of impaired renal blood flow, leading to nephrosclerosis/glomerulosclerosis. Recurrent cholesterol emboli from atherosclerotic plaques may contribute to injury in the atherosclerotic form.
  - Antihypertensive medications lead to a decrease in blood pressure (BP), which, in the presence of renal artery stenosis, results in decreased afferent arteriolar pressure and a drop in glomerular filtration rate (GFR). RAS blockers such as angiotensin-converting enzyme inhibitors (ACE-Is) and angiotensin-receptor blockers cause efferent arteriolar dilatation, thus further decreasing GFR (Fig. 15.2A and B). A marked fall in GFR when RAS blockers are begun should raise suspicion for RAS.

- Diagnosis:
  - *Plasma renin activity:* Not helpful, because it is inadequately sensitive and specific and is affected by antihypertensive medications.
  - *Renal vein renin sampling:* Classic test; an increase in renin from the affected kidney with contralateral renin suppression is expected with unilateral stenosis; however, difficult to interpret with bilateral stenosis; invasive; now rarely performed (Simon & Coleman, 1994).
  - *ACE-I–augmented renal scintigraphy:* The fall in GFR in the affected kidney is detected; can predict response to intervention; however, now performed rarely (Taylor, 2000).
  - *Doppler ultrasound:* Compares peak systolic velocity of the renal arteries (stenosis leads to an increase in velocity); operator-dependent; in some centers, it is screening procedure of choice (Olin et al., 1995; Radermacher et al., 2001).
  - *Magnetic resonance angiography (MRA) (with or without gadolinium):* Requires breath holding, long scan times, and may be uncomfortable for patients with claustrophobia; gadolinium contrast contraindicated with severe CKD (eGFR <30 mL/min/1.73 m^2) or end-stage kidney disease (ESKD).

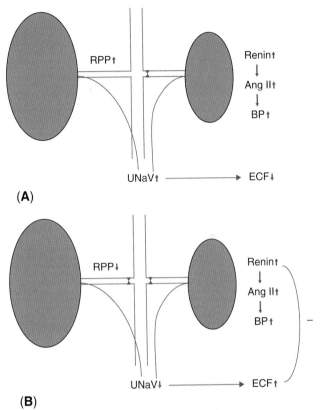

FIGURE 15.1. A: Unilateral renal artery stenosis. **B:** Bilateral renal artery stenosis. Ang II, angiotensin II; BP, blood pressure; ECF, extracellular fluid; RPP, renal perfusion pressure; UNaV, urinary sodium excretion.

Contraindicated in some patients (i.e., pacemakers, metal vascular clips) and hard to interpret in patients with previous stents (Cheung et al., 2006).
- *Computed tomography (CT) angiography with contrast:* Best for fibromuscular dysplasia; can involve substantial contrast load (Olbricht et al., 1995).
- *Selective angiography:* Gold standard, but invasive. Advantages are that it can measure pressure gradient and allow for immediate intervention with angioplasty ± stent.
- Treatment:
  - *Surgery:* Risks include bleeding, infection, MI, cerebrovascular accident (CVA), atheroembolism, and acute renal failure. Mortality is 1% to 6%. Excellent patency. Now rarely done in most centers.

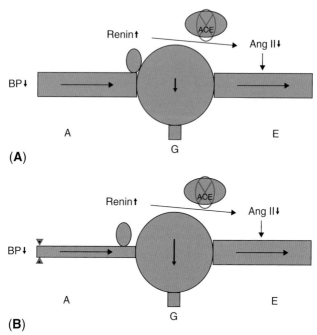

(A)

(B)

FIGURE 15.2. A: Inhibition of renin–angiotensin system (RAS) dilates efferent arterioles and lowers glomerular capillary pressure. **B:** In the presence of renal artery stenosis, there is a greater drop in glomerular capillary pressure after RAS inhibition. A, afferent arteriole; ACE, angiotensin-converting enzyme; Ang II, angiotensin II; BP, blood pressure; E, efferent arteriole; G, glomerulus.

- *Percutaneous transluminal angioplasty (PTA):* Procedure of choice for fibromuscular dysplasia. It can be repeated if stenosis recurs. Stenting is not used in fibromuscular dysplasia because PTA provides up to 100% cure rate.
- *Stent placement:* Stenting is appropriate for atherosclerotic renal artery stenosis because it maintains patency despite elastic recoil. Definite indications include (1) poor response to PTA, (2) early restenosis after angioplasty, and (3) renal artery dissection. However, the benefit of peripheral revascularization comes with risks as well; in atherosclerotic renal artery stenosis, the likelihood of cure is variable and there is widespread variability in the reporting of outcomes (Ives et al., 2003). A major clinical trial of stenting versus medical therapy in atherosclerotic renal artery disease is currently being performed (Cooper et al., 2006).
- *Medical therapy:* control diabetes, control lipids, and maximally manage coronary artery disease
  - Fibromuscular dysplasia: Medical therapy is inferior to intervention.

- Atherosclerosis: control BP and risk factors for CVA and MI (antiplatelet drugs, statins, smoking cessation); need to follow serum creatinine; otherwise, unexplained progressive renal insufficiency warrants consideration for intervention

RENAL ARTERY EMBOLISM

- Presentation: Variable with abdominal pain, gross hematuria, flank tenderness, fever, and hypertension. Anuria is present in bilateral renal thromboembolism and solitary kidney with renal thromboembolism.
- Etiology: The most common cause is atrial fibrillation, which is known to be associated with a four- to sevenfold higher risk of peripheral emboli. Renal thromboembolism constitutes 2% of peripheral emboli caused by atrial fibrillation. Other causes include bacterial endocarditis, heart tumors, mural thrombus (dilated cardiomyopathy), repair of aortic aneurysms, and revascularization of renal artery stenosis (Cheng et al., 2003).
- Laboratory:
  - Elevated lactate dehydrogenase (LDH), aspartate aminotransferase (AST) (renal infarction)
  - Hematuria
  - Decreased urinary sodium (because of renal hypoperfusion)
- Diagnosis:
  - CT with contrast will demonstrate lack of kidney enhancement. However, the use of contrast carries with it the risk of renal failure.
  - Magnetic resonance imaging (MRI) will usually visualize renal arteries. However, MRA with gadolinium may be necessary for visualization (note that gadolinium is contraindicated with GFR <30 mL/min).
  - Renal isotopic flow scans will demonstrate absent or reduced perfusion.
  - Doppler ultrasound studies are generally not useful.
  - Angiography is the gold standard but is invasive; this is only used if intervention is contemplated. Again, the use of contrast carries with it the risk of renal failure.
- Treatment:
  - Kidneys can tolerate lack of blood flow for only 60 to 90 minutes without tubular injury. In the absence of collateral circulation (which is typical of renal artery embolism), prolonged ischemia results in renal infarction.
  - Surgical embolectomy restores kidney function 60% to 70% of the time but is associated with an unacceptably high mortality and is now rarely performed.
  - Intra-arterial thrombolysis is usually successful if performed promptly. Systemic thrombolysis is not indicated.
  - Angioplasty/stenting with thrombolysis can be successful in restoring renal perfusion.

RENAL INFARCTION

- **Pathogenesis:** Occurs because of occlusion of the main renal, branch, interlobular, or arcuate arteries. It may also occur with renal vein occlusion.
- **Diagnosis:** CT will demonstrate nonenhancing wedge-shaped nonperfused areas. Infarction is characterized by the cortical rim sign in which the entire kidney is nonenhancing except for the outer cortex, which is perfused by capsular branches (Kamel & Berkowitz, 1996).
- **Pathology:**
  - **Gross appearance:** Initially, the infarct is red and pyramidal. It then develops a grayish hue with a red rim because of parenchymal congestion. Necrotic tissue is ultimately replaced by collagen and results in a V-shaped scar. Infarctions are cortical and usually spare the medulla.
  - **Microscopic appearance:** Initially, there is congestion. This is followed by cytoplasmic and nuclear degradation such that the cytoplasm looks homogeneous and eosinophilic and the nuclei undergo condensation and karyorrhexis. The periphery of the infarct becomes infiltrated with neutrophils. Finally, the necrotic area collapses and is replaced with a scar.
- **Treatment:** Treatment includes prevention of recurrence by anticoagulation or correction of the underlying cause.

NONTRAUMATIC RENAL ARTERY THROMBOSIS

- **Presentation:** As opposed to renal artery embolism (see above), this condition is usually insidious in onset because of the presence of collateral circulation.
- **Etiology:**
  - Vascular disease
    - Atherosclerosis
    - Renal artery aneurysm
    - Fibromuscular dysplasia
    - Aortic dissection
  - Hypercoagulable states
    - Antiphospholipid syndrome
    - Heparin-induced thrombocytopenia (platelet aggregation leading to platelet thrombi)
    - Factor V Leiden mutation (platelet thrombi)
    - Antithrombin III deficiency (seen in nephrotic syndrome)
    - Methylenetetrahydrofolate reductase mutation (platelet thrombi)
    - Hyperhomocysteinemia

TRAUMATIC RENAL ARTERY THROMBOSIS

- **Presentation:** history of trauma, flank and abdominal pain, nausea, vomiting, fever, hypertension, anemia, and hematuria

- Etiology: Blunt abdominal trauma, most commonly motor vehicle accidents, results in stretch injury, contusion, or avulsion and is associated with 44% mortality (Dinchman & Spirnak, 1995).
- Laboratory (similar to renal artery embolism):
  - Elevated LDH, AST (renal infarction)
  - Hematuria
  - Decreased urinary sodium (because of renal hypoperfusion)
- Diagnosis:
  - CT with contrast will demonstrate lack of kidney enhancement and abrupt termination of the renal artery. However, the use of contrast carries with it the risk of renal failure.
  - MRI will usually visualize renal arteries. However, MRA with gadolinium may be necessary for visualization (note that gadolinium is contraindicated with GFR <30 mL/min).
  - Renal isotopic flow scans will demonstrate absent or reduced perfusion.
  - Doppler ultrasound studies are generally not useful.
  - Angiography is the gold standard but is invasive; this is only used if intervention is contemplated. Again, the use of contrast carries with it the risk of renal failure.
- Treatment:
  - Treatment is similar to embolism. If renal artery thrombosis is treated within 12 hours, results are usually successful. After 18 to 24 hours, renal infarction is expected.
  - Surgical revascularization may not be better than observation and medical management. However, surgery is definitely indicated in bilateral renal artery thrombosis and in solitary kidney. Surgical procedures include thrombectomy, resection of the injured arterial segment, bypass, and endovascular stents for intimal tears.

RENAL VEIN THROMBOSIS

- Presentation:
  - Acute: Flank pain, macroscopic hematuria, and loss of renal function. Can mimic renal colic or pyelonephritis.
  - Chronic: May have few or no symptoms. There may be gradual decline in renal function. May present with pulmonary emboli.
- Etiology:
  - Nephrotic syndrome (increased hepatic synthesis of clotting factors; loss of antithrombin III in urine; hypoalbuminemia leads to increased platelet aggregation and decreased systemic fibrinolysis) (Sagripanti & Barsotti, 1995)
  - Oral contraceptives (hypercoagulable state)
  - Steroids (increased Factor VIII and decreased fibrinolysis)
  - Genetic procoagulant states (i.e., Factor V Leiden)
  - Trauma
  - Tumors

- Diagnosis:
  - Ultrasound with Doppler color flow is the initial study of choice.
  - CT with contrast—usually diagnostic but should follow ultrasound if necessary owing to need for contrast
  - MRI can sometimes visualize the thrombus without gadolinium.
  - Inferior venacavography with selective catheterization of the renal vein with or without epinephrine is gold standard but rarely necessary.
- Treatment:
  - Anticoagulation: Heparin or low–molecular-weight heparin should be used as a bridge while warfarin is used to achieve a therapeutic International Normalized Ratio. Warfarin should be used for as long as the patient is nephrotic or has low albumin. Aspirin is also indicated.
  - Thrombolysis is more rapid and may lead to a more complete resolution. However, there is a higher risk of bleeding.

VIGNETTE 1

A 25-year-old African American woman with resistant hypertension on therapeutic doses of metoprolol, amlodipine, and hydrochlorothiazide presents to your clinic for hypertension evaluation. She complains of occasional dizziness and mild headache. She also has intermittent left-sided nonradiating chest pain unrelated to exertion. She denies visual changes, dyspnea, palpitations, or abdominal pain. She denies a family history of hypertension. On physical examination, vital signs include BP, 180/115 mm Hg; pulse, 88 beats/min; respiratory rate, 20 breaths/min; temperature, 37°C. Funduscopic examination is normal. She has an epigastric bruit. There is no edema. The remainder of the examination is normal.

Blood chemistry:
Sodium: 140 mmol/L
Potassium: 4 mmol/L
Chloride: 110 mmol/L
Total CO_2: 26 mmol/L
Urea nitrogen: 15 mg/dL (urea: 5.4 mmol/L)
Creatinine: 0.9 mg/dL (80 mcmol/L)
Glucose: 115 mg/dL (6.7 mmol/L)

Urinalysis:
Color: yellow

pH: 5.5
Specific gravity: 1.025
Protein: 1+
Blood: negative
Glucose: negative
Ketones: negative
Bilirubin: negative
Urobilinogen: negative
WBCs: 2/hpf
RBCs: 0/hpf
Bacteria: none

Electrocardiogram (EKG) left bundle branch block, no old EKGs for comparison

2-D echo, ejection fraction: 55%, right ventricular systolic pressure: 28 mm Hg

Thyroid-stimulating hormone: 2.5 mIU/L

24-Hour urinary free cortisol: 75 mcg/24 hour (207 nmol/24 hour) (normal)

Plasma normetanephrine: 200 pmol/L (normal < 900)

Plasma metanephrine: 70 pmol/L (normal < 500)

Plasma renin activity (supine): 1.0 ng/mL/h (normal < 1.6)

Plasma aldosterone (supine): 10 ng/dL (280 pmol/L) (normal < 16[443])

Renal ultrasound: normal kidney size (Doppler not done)

Lisinopril is started at a dose of 10 mg daily which is rapidly titrated to 40 mg orally daily, over the next week.

One week later, the blood chemistries are as follows:
Sodium: 136 mmol/L
Potassium: 4.1 mmol/L
Chloride: 110 mmol/L
Total CO_2: 20 mmol/L
Urea nitrogen: 20 mg/dL (urea: 7.1 mmol/L)
Creatinine: 1.9 mg/dL (168 mcmol/L)
Glucose: 120 mg/dL (6.7 mmol/L)

Q: Which of the following does not support the diagnosis of renal artery stenosis in this case?

1. Normal plasma renin activity
2. Epigastric bruit
3. Worsening of renal function with lisinopril
4. Hypertension resistant to multiple antihypertensives
5. Normal renal ultrasound
6. None of the above

A: In this young female patient with resistant hypertension, an epigastric bruit, and worsening of renal failure upon addition of an ACE-I, the most likely diagnosis is renal artery stenosis due to fibromuscular dysplasia. ACE-Is can worsen renal perfusion in renal artery stenosis by dilating the efferent arterioles; acute renal failure is more likely to be evident if there is bilateral renal artery involvement. Normal plasma renin activity does not exclude the diagnosis, especially in patients taking a beta-blocker, which inhibits renin release from the juxtaglomerular cells. (Moreover, in bilateral renal artery stenosis, patients are typically hypervolemic; thus, plasma renin levels are often normal.) Normal kidney sizes on ultrasound also do not exclude the diagnosis, which will only show a decrease in kidney size if there has been time for ischemic damage to one or both the kidneys. The other secondary causes of secondary hypertension to consider would be hyperthyroidism, pheochromocytoma, Cushing syndrome, and hyperaldosteronism, but there is no clinical or laboratory evidence for these conditions. Renal angiography in this patient revealed high-degree fibromuscular dysplasia in both the renal arteries and BP improved after bilateral angioplasty.

15

A 77-year-old man with known coronary artery disease, who 5 years previously had undergone cardiac catheterization with placement of stents in the right coronary and left anterior descending arteries, presents for evaluation of hypertension resistant to multiple antihypertensives and progressive worsening of renal function over the past 2 years. He denies visual changes, chest pain, palpitations, abdominal pain, nausea, vomiting, diarrhea, or constipation. Medications include aspirin, clopidogrel, metoprolol, and amlodipine. Vital signs include pulse, 90 beats/min and regular; BP, 175/99 mm Hg; respiratory rate, 22 breaths/min; temperature, 37°C. Physical examination reveals a cardiac gallop, bibasilar rales, bilateral carotid and epigastric bruits, 1+ edema, and diminished pulses in the lower extremities.

Blood chemistry:
Sodium: 145 mmol/L
Potassium: 4.5 mmol/L
Chloride: 115 mmol/L
Total CO_2: 20 mmol/L

Urea nitrogen: 35 mg/dL (urea: 12.5 mmol/L)
Creatinine: 2.2 mg/dL (194 mcmol/L)
Glucose: 90 mg/dL (5 mmol/L)
Urinalysis: normal

Renal ultrasound—right kidney: 10.0 cm; left kidney: 8.6 cm
MRA renal arteries—left renal artery stenosis: 80%; normal right renal artery

The primary care physician is concerned about using an ACE-I because of progressive renal insufficiency in the presence of renal artery stenosis.

Q: Which of the following statements about ACE-Is in this patient is false?

1. They may initially worsen renal failure.
2. They are the preferred antihypertensive agents to treat renal artery stenosis.
3. They are contraindicated because of renal artery stenosis.
4. They are secondary therapy to be used only if the patient refuses intervention (angioplasty and stent placement).

A: This patient has unilateral left renal artery stenosis. In unilateral renal artery stenosis, decreased perfusion of the affected kidney increases renin secretion and the systemic as well as intrarenal renin–angiotensin–aldosterone system is upregulated. Although the renal artery is normal to the contralateral kidney, uncontrolled hypertension may over time lead to ischemic damage (nephrosclerosis) in that kidney. In this patient with coronary atherosclerosis and advanced age, the etiology of the renal artery stenosis is likely to be atherosclerotic. The role of renal angioplasty and stent placement in such patients is controversial because no improvement in patient outcomes has been shown and there is substantial risk of these procedures to the patient. RAS inhibitors are indicated in unilateral renal artery stenosis, and providing that the contralateral kidney has no stenosis will not usually cause much of a decrease in renal function (although some initial worsening because of control of BP and decreased renal perfusion to the affected kidney is typical).

References

Cheng KL, Tseng SS, Tarng DC. Acute renal failure caused by unilateral renal artery thromboembolism. *Nephrol Dial Transplant.* 18:833–835, 2003.

Cheung CM, Shurrab AE, Buckley DL. MR-derived renal morphology and renal function in patients with atherosclerotic renovascular hypertension. *Kidney Int.* 69:715–722, 2006.

Cooper CJ, Murphy TP, Matsumoto A, et al. Stent revascularization for the prevention of cardiovascular and renal events among patients with renal artery stenosis and systolic hypertension: rationale and design of the CORAL trial. *Am Heart J.* 152(1):59–66, 2006.

Dinchman KH, Spirnak JP. Traumatic renal artery thrombosis: evaluation and treatment. *Semin Urol.* 13(1):90–93, 1995.

Ives NJ, Wheatley K, Stowe R, et al. Continuing uncertainty about the value of percutaneous revascularization in atherosclerotic renovascular disease: a meta-analysis of randomized trials. *Nephrol Dial Transplant.* 18:298–304, 2003.

Kamel IR, Berkowitz JF. Assessment of the cortical rim sign in posttraumatic renal infarction. *J Comput Assist Tomogr.* 20:803–806, 1996.

Olbricht CJ, Paul K, Prokop M, et al. Minimally invasive diagnosis of renal artery stenosis by spiral computed tomography angiography. *Kidney Int.* 48:1332–1337, 1995.

Olin JW, Piedmonte MR, Young JR, et al. The utility of duplex ultrasound scanning of the renal arteries for diagnosing significant renal artery stenosis. *Ann Intern Med.* 122:833–838, 1995.

Pickering TG. Renovascular hypertension: etiology and pathophysiology. *Semin Nucl Med.* 19(2):79–88, 1989.

Radermacher J, Chavan A, Bleck J, et al. Use of Doppler ultrasonography to predict the outcome of therapy for renal artery stenosis. *N Engl J Med.* 344:410–417, 2001.

Sagripanti A, Barsotti G. Hypercoagulability, intraglomerular coagulation, and thromboembolism in nephrotic syndrome. *Nephron.* 70(3):271–281, 1995.

Simon G, Coleman CC. Captopril-stimulated renal vein renin measurements in the diagnosis of atherosclerotic renovascular hypertension. *Am J Hypertens.* 7:1–6, 1994.

Taylor A. Functional testing: ACEI renography. *Semin Nephrol.* 20:437–444, 2000.

16

Microvascular Diseases of the Kidney

CASE STUDY 16.1

A 65-year-old male with a past medical history of hyperlipidemia, vitamin D deficiency, hypertension, atrial fibrillation, and tobacco smoking is admitted for shortness of breath and is found to have a left lower lobe pneumonia. He relates easy bruising from needlesticks and has been having nosebleeds for the past year. He denies chest pain, palpitations, abdominal pain, dark urine, urinary frequency or urgency, or diarrhea. Medications on admission are atorvastatin, omeprazole, diltiazem, and vitamin D. On examination, his blood pressure (BP) is 220/115 mm Hg. He has left-sided chest rales and no edema. There is no abdominal bruit.

Blood chemistry:
Sodium: 128 mmol/L
Potassium: 4.1 mmol/L
Chloride: 91 mmol/L
Bicarbonate: 20 mmol/L
Urea nitrogen: 59 mg/dL (urea: 21 mmol/L)
Creatinine: 4.5 mg/dL (398 mcmol/L)

Complete blood count:
WBCs: 11,000/mm^3
Hemoglobin: 8.2 g/dL (82 g/L)
Hematocrit: 23%
Platelets: 65,000/mm^3
Reticulocytes: 5%
Haptoglobin <10 mg/dL (1 mcmol/L) (low)
Lactate dehydrogenase (LDH) : 544 U/L (9 mckat/L) (elevated)

The peripheral smear shows many schistocytes. A Coombs test is negative. The prothrombin time (PT), partial thromboplastin time, and fibrinogen are normal.

Urinalysis:
Color: yellow
pH: 5.5
Specific gravity: 1.025
Protein: 2+
Blood: 3+
Glucose: negative
Ketones: negative
Bilirubin: negative

Urobilinogen: negative
WBCs: 2/hpf
RBCs: 10 to 20/hpf
Bacteria: none

Question 16.1.1: What is the differential for microangiopathic hemolytic anemia and thrombocytopenia?

- These laboratory findings suggest the presence of thrombotic microangiopathy (TMA), which is a specific pathologic lesion of arterioles and capillaries with resultant microvascular thrombosis caused by endothelial injury. The differential of TMA includes:
  - Thrombotic thrombocytopenic purpura (TTP)
  - Hemolytic-uremic syndrome (HUS)
  - Hypertensive emergency
  - Scleroderma renal crisis (SRC)
  - Disseminated intravascular coagulation (DIC)
  - Other (pregnancy, infection, malignancy, collagen vascular disease, antiphospholipid antibody syndrome, organ transplantation)

Question 16.1.2: What is thrombotic microangiopathy?

THROMBOTIC MICROANGIOPATHY

- Definition: Alteration in the microvasculature with detachment of the endothelium, deposition of amorphous material in the subendothelial space, platelet aggregation, and microthrombosis. The most prominent TMAs are TTP and HUS. Because the distinction between these two entities remains unclear, they are often referred to as a single entity, TTP/HUS.

Question 16.1.3: What are the laboratory manifestations of TTP/HUS?

- Laboratory:
  - Thrombocytopenia (due to platelet aggregation in small blood vessels)
  - Low serum haptoglobin (due to hemolytic anemia)
  - Elevated reticulocyte count (hemolysis)
  - Schistocytes on peripheral smear (hemolysis)
  - Elevated LDH (hemolysis)
  - Elevated indirect bilirubin (hemolysis) (this is a low sensitivity test in this disorder)
  - Negative Coombs test (not immune-mediated)
  - Normal PT/PTT/fibrinogen (except in DIC)
  - Microscopic hematuria (may or may not be present)
  - Proteinuria (nephrotic or subnephrotic)

CASE STUDY 16.1 CONTINUED

A bone marrow examination shows erythroid hyperplasia and increased megakaryocytes. A kidney biopsy is performed. Subsequent laboratory testing reveals the following:
Stool culture for enterotoxigenic *Escherichia coli* (ETEC): negative

Human immunodeficiency virus (HIV) screen: nonreactive

Cytomegalovirus (CMV) antibody (immunoglobulin M [IgM]): negative

Anti-scleroderma (anti-SCL-70) antibody: negative

Anti-RNA polymerase III antibodies: negative

Antinuclear antibodies (ANAs) positive, speckled, with ANA titer of 1:1,280

Extractable nuclear antigen (ENA) antibodies: negative

Antineutrophil cytoplasmic antibodies (C-ANCA and P-ANCA): negative

Anti–glomerular basement membrane antibodies: negative

Hepatitis panel: nonreactive

Total complement, C3, C4 all within normal limits

Serum free light chains: normal

ADAMTS13 activity: 74% (normal) (see Question 16.1.5)

Factor H autoantibodies: positive

Question 16.1.4: What are the kidney biopsy findings in TMA?

- Pathology:
  - Light microscopy/immunofluorescence:
    - Glomeruli: Capillary wall thickening, endothelial cell swelling, lumen obliteration
    - Fibrinogen stains along glomerular capillary walls and in arterial thrombi
    - TTP—Microthrombi are composed of platelet aggregates and a thin layer of fibrin and strongly stain for von Willebrand Factor (vWF).
    - HUS—Microthrombi are composed prominently of fibrin.
  - Electron microscopy—Swelling of glomerular endothelial cells and detachment from the glomerular basement membrane. Electron lucent material fills space between the basement membrane and the detached endothelial cells.

CASE STUDY 16.1 CONTINUED

The biopsy findings in this patient show microvascular thrombi, endothelial injury, schistocytes, mucoid degeneration, and intimal hyperplasia ("onion skinning"). There are no immune complexes. There is ~50% interstitial fibrosis. This is interpreted as TMA with severe hypertensive changes.

Question 16.1.5: What is the pathogenesis of TTP/HUS?

- TTP: ADAMTS13 (*A D*isintegrin-like *A*nd *M*etalloprotease with *T*hrombo*S*pondin type 1 repeats) cleaves large vWF multimers and prevents thrombosis. TTP is due to deficiency in ADAMTS13 (hereditary) or autoantibodies to ADAMTS13 (sporadic) (Shelat et al., 2006; Tsai, 2003). There is some literature to suggest that the differentiation between TTP and HUS can be made with the ADAMTS13 assay, with ADAMTS13 deficiency seen in TTP but normal in HUS. However, this test is not often available at the time of patient presentation. Moreover, this clear distinction is not universally accepted and currently cannot be relied upon to guide therapy (see below).

- TTP/HUS is also associated with the following drugs or conditions (ADAMTS13 is usually normal):
  - Mitomycin C
  - Chemotherapy
  - Ticlopidine
  - Clopidogrel
  - Cyclosporine
  - Vascular endothelial growth factor (VEGF) antagonists (e.g., sunitinib)
  - Bone marrow transplant
  - Pregnancy
- D+ HUS (diarrhea plus HUS)

  Most D+ HUS is sporadic and is caused by *E. coli* 0157:H7. Verocytotoxins, including Shiga-like toxins, bind glycolipid receptors on membranes of renal endothelial, mesangial, and tubular epithelial cells and cause apoptosis, block protein synthesis, and alter cell adhesion enabling leukocyte-dependent inflammation (Tarr et al., 2005).

- D− HUS (diarrhea minus HUS)

  D− HUS can be hereditary (caused by deficient factor H or deficient membrane cofactor protein [MCP]) or sporadic (caused by autoantibodies to factor H or MCP) (Caprioli et al., 2003; Dragon-Durey et al., 2005). Factor H is a cofactor for C3b-cleaving enzyme (factor I). MCP is also involved in the regulation of C3 activation. A deficiency in factor H or MCP leads to uncontrolled complement activation.

Question 16.1.6: What are the symptoms of TTP/HUS?

Classically, TTP is presented as a pentad: (1) thrombocytopenia; (2) microangiopathic hemolytic anemia; (3) fever; (4) neurologic features such as headaches, cranial nerve palsies, confusion, stupor, and coma; and (5) renal manifestations (proteinuria, hematuria, azotemia). However, many patients present with only thrombocytopenia and microangiopathic hemolytic anemia with or without renal failure. HUS has more prominent renal manifestations and may present with or without diarrhea (D).

- D+ HUS—Ninety percent of HUS presents with bloody diarrhea caused by Shiga-like toxin produced by ETEC. Symptoms start 2 to 12 days after consumption of contaminated food. Renal failure occurs in up to 70% of cases.
- D− HUS—represents 5% to 10% of HUS. There is no diarrhea, and Shiga-like toxin is not involved. It may be familial or sporadic. There is up to 25% mortality, and half may progress to end-stage kidney disease (ESKD). Fever and neurologic symptoms occur in 30% of patients.

Question 16.1.7: What is the treatment of TTP/HUS?

- Acute TTP

Plasma infusion is used for hereditary TTP and plasma exchange for acquired TTP (which requires antibody removal). Plasmapheresis is also frequently used in HUS with less predictable response. Plasma exchange is generally performed daily until platelet count normalizes or there is resolution of neurologic symptoms. Fresh-frozen plasma may help by replacing proteases. Corticosteroids suppress immunity and can control the autoimmune process.

■ Chronic TTP

Low levels of inhibitors to ADAMTS13 may persist and may cause frequent relapses. In these cases, the following options are available:

■ Antiplatelet agents
■ Vincristine
■ Cyclophosphamide
■ Staphylococcal protein A columns
■ High-dose immunoglobulins
■ Rituximab

■ HUS

Treatment is directed at the underlying pathogenesis.

Dialysis is frequently required. Renal transplantation is safe in D+ HUS. In D− HUS, 1-year graft survival is <30%, and there is 50% recurrence in the graft. Because factor H is made in the liver, a combined kidney–liver transplant is the best option in HUS due to complement deficiency.

Question 16.1.8: What is the treatment of drug-induced TMA?

Drug-induced TMA is treated by decreasing the dose of the drug or stopping it altogether if necessary. There is no benefit of plasmapheresis.

Question 16.1.9: What is the treatment of atypical HUS?

Eculizumab is a monoclonal antibody that binds C5 and inhibits its cleavage to C5a and C5b and preventing the generation of the terminal complement complex C5b-9.

CASE STUDY 16.1 CONCLUDED

This patient is diagnosed to have atypical HUS due to factor H autoantibodies and is treated with plasmapheresis and eculizumab.

SYSTEMIC SCLEROSIS (SCLERODERMA)

■ Definition:
  ■ Scleroderma is a rare disease characterized by autoantibodies, increased collagen production, and endothelial cell abnormalities that result in vasospasm, cutaneous induration, azotemia, hypertension, and extrarenal manifestations.
■ Pathogenesis:
  ■ Vasospasm may be related to elevated renin. Increased transforming growth factor-beta (TGF-β) and decreased interferon-gamma contribute to increased collagen synthesis

(Rosenbloom et al., 1986; Smith & LeRoy, 1990). Damage to endothelial cells leads to platelet aggregation, release of platelet-derived growth factor and TGF-β, and subsequent subintimal proliferation and fibrosis.

- In SRC (see below), an initial trigger (like cold weather, stress, or hormonal change) causes Raynaud phenomenon, cortical ischemia, and release of renin and angiotensin II, which leads to further renal vasoconstriction.

- Symptoms and signs:
  - Extrarenal manifestations
    - Thick skin
    - Sclerodactyly
    - Raynaud phenomenon
    - Telangiectasias
    - Arthralgias/arthritis
    - Myopathy
    - Esophageal dysmotility
    - Pulmonary fibrosis
    - Myocardial fibrosis
  - Renal involvement
    - Slowly progressing form of chronic kidney disease (CKD) in systemic sclerosis involves subnephrotic proteinuria and hypertension.
    - SRC is typically characterized by malignant hypertension and acute oliguric azotemia. Symptomatology may include headaches, blurred vision, encephalopathy, seizures, and left ventricular failure. Some patients may be normotensive.

- Laboratory findings
  - Positive ANAs
  - Anticentromere antibodies are positive in 5% of patients
  - Anti-SCL-70 antibodies are positive in 70% of patients with systemic sclerosis
  - Anti-RNA polymerase 3 (POL3) antibodies are most strongly associated with scleroderma renal disease (Okano et al., 1993)
  - SRC:
    - Subnephrotic proteinuria
    - Microscopic hematuria
    - Elevated plasma renin
    - Microangiopathic hemolytic anemia
    - Thrombocytopenia

- Pathology
  - Slowly progressing scleroderma renal disease—subintimal proliferation and luminal narrowing in small- and medium-sized arteries
  - SRC—Luminal narrowing, tissue ischemia, adventitial and periadventitial fibrosis, and fibrinoid necrosis. Lymphocytes and inflammatory cells are absent.

- Management
  - Angiotensin-converting enzyme (ACE) inhibitors have remarkably improved survival in SRC. Before ACE inhibitors, 1-year survival was 10%. After ACE inhibitors, 5-year survival has improved to 65%.

- Systemic sclerosis patients may progress to ESKD and require dialysis. With dialysis, there is 30% survival at 3 years. Some patients with SRC will improve enough with ACE inhibitors to discontinue dialysis.
- Penicillamine can be used with kidney disease. Corticosteroids (high dose and even low dose) may be a risk factor for SRC.
- Renal transplantation has been performed in scleroderma patients with ESKD.

RENAL VASCULITIS

See Chapter 10.

VIGNETTE 1

A 45-year-old man with coronary artery disease undergoes cardiac catheterization and stenting of the left anterior descending artery with initiation of clopidogrel (Plavix) in addition to metoprolol, lisinopril, and pravastatin. He now presents for evaluation of thrombocytopenia and renal failure. His family says that he is a little confused. He also has been fatigued and looks pale. He has a slight fever that is accompanied by headaches. On examination, his vital signs are normal. He has purpuric lesions on his lower extremities.

Blood chemistry:
Sodium: 140 mmol/L
Potassium: 5.2 mmol/L
Chloride: 104 mmol/L
Total CO_2: 26 mmol/L
Urea nitrogen: 30 mg/dL
  (urea: 10.7 mmol/L)
Creatinine: 2.0 mg/dL
  (177 mcmol/L)
Glucose: 100 mg/dL (5.6 mmol/L)
Coombs test: negative
PT: 11 seconds
Partial thromboplastin time:
  30 seconds

Urinalysis:
Color: yellow
pH: 5.5
Specific gravity: 1.025
Protein: 2+
Blood: 3+

Glucose: negative
Ketones: 1+
Bilirubin: 2+
Urobilinogen: 2+
WBCs: 2/hpf
RBCs: 10/hpf
Bacteria: none

Complete blood count:
WBCs: 12,000/mm^3
Hemoglobin: 9 g/dL (90 g/L)
Hematocrit: 27 g/dL
Platelets: 40,000/mm^3
Schistocytes: prominent
Reticulocyte count: 3%
LDH: 200 U/L (elevated)
Haptoglobin: 30 mg/dL (0.3 g/L)
  (low)
Bone marrow, erythroid hyperplasia, increased megakaryocytes

Q: What is the pathophysiology of renal failure in this patient?

1. Verocytotoxins bind glycolipid receptors on membranes and cause apoptosis, block protein synthesis, and alter cell adhesion enabling leukocyte-dependent inflammation.
2. A deficiency in or autoantibodies to factor H or MCP leads to uncontrolled complement activation.
3. A deficiency in or autoantibodies to ADAMTS13 causes widespread thrombosis.
4. Plavix can cause medication-induced TTP.
5. Both 3 and 4.

A: This patient has the classic pentad associated with TTP: (1) thrombocytopenia, (2) microangiopathic hemolytic anemia, (3) fever, (4) neurologic manifestations (headaches and confusion), and (5) renal failure. The elevated reticulocyte count, schistocytes, hyperkalemia, elevated LDH, and bilirubinuria all are consistent with hemolytic anemia. The Coombs test is negative; hence, this is not due to antibodies against RBC antigens. The low haptoglobin is also characteristic of hemolysis. The normal coagulation profile rules out processes such as DIC.

HUS associated with diarrhea is usually caused by *E. coli* 0157:H7 and Shiga-like toxins, which bind glycolipid receptors on membranes and cause apoptosis, block protein synthesis, and alter cell adhesion enabling leukocyte-dependent inflammation. HUS not associated with diarrhea caused by a deficiency in or autoantibodies to factor H or MCP leads to uncontrolled complement activation. TTP is due to deficiency in ADAMTS13 or is due to autoantibodies to ADAMTS13. ADAMTS13 cleaves large vWF multimers and prevents thrombosis. Some antiplatelet medications, such as ticlopidine and clopidogrel, have been associated with HUS/TTP, though drug-dependent antibody production to ADAMTS13 does not appear to be involved.

VIGNETTE **2**

16

A 55-year-old woman with known systemic sclerosis (scleroderma) presents with accelerated hypertension and renal failure. She complains of some orthopnea and paroxysmal nocturnal dyspnea, shortness of breath, headaches, and blurred vision. Physical examination shows thick skin, sclerodactyly, blanching of the fingers, telangiectasias, and weakness in all four extremities. Vital signs are as follows: pulse, 90 beats/min; BP, 180/110 mm Hg; respiratory rate, 22 breaths/min; temperature, 37.5°C. Labs are positive for ANA (1:640 titer) and anti-RNA POL3 (1:320 titer). There is thrombocytopenia and microangiopathic hemolytic anemia, and the plasma renin is elevated.

Q: Which of the following statements about SRC is false?

1. Penicillamine causes marked improvement in renal failure.
2. Renin-induced vasospasm and vasoconstriction cause hypertensive crisis.
3. ACE inhibitors are the mainstay of treatment even in dialysis-dependent patients.
4. Half of the patients with SRC will be able to discontinue dialysis in 3 to 18 months if ACE inhibitor is continued.

A: Penicillamine is a treatment for scleroderma of the skin. However, penicillamine does not improve renal function. The pathogenesis of scleroderma involves excessive renin secretion, vasospasm and renal vasoconstriction, increased collagen production, and endothelial injury from cytotoxic serum. Although autoantibodies have been demonstrated in scleroderma, an immunologic mechanism of disease causation has not been proven.

The mainstay of treatment for SRC is ACE inhibitor treatment. SRC can progress to ESKD; dialysis leads to 33% survival in 3 years. However, half the patients on dialysis may be able to come off dialysis in 3 to 18 months if ACE inhibitor therapy is continued.

References

Caprioli J, Castelletti F, Bucchioni S, et al. Complement factor H mutations and gene polymorphisms in haemolytic uremic syndrome: the C-257T, the A2089G and the G2881T polymorphisms are strongly associated with the disease. *Hum Mol Genet.* 12:3385–3395, 2003.

Dragon-Durey MA, Loirat C, Cloarec S, et al. Anti-factor H autoantibodies associated with atypical hemolytic uremic syndrome. *J Am Soc Nephrol.* 16:555–563, 2005.

Okano Y, Steen VD, Medsger TA Jr. Autoantibody reactive with RNA polymerase III in systemic sclerosis. *Ann Intern Med.* 119(10):1005–1013, 1993.

Rosenbloom J, Feldman G, Freundlich B, et al. Inhibition of excessive scleroderma fibroblast collagen production by recombinant gamma-interferon. Association with a coordinate decrease in types I and III procollagen messenger RNA levels. *Arthritis Rheum.* 29:851–856, 1986.

Shelat SG, Smith P, Ai J, et al. Inhibitory autoantibodies against ADAMTS-13 in patients with thrombotic thrombocytopenic purpura bind ADAMTS-13 protease and may accelerate it clearance in vivo. *J Thromb Haemost.* 4(8):1707–1717, 2006.

Smith EA, LeRoy EC. A possible role for transforming growth factor beta in systemic sclerosis. *J Invest Dermatol.* 95:125S–127S, 1990.

Tarr PI, Gordon CA, Chandler WL. Shigo-toxin producing *Escherichia coli* and haemolytic uremic syndrome. *Lancet.* 365:1073–1086, 2005.

Tsai HM. Is severe deficiency of ADAMTS-13 specific for thrombotic thrombocytopenic purpura? Yes. *J Thromb Haemost.* 1(4):625–631, 2003.

17 Nephrolithiasis

INTRODUCTION

- Renal stone disease (nephrolithiasis) occurs in 12% of men and 5% of women (lifetime risk).
- The major types of stones are calcium (70%–80%, oxalate more common than phosphate), uric acid (5%–10%), cystine (<1%), and magnesium ammonium phosphate (struvite) (10%). Combined calcium/urate stones are also often seen.
- A patient with a calcium-containing stone episode has an overall 50% chance of recurrence within 10 years, which is higher for men than for women (Fig. 17.1).

CALCIUM STONES

Idiopathic Hypercalciuria
Idiopathic hypercalciuria is the most common etiology of calcium stones.
- Autosomal dominant
- Multigenic

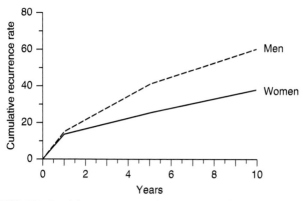

FIGURE 17.1. Cumulative recurrence rate for stone disease (Uribarri et al., 1989). (Reproduced with permission from Emmett M, Szerlip H. Pathogenesis of metabolic alkalosis. *UpToDate*. Waltham, MA. https://www.uptodate.com/contents/pathogenesis-of-metabolic-alkalosis/print. Accessed November 29, 2018. Copyright © 2018 UpToDate, Inc. For more information visit www.uptodate.com and Preminger GM, Curhan GC. The first kidney stone and asymptomatic nephrolithiasis in adults. *UpToDate*. Waltham, MA. https://www.uptodate.com/contents/the-first-kidney-stone-and-asymptomatic-nephrolithiasis-in-adults. Accessed November 29, 2018. Copyright © 2018 UpToDate, Inc. For more information visit www.uptodate.com.)

- Exact pathogenesis uncertain, but may have different etiologies (renal phosphorus and/or calcium leak, intestinal hyperabsorption, increased bone resorption)

Risk Factors for Calcium Stones
- Lower urinary volume
- Higher urinary calcium excretion (Table 17.1) (Marshall et al., 1972)
- Higher urinary oxalate excretion (calcium oxalate stones)
- Higher urinary uric acid excretion
- Lower urinary citrate excretion
- Higher urinary pH (calcium phosphate stones)
- Anatomic abnormalities (medullary sponge kidney, horseshoe kidney)

Prevalence of Urinary Biochemical Abnormalities in Patients with Calcium Stones (Levy et al., 1995)
- Hypercalciuria—61%, including some patients with primary hyperparathyroidism
- Hyperuricosuria—36%
- Hypocitraturia—28% idiopathic and 3.3% due to type 1 (distal) renal tubular acidosis (RTA) or chronic diarrhea
- Low urine volume (<1 L/day)—15%
- Hyperoxaluria—8%, including enteric and primary forms and markedly increased oxalate intake

Dietary Risk Factors for Calcium Stones
- Lower fluid intake (increases urinary calcium and oxalate concentration)
- Lower dietary calcium (increases oxalate absorption and urinary oxalate excretion)
- Higher dietary oxalate (increases urinary oxalate excretion)
- Lower dietary potassium (may increase urinary calcium excretion)
- Higher animal protein intake (increases calcium and uric acid excretion, lowers urine pH, thus decreasing citrate excretion)
- Higher sodium intake (increases calcium excretion)
- Higher sucrose intake (may increase calcium excretion)
- Vitamin C intake (increases oxalate excretion)
- Vitamin D intake (increases calcium excretion)

Medical Conditions Associated with Calcium Stones
- Hypercalcemia (especially primary hyperparathyroidism and granulomatous disorders such as sarcoidosis)

TABLE 17.1	Risk of Calcium Stone Formation Relative to Urinary Calcium Excretion	
24-h Calcium (mg/d)		**Relative Stone Risk**
<100		1.0
100–199		1.5
200–299		2
>300		2.5

- Hypercalciuria
  - Idiopathic (primary)
  - Secondary
    - Hyperparathyroidism (also have hypercalcemia)
    - Granulomatous disorders (especially sarcoidosis) because of increased conversion of 25-hydroxyvitamin D to 1,25-dihydroxyvitamin D by activated macrophages (may not have hypercalcemia)
    - RTA, classic distal type—failure of H+ excretion results in acidemia, leading to calcium release from bone and hypercalciuria; alkaline urine leads to calcium phosphate stones
- Hyperoxaluria
  - Increased dietary oxalate
  - High-dose vitamin C (metabolized to oxalate)
  - Enteric hyperoxaluria (malabsorption syndromes such as inflammatory bowel disease, leading to decreased calcium oxalate binding in the gut coupled with bile salt–induced increase in oxalate absorption) (Chadwick et al., 1973; Smith et al., 1972); bariatric surgery (Roux-en-Y gastric bypass) can cause hyperoxaluria, nephrolithiasis, and, occasionally, irreversible renal failure (Nasr et al., 2008)
- Hyperuricosuria (gout, high animal protein intake; uric acid can serve as nidus for calcium stone formation, leading to calcium and mixed calcium/urate stones as well as pure uric acid stones) (Coe et al., 1975)

Inhibitors of Stone Formation
- Citrate (impairs calcium oxalate lattice formation) (Ettinger et al., 1997; Nicar et al., 1987)
  - Filter and reabsorb by proximal tubule
  - Amount reabsorbed depends on tubular and intracellular pH

$$\text{Citrate}^{(2-)} + \text{HCO}_3^- \rightarrow \text{Citrate}^{(3-)} + \text{CO}_2 + \text{H}_2\text{O}$$

  - Decreased tubular and intracellular pH will increase citrate reabsorption and decrease urinary citrate excretion; treatment with alkali will have opposite effect. Hypokalemia will decrease intracellular pH and urinary citrate excretion.
- Glycoprotein inhibitors
  - Tamm-Horsfall protein (uromodulin)
  - Nephrocalcin
  - Uropontin

Treatment of Calcium Stones
- Increase fluid intake (Pak et al., 1980)
- Dietary interventions (decrease protein and sodium intake) (Muldowney et al., 1982)
- Thiazide diuretics (if at high risk for recurrence, coexistent medical conditions, or recurrent/multiple stones) (Laerum & Larsen, 1984)
- Potassium citrate (if urinary citrate low) (Ettinger et al., 1997)
- Allopurinol (if coexistent hyperuricosuria unresponsive to dietary restriction) (Ettinger et al., 1986)

URIC ACID STONES

Risk Factors for Uric Acid Stones

- Low urine pH and urine volume
- Gout and/or hyperuricosuria (in some patients) (Yü & Gutman, 1967)

$$H(^+) + Urate(^-) \leftrightarrow Uric\ acid,\ pK\ 5.75$$

- Thus, at urine pH 5.75, half of urine uric acid is in relatively insoluble uric acid form.
- Type 2 diabetes increases the risk for uric acid stones (Daudon et al., 2006).

Prevention and Treatment of Uric Acid Stones

- Raising urine pH to >6.5 with alkali will markedly increase urate to uric acid ratio and decrease stone risk (Pak et al., 1986).
- Increasing fluid intake also of benefit by decreasing urine uric acid concentration

CYSTINE STONES

Cystinuria

- Rare
- Autosomal dominant
- Due to abnormality of amino acid transport
- Treatment is urinary alkalinization and increased fluid intake.

STRUVITE STONES

Struvite stones are also called infection stones (Rodman, 1999).

- Are composed of calcium carbonate apatite and magnesium ammonium phosphate
- Form only in the presence of urea-splitting organisms (e.g., *Proteus* species)—urea is split into ammonia and carbon dioxide, resulting in alkaline urine that promotes calcium phosphate or magnesium ammonium phosphate crystallization
- Difficult to eradicate even with interventional/surgical procedures
- Can cause end-stage kidney disease
- Urinary diversion—Patients with a partially obstructed ileal conduit develop urinary stasis and can develop chronic metabolic acidosis (due to chloride–bicarbonate exchange by the ileal mucosa), leading to hypercalciuria and hypocitraturia. Persistent infections with urease-producing bacteria can lead to the formation of struvite stones (see above).

UROLOGIC CONSULTATION

Acute Stone Management

- Likelihood of stone passage depends on size (Miller & Kane, 1999).
  - <2 mm—only 5% require intervention; most pass spontaneously with average time to stone passage of 8 days (95% pass within 31 days)

- 2- to 4-mm stones—17% require intervention; the rest pass spontaneously with average time to stone passage of 12 days (95% pass within 40 days)
- 4- to 6-mm stones—only 50% pass spontaneously with average time to stone passage of 22 days (95% of these pass within 39 days)
- Spontaneous passage rate also depends on stone location (48% for stones in the proximal ureter, 60% for midureteral stones, 75% for distal stones, and 79% for ureterovesical junction stones).

Urologic Consultation

- Urgent: urosepsis, acute renal failure, anuria, and/or persistent pain, nausea, or vomiting
- Outpatient: stone >10 mm in diameter and in patients who fail to pass the stone after a trial of conservative management, particularly if the stone is >4 mm
- For stones <10 mm
    - Proximal—Extracorporeal shock wave lithotripsy (ESWL) or ureteroscopy/stone removal
    - Distal—Ureteroscopy is better than ESWL
- For stones >10 mm—Ureteroscopy is better than EWSL
- Stent necessary if ureteral injury, stricture, solitary kidney, renal failure, or large stones
- Complex stones >2 cm—Percutaneous nephrolithotomy
- If patient is septic, defer definitive treatment and place nephrostomy tube or stent

VIGNETTE **1**

A 50-year-old white male construction worker with a long history of back pains undergoes magnetic resonance imaging, which discloses renal calculi. He is referred to a urologist, where computed tomography (CT) reveals bilateral stones. He undergoes ESWL on two occasions. Follow-up ultrasound reveals a residual 7-mm stone in the right kidney (Fig. 17.2). Stone analysis on the gravel that is obtained after ESWL shows calcium oxalate. He is subsequently referred by the urologist to a nephrologist. Family history is remarkable for a brother and a cousin with stones. Medications include occasional acetaminophen. Diet is only remarkable for a recent decrease in dairy product intake. There is no history of gout or diarrhea. Physical examination is entirely normal. Plasma electrolytes, urea nitrogen, and creatinine, calcium ×3 are normal. Urinalysis shows crystals (Fig. 17.3). A 24-hour urine values are as follows:

Calcium × 3 = 250, 258, 245 mg (normal <300 for male; <250 for female) (6.25, 6.45, 6.125 mmol)

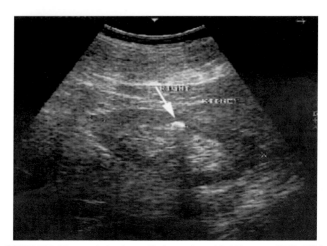

FIGURE 17.2. Ultrasound showing residual stone (*arrow*) in kidney post-ESWL. ESWL, extracorporeal shock wave lithotripsy. (Reproduced with permission from Curhan GC. Prevention of recurrent calcium stones in adults. *UpToDate*. Waltham, MA. https://www .uptodate.com/contents/prevention-of-recurrent-calcium-stones-in-adults. Accessed November 29, 2018. Copyright © 2018 UpToDate, Inc. For more information visit www.uptodate. com and Emmett M, Szerlip H. Causes of metabolic alkalosis. *UpToDate*. Waltham, MA. https://www.uptodate.com/contents/causes-of-metabolic-alkalosis. Accessed November 29, 2018. Copyright © 2018 UpToDate, Inc. For more information visit www.uptodate.com.)

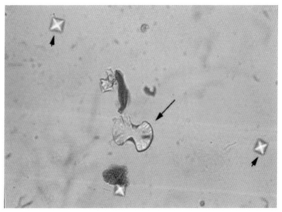

FIGURE 17.3. Urinalysis showing calcium oxalate crystals (*arrows*). (Reproduced with permission from Emmett M, Szerlip H. Pathogenesis of metabolic alkalosis. *UpToDate*. Waltham, MA. https://www.uptodate.com/contents/pathogenesis-of-metabolic-alkalosis/ print. Accessed November 29, 2018. Copyright © 2018 UpToDate, Inc. For more information visit www.uptodate.com and Preminger GM, Curhan GC. The first kidney stone and asymptomatic nephrolithiasis in adults. *UpToDate*. Waltham, MA. https://www.uptodate .com/contents/the-first-kidney-stone-and-asymptomatic-nephrolithiasis-in-adults. Accessed November 29, 2018. Copyright © 2018 UpToDate, Inc. For more information visit www.uptodate.com.)

Uric acid × 3 = 600, 592, 718 mg (<800 for male; <750 for female)
(3.6, 3.6, 4.3 mmol)

Sodium × 3 = 212, 182, 200 mmol

Creatinine × 3 = 1,793; 2,011; 2,050 mg (15.9, 17.8, 18.1 mmol)

Volume × 3 = 1,200; 1,100; 1,100 mL

Citrate, 539 mg (normal >320; usual, 450–600 for male; 650–800 for
female) (2.8 mmol)

Oxalate, 20 mg (normal < 45) (222 mcmol)

He is treated with hydrochlorothiazide, 25 mg, every morning,
to decrease calcium excretion. He is also instructed to decrease his
sodium and protein intake and to increase his fluid intake. Three
months later, the urine values are as follows: volume, 2,400 mL; calcium, 254 mg (6.35 mmol); sodium, 269 mmol; creatinine, 2,400 mg
(17.7 mmol). He is instructed to use a salt substitute (Morton Lite
salt). Two months later, the urine values are as follows: volume,
2,000 mL; calcium, 150 mg (3.75 mmol); sodium, 151 mmol; creatinine, 1,890 mg (16.7 mmol).

As can be seen, initially, the expected hypocalciuric effect of hydrochlorothiazide is not seen, probably because of the high sodium
intake and excretion (sodium and calcium compete for reabsorption
by the renal tubules, so a high-salt diet will blunt or prevent the hypocalciuric effect of thiazides). Once salt is restricted, the hypocalciuric
effect becomes evident.

VIGNETTE 2

A 60-year-old white man is admitted to the ENT service for a nasal polypectomy. Eleven years ago, he had donated his left kidney
to a brother suffering from end-stage kidney disease. There is no
personal or family history of nephrolithiasis or gout. Physical examination reveals nasal polyps and mild hypertension. The plasma
urea nitrogen and creatinine are 125 mg/dL (urea, 44.6 mmol/L)
and 12 mg/dL (1,061 mcmol/L), respectively. Urinalysis reveals a
urine pH 5.0 and crystals (Fig. 17.4). Plasma uric acid is 8.7 mg/
dL (517 mcmol/L). Plasma calcium and phosphorus are 9.3 mg/dL
(2.3 mmol/L) and 8.2 mg/dL (2.6 mmol/L), respectively. Ultrasound

FIGURE 17.4. Urinalysis showing uric acid crystals. (Reproduced with permission from Preminger GM, Curhan GC. The first kidney stone and asymptomatic nephrolithiasis in adults. *UpToDate*. Waltham, MA. https://www.uptodate.com/contents/the-first-kidney-stone-and-asymptomatic-nephrolithiasis-in-adults. Copyright © 2018 UpToDate, Inc. For more information visit www.uptodate.com.)

of the solitary right kidney reveals hydronephrosis and multiple stones. Retrograde pyelography shows three radiolucent stones almost obstructing the ureter. A ureteral stent is placed, and the renal pelvis is irrigated with $NaHCO_3$. The stones resolve, and the plasma urea nitrogen and creatinine decrease to 14 and 1.4 mg/dL, respectively (urea, 5 mmol/L and creatinine, 124 mcmol/L). A 24-hour urinary uric acid excretion is normal. The patient receives sodium citrate and nightly acetazolamide to maintain the urine pH >6.5 and has no stone recurrence.

VIGNETTE 3

17

A 24-year-old man presents with vague flank discomfort. Family history is positive for a sister with kidney stones. Physical examination is remarkable for a BP of 140/90 mm Hg and minimal right costovertebral angle tenderness. A renal ultrasound reveals a moderately radio-opaque 2-cm stone in the right kidney. Urinalysis reveals pH 5.0 and multiple hexagonal crystals (Fig. 17.5). A 24-hour urinary calcium is normal. The patient is treated with increased fluid intake, potassium citrate, and nightly acetazolamide. Six months later, the stone has decreased to half its original size.

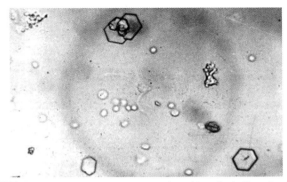

FIGURE 17.5. Hexagonal cystine crystals in a patient with cystinuria. (Reproduced with permission from Preminger GM, Curhan GC. The first kidney stone and asymptomatic nephrolithiasis in adults. *UpToDate*. Waltham, MA. https://www.uptodate.com/contents/the-first-kidney-stone-and-asymptomatic-nephrolithiasis-in-adults. Accessed November 29, 2018. Copyright © 2018 UpToDate, Inc. For more information visit www.uptodate.com.)

VIGNETTE **4**

17

A 40-year-old C5 quadriplegic man with a chronic indwelling urinary catheter presents with urosepsis. His spinal cord injury has been sustained at age 17 during a football practice. After administering antibiotics, a CT is done, which reveals bilateral staghorn calculi. Urinalysis reveals a urine pH of 9.0 and coffin-lid crystals (Fig. 17.6).

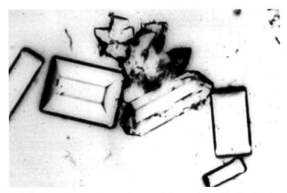

FIGURE 17.6. Urinalysis showing struvite crystals in a patient with chronic urinary tract infection and infection stones. (Reproduced with permission from Wald R. Urinalysis in the diagnosis of kidney disease. *UpToDate*. Waltham, MA. https://www.uptodate.com/contents/urinalysis-in-the-diagnosis-of-kidney-disease. Accessed November 29, 2018. Copyright © 2018 UpToDate, Inc. For more information visit www.uptodate.com.)

Urine culture has grown multiple organisms, including *Proteus*, *Pseudomonas*, *Providencia*, and *Enterococcal* species. He undergoes left ESWL ×2 and right ESWL. The patient has refused sphincterotomy, preferring to continue to use the urinary catheter.

References

Chadwick VS, Modha K, Dowling RH. Mechanism for hyperoxaluria in patients with ileal dysfunction. *N Engl J Med*. 1973;289:172–176.

Coe FL, Lawton RL, Goldstein RB, et al. Sodium urate accelerates precipitation of calcium oxalate in vitro. *Proc Soc Exp Biol Med*. 1975;149:926–929.

Daudon M, Traxer O, Conort P, et al. Type 2 diabetes increases the risk for uric acid stones. *J Am Soc Nephrol*. 2006;17:2026–2033.

Ettinger B, Pak CY, Citron JT, et al. Potassium-magnesium-citrate is an effective prophylaxis against recurrent calcium oxalate nephrolithiasis. *J Urol*. 1997;158:2069–2073.

Ettinger B, Tang A, Citron JT, et al. Randomized trial of allopurinol in the prevention of calcium oxalate calculi. *N Engl J Med*. 1986;315:1386–1389.

Laerum E, Larsen S. Thiazide prophylaxis of urolithiasis: a double-blind study in general practice. *Acta Med Scand*. 1984;215:383–389.

Levy FL, Adams-Huet B, Pak CY. Ambulatory evaluation of nephrolithiasis: and update of a 1980 protocol. *Am J Med*. 1995;98(1):50–59.

Marshall RW, Cochran M, Robertson WC, et al. The relation between the concentration of calcium salts in the urine and renal stone composition in patients with calcium-containing renal stones. *Clin Sci*. 1972;43:433–441.

Miller OF, Kane CJ. Time to stone passage for observed ureteral calculi: a guide for patient education. *J Urol*. 1999;162:688–691.

Muldowney FP, Freaney R, Moloney MF. Importance of dietary sodium in the hypercalciuria syndrome. *Kidney Int*. 1982;22:292–296.

Nasr SH, D'Agati VD, Said SM, et al. Oxalate nephropathy complicating Roux-en-Y gastric bypass: an underrecognized cause of irreversible renal failure. *Clin J Am Soc Nephrol*. 2008;3(6):1676–1683.

Nicar MJ, Hill K, Pak CY. Inhibition by citrate of spontaneous precipitation of calcium oxalate in vitro. *J Bone Miner Res*. 1987;2:215–220.

Pak CY, Sakhaee K, Crowther C, et al. Evidence justifying a high fluid intake in treatment of nephrolithiasis. *Ann Intern Med*. 1980;93:36–39.

Pak CY, Sakhaee K, Fuller C. Successful management of uric acid nephrolithiasis with potassium citrate. *Kidney Int*. 1986;30:422–428.

Rodman JS. Struvite stones. *Nephron*. 1999;81(1)(suppl):50–59.

Smith LH, Frueth AJ, Hoffman AF. Acquired hyperoxaluria, nephrolithiasis and intestinal disease. *N Engl J Med*. 1972;286:1371–1375.

Uribarri J, Oh, MS, Carroll HJ. The first kidney stone. *Ann Intern Med*. 1989;111:1006–1009.

Yü TF, Gutman AB. Uric acid nephrolithiasis in gout. *Ann Intern Med*. 1967;67:1133–1148.

18 Cystic Renal Diseases

CASE STUDY

A 65-year-old male with a history of cigarette smoking presents for evaluation of an incidental finding of four cysts in each kidney on an abdominal ultrasound (US) done for abdominal aortic aneurysm screening. The kidneys are of normal size with normal echogenicity. The cysts vary in size from 1 to 3 cm in diameter; all are of water density and have thin walls without septa, calcifications, or solid components.

Question 18.1.1: What is a renal cyst? How are they formed? What symptoms can they cause?

- Definition: A cyst is a sac of clear, serous fluid (ultrafiltrate of plasma) that is lined by a single layer of epithelial cells.
- Pathophysiology: Renal cysts are derived from progressive dilatation and detachment of diverticula in the distal convoluted tubule and collecting duct. Incidental cysts may be solitary or multiple, and their frequency increases with age (up to 50% of patients aged 40–50 years will show cysts).
- Symptoms: Patients are usually asymptomatic. They may have abdominal or flank discomfort. Some patients present with gross hematuria or symptoms and signs of infection. Hypertension is rare. If there are multiple cysts and renal function is impaired, consider acquired cystic disease (see below).

Question 18.1.2: What is the differential diagnosis of renal cysts?

The differential diagnosis includes the following:

1. Incidental renal cysts
2. Acquired cystic kidney disease
3. Polycystic kidney disease (PKD) without a positive family history (sporadic)
4. Familial autosomal dominant polycystic kidney disease (ADPKD)

Question 18.1.3: What features are suggestive of incidental renal cysts?

The diagnosis of incidental cysts is supported by:
- Incidental finding of simple cyst(s) on US, computed tomography (CT) of the abdomen, or magnetic resonance imaging (MRI) of the abdomen (see below)

- Absence of liver cysts
- Absence of family history

> **Question 18.1.4:** How do you distinguish benign renal cysts from malignant renal cysts?

- Imaging studies can usually distinguish between benign and malignant cysts.
  - US criteria for benign lesions:
    - Round and sharply demarcated with smooth walls
    - No echoes (anechoic) within the mass
    - Strong posterior wall echo indicating good transmission through the cyst and enhanced transmission beyond the cyst
  - CT criteria (Bosniak classification): Cysts can be classified based on morphologic and contrast enhancement characteristics (Israel & Bosniak, 2005).
    - Category I: Benign simple cyst with a thin wall without septa, calcifications, or solid components; water density; no contrast enhancement; no follow-up needed
    - Category II: Benign cystic lesions in which there may be a few thin septa; the wall or septa may contain fine calcification or a short segment of slightly thickened calcification; <3 cm in diameter, well-marginated, and nonenhancing; no follow-up needed
    - Category IIF: Multiple thin septa or minimal smooth thickening of the septa or wall, which may contain calcification that may also be thick and nodular; no measurable contrast enhancement; may be more than 3 cm in diameter; require follow-up to ascertain that they are nonmalignant
    - Category III: Indeterminate cystic masses with thickened irregular or smooth walls or septa; measurable enhancement is present. Risk of malignancy is ~50% (cystic renal cell carcinoma [RCC] and multiloculated cystic RCC); require further imaging and consideration of surgery
    - Category IV: These lesions have all the characteristics of Category III cysts, plus they contain enhancing soft-tissue components that are adjacent to and independent of the wall or septum; these lesions are very likely malignant and require surgery

> **Question 18.1.5:** What is the management of renal cysts?

- If patient is symptomatic or develops significant obstruction, percutaneous aspiration and obliteration with a sclerosing agent may be needed.
- If the cyst becomes larger than 500 mL, consider drainage even in the absence of symptoms.
- Infected cysts may require surgery.
- Cysts that are likely malignant generally require surgery (see above).

CASE STUDY 18.1 CONTINUED

Incidental renal cysts is a diagnosis of exclusion. In this patient, plasma creatinine is 1.0 mg/dL (88.4 mmol/L). The absence of kidney disease rules out acquired cystic kidney disease (ACKD).

Question 18.1.6:   **What is ACKD?**

ACQUIRED CYSTIC KIDNEY DISEASE

- Definition: Noninherited small cysts that are distributed throughout the renal cortex and medulla of patients with kidney disease, especially end-stage kidney disease (ESKD).
- Pathophysiology: Uremia causes epithelial hyperplasia that promotes the development of cysts and tumors. However, a relationship between cyst formation and efficacy of dialysis has not been established. Transplantation stops the progression of cyst formation and may cause regression. Cysts can recur in rejected kidneys; cyclosporine may cause cyst formation.
- Symptoms: Gross hematuria, flank pain, renal colic, fever, palpable renal mass, and rising hematocrit may be present, though most patients are asymptomatic.

Question 18.1.7:   **How is ACKD diagnosed? Is ACKD premalignant? What is the follow-up and treatment of ACKD?**

- Diagnosis
  - Incidental finding on US, CT of the abdomen, or MRI of the abdomen
  - As opposed to incidental cysts, which do not increase the risk of malignancy, RCC is three times more common in ACKD than in the general population; RCC is six times more common in the presence of large cysts. However, RCC associated with ACKD has lower risk of metastasis and carries a better prognosis.
- Follow-up and treatment:
  - Patients with ACKD require follow-up. Generally, US or CT of the abdomen should be performed at 1- to 2-year intervals in patients who would be surgical candidates if a malignancy is found.
  - Bleeding should be treated with bed rest and analgesia. Persistent bleeding is associated with a high risk of RCC and warrants nephrectomy.
  - Renal masses >3 cm should be treated with nephrectomy. A renal mass that is <3 cm can also be treated with nephrectomy or it may be observed with annual CT.
  - Nephrectomy should be bilateral in ESKD patients because RCC in the setting of ACKD is usually multicentric and bilateral.

Question 18.1.8:   **Could this be ADPKD if family history is absent (i.e., sporadic ADPKD)?**

Probably not. In the absence of a family history of ADPKD, >10 cysts (arbitrarily) in each kidney is needed to make a diagnosis of ADPKD. Very large kidneys or concomitant liver cysts also suggest ADPKD.

CASE STUDY 18.1 CONTINUED

This patient does have a family history of ADPKD in his father and brother.

Question 18.1.9: What are the criteria to diagnose ADPKD in this patient with a family history of ADPKD?

- US criteria (Ravine et al., 1994) in patients with 50% risk
  - <30 years—At least two unilateral or bilateral cysts
  - 30 to 59 years—At least two cysts in each kidney
  - >60 years—At least four cysts in each kidney

CASE STUDY 18.1 CONCLUDED

Because this patient is 65 years old, has a family history of AD-PKD, and has four cysts in each kidney, a diagnosis of ADPKD is appropriate. This could be confirmed by genetic testing, though this is not usually needed.

AUTOSOMAL DOMINANT POLYCYSTIC KIDNEY DISEASE

- Definition: Multiple cysts that are found on imaging of the kidneys usually in a patient with autosomal dominant family history of polycystic kidneys. Five percent of patients do not have a family history.
- Genetics and pathophysiology: ADPKD is due to a gene mutation in either the PKD1 or PKD2 loci. PKD1 encodes for polycystin-1 (PC1) (Thivierge et al., 2006), and PKD2 encodes for polycystin-2 (PC2) (Wu et al., 1998); both of these proteins are in the plasma membrane overlying cilia. Polycystins cause amplified calcium release (Koulen et al., 2002), which probably modulates signaling pathways (such as cyclic adenosine monophosphate, receptor tyrosine kinase, and extracellular signal-regulated kinase) that regulate cellular differentiation, proliferation, and apoptosis.
- Symptoms and signs: Early ADPKD is characterized by impaired urine concentrating capacity, vasopressin resistance, defective medullary trapping of ammonia, low urine pH, and stone formation. Patients with ADPKD invariably have hypertension because of activation of the renin–angiotensin–aldosterone system (RAAS) (Chapman et al., 1990) and heightened sympathetic activity (Klein et al., 2001). They may present with abdominal pain, cyst hemorrhage, cyst infection, or stones.
- In mid-to-late stage of the disease, ADPKD is characterized by mild-to-moderate proteinuria. Renal failure does not occur until the fourth to sixth decades because of compensatory adaptation.
- Risk factors for progression of renal failure are as follows:
  - Male
  - Kidney size
  - Cyst volume
  - Diagnosis before 30 years
  - First hematuria before 30 years

- Hypertension before 35 years
- Hyperlipidemia
- Low high-density lipoprotein
- Sickle cell trait
- Low renal blood flow

- Extrarenal manifestations of ADPKD are as follows:
  - Polycystic liver disease 90%
  - Pancreatic cysts 5%
  - Arachnoid cysts 8%
  - Seminal vesicle (not ovarian) cysts 40%
  - Intracerebral aneurysms 10%
  - Thoracic aortic aneurysms (rare)
  - Coronary artery aneurysms (rare)
  - Mitral valve prolapse 25%
  - Aortic insufficiency
  - Colon diverticulitis

- Pathology: ADPKD kidneys are moderately to massively enlarged (up to ×20 normal). Cysts arise from the collecting ducts but can arise from all segments of the nephron. By the time of ESKD, noncystic parenchyma is scant, probably due to apoptosis. Ninety percent of patients with ADPKD have liver cysts. These cysts enclose fluid resembling bile with a single layer of epithelium that resembles the biliary tract. These liver cysts form when biliary ductules proliferate and dilate and then detach from the biliary system.

- Diagnosis:
  - Family history in 95% of patients
  - US criteria (Ravine et al., 1994) in patients with 50% risk
    - <30 years—At least two unilateral or bilateral cysts
    - 30 to 59 years—At least two cysts in each kidney
    - >60 years—At least four cysts in each kidney
  - Genetic testing (if imaging equivocal)
    - Linkage analysis, which uses microsatellite markers flanking PKD1 and PKD2, is the best, but it requires family members to be willing to be tested.
    - Direct DNA analysis has many obstacles because PKD1 and PKD2 are large, complex, and heterogeneous.
    - Mutation analysis is not useful because most mutations are unique, one-third are missense, and it is hard to prove their pathogenicity.

- Treatment:
  - Hypertension: The goal is to keep blood pressure below 130/80 mm Hg. Angiotensin-converting enzyme (ACE) inhibitors and angiotensin-receptor blockers (ARBs) are preferred to other agents because the RAAS pathway is implicated in the causation of hypertension in ADPKD (Chapman et al., 1990).
  - Pain:
    - Look for cause
    - Avoid narcotics
    - Reassurance
    - Lifestyle
    - Tricyclic antidepressants

- Pain clinic, if necessary
- Aspiration and the use of sclerosing agents may be necessary if the cysts are large enough to cause pain.
- Laparoscopic or surgical cyst fenestration
- Laparoscopic renal denervation
- Sympathosplanchnicectomy
- Arterial embolization
- Nephrectomy

- Hemorrhage:
  - Bed rest
  - Analgesia
  - Hydration
  - If hematoma or decreased hematocrit or hemodynamic stability develops, hospitalization, transfusion, CT of the abdomen, and/or arterial embolization may be necessary.
- Infection:
  - Poor penetration of some antibiotics (e.g., aminoglycosides) into cysts
  - Abscess drainage
  - Nephrectomy
- Nephrolithiasis:
  - Treatment is the same as in non-ADPKD (see Chapter 17).
- ESKD:
  - Dialysis (peritoneal dialysis [PD] is usually possible) or transplant (bilateral nephrectomy may be necessary prior to transplant)

AUTOSOMAL RECESSIVE POLYCYSTIC KIDNEY DISEASE

- Definition: Autosomal recessive polycystic kidney disease (ARPKD) is usually diagnosed in infancy, and 30% of the affected infants die in utero. The prevalence of the disease is 1:20,000.
- Pathophysiology: In analogy to the polycystins in ADPKD, ARPKD is caused by mutations in *PKHD1* (Bergmann, 2004), which encodes the gene for fibrocystin. Fibrocystin is also localized in cilia and is closely related to calcium homeostasis (Nagano et al., 2005).
- Symptoms and signs: Thirty percent of affected individuals die in utero. Those who survive to childhood may have stable renal function for many years and reach adulthood. However, they may experience growth failure, anemia, renal osteodystrophy, liver failure, splenomegaly, and cytopenias. Adults with ARPKD will have portal hypertension and bile duct dilatation with normal kidneys or mild collecting duct ectasias. Adults can manifest proteinuria, nephrolithiasis, and renal insufficiency.
- Diagnosis:
  - Sonography in utero or shortly after birth is the main method of diagnosing ARPKD.

- There is usually a positive family history.
  - Direct DNA diagnosis is complicated by marked allelic heterogeneity and uncertain missense mutations. However, analysis of mutations does improve the accuracy of diagnosis. If two clearly pathogenic mutations are identified, the diagnosis of ARPKD is considered reliable. If one mutation is identified and genetic linkage is sound, the diagnosis is considered reliable. Mutation analysis has allowed 72% definite assignment and 25% improved risk assignment.
- Treatment:
  - In infants, PD and/or transplant are preferred.
  - Patients with bile duct dilatation and recurrent cholangitis should be treated with a combined kidney and liver transplantation.

MEDULLARY CYSTIC DISEASE (NEPHRONOPHTHISIS)

- Definition: Autosomal dominant disease with cysts at the corticomedullary junction that usually presents in adolescence or early adulthood.
- Pathology: Kidneys are small to normal. Cysts are present at the corticomedullary junction. There is interstitial fibrosis.
- Symptoms: Polydipsia, polyuria, sodium wasting, and gout
- Treatment: Transplant is a preferred option.

MEDULLARY SPONGE KIDNEY

- Definition: Dilated collecting ducts and cysts confined to medullary pyramids.
- Pathophysiology: Medullary sponge kidney is probably usually acquired, but a familial form has been described. Associated with formation of calcium stones (13%), probably due to urinary stasis and anatomic abnormality. Also associated with primary hyperparathyroidism, Ehlers-Danlos syndrome.
- Symptoms: Patients may present with gross or microscopic hematuria, urinary tract infection, renal colic due to calcium oxalate or calcium phosphate stones.
- Diagnosis:
  - Plain X-rays—Dilated collecting ducts without ureteral obstruction. May see renal calculi or nephrocalcinosis.
  - CT of the abdomen—Cortical layer is free of cysts.
  - Absence of family history (usually)
  - Renal tubular acidosis (RTA) often present
- Treatment:
  - Treat stones and/or urinary tract infections.
  - Alkali for RTA may promote calcium phosphate stones.

A 50-year-old woman with a history of ovarian cysts presents for evaluation of incidental simple 1-cm renal cysts (one on each kidney) that are found on CT scan of the abdomen/pelvis, which is done for the purpose of evaluating the pelvis in the workup of menorrhagia. There is no contrast enhancement of the cysts. The kidneys are of normal size. The patient does not have any liver cysts. There is no known family history of renal cystic disease. She is otherwise asymptomatic and does not have abdominal or flank discomfort, gross hematuria, or difficulty with urinary stream. Blood pressure is normal. Physical examination is normal, and renal function is not impaired.

Q: What is the best next step?

1. Reassure the patient
2. Periodic surveillance US
3. Periodic surveillance CT with contrast
4. Genetic testing to exclude ADPKD
5. Referral to a urologist

A: In this 50-year-old woman with normal size kidneys containing only two small cysts, absence of liver cysts, and no family history, ADPKD is excluded. Incidental renal cysts are commonly found in patients ≥50 years of age undergoing abdominal imaging for various reasons. These cysts appear to be Bosniak Category I to II cysts, and therefore, follow-up is not needed.

A 45-year-old man with no family history of renal cystic disease presents for detection of bilateral renal cysts that are detected on CT scan of the abdomen, which is done because abdominal palpation is significant for palpably large kidneys. Both kidneys are 15 cm in length, and each has three cysts. He does have two hepatic cysts. He rejects testing for inherited PKD. By CT scan criteria, he is thought to have adult PKD. He is asymptomatic except for polyuria. Physical examination is significant for blood pressure of 150/100 mm Hg. Renal function is normal.

Q: Which of the following regarding the pathophysiology of hypertension in this patient is false?

1. There is increased sympathetic activity.
2. The RAAS is activated due to ischemia caused by cyst expansion.
3. There is disruption of polycystin function in the vasculature.
4. There is impaired nitric oxide endothelium–dependent vasorelaxation.
5. None of the above.

A: This patient, despite lack of family history and lack of genetic data, is a candidate for the diagnosis of adult dominant PKD. Hypertension in ADPKD is due to RAAS activation caused by cyst expansion–related stretching and compression of blood vessels and resultant ischemia. Hence, ACE inhibitor or an ARB would be ideal therapeutic choices for the treatment of blood pressure in this patient. In ADPKD, hypertension is also associated with increased sympathetic activity. Polycystin disruption in the vasculature and impaired nitric oxide–related vasorelaxation are other factors that contribute to hypertension. Insulin resistance and plasma endothelin-1 may also play a role.

References

Bergmann C, Senderek J, Küpper F, et al. PKHD1 mutations in autosomal recessive polycystic kidney disease (ARPKD). *Hum Mutat.* 2004;23(5):453–463.

Chapman AB, Johnson H, Gabow PA, et al. The renin–angiotensin–aldosterone system and autosomal dominant polycystic kidney disease. *N Engl J Med.* 1990;323:1091–1096.

Israel GM, Bosniak MA. An update of the Bosniak renal cyst classification system. *Urology.* 2005;66(3):484–488.

Klein IH, Ligtenberg G, Oey PL, et al. Sympathetic activity is increased in polycystic kidney disease and is associated with hypertension. *J Am Soc Nephrol.* 2001;12:2427–2433.

Koulen P, Cai Y, Geng L, et al. Polycystin-2 is an intracellular calcium release channel. *Nat Cell Biol.* 2002;4:191–197.

Nagano J, Kitamura K, Hujer KM, et al. Fibrocystin interacts with CAML, a protein involved in Ca^{2+} signaling. *Biochem Biophys Res Commun.* 2005;338(2):880–889.

Ravine D, Gibson RN, Walker RG, et al. Evaluation of ultrasonographic diagnostic criteria for autosomal dominant polycystic kidney disease. *Lancet.* 1994;343:824–827.

Thivierge C, Kurgegovic A, Couillard M, et al. Overexpression of PKD1 causes polycystic kidney disease. *Mol Cell Biol.* 2006;26:1538–1548.

Wu G, D'Agati V, Cai Y, et al. Somatic inactivation of PKD2 results in polycystic kidney disease. *Cell.* 1998;93:177–188.

19 Renal Replacement Therapies

RENAL REPLACEMENT THERAPY

■ As the name implies, renal replacement therapy (RRT) involves the use of procedures to do the work of the kidneys when the native kidneys are unable to sustain life. RRT removes toxins from the blood, corrects serum electrolytes, restores acid–base balance, and achieves euvolemia. These processes are achieved through diffusion, convection, and ultrafiltration (UF).
   ■ Diffusion is defined as the net movement of molecules down their concentration gradient (from an area of high concentration to an area of low concentration).
   ■ Convection implies that solute removal through a membrane is facilitated by a moving stream of fluid, independent of the concentration gradient.
   ■ UF is the movement of fluid across a semipermeable membrane in which colloidal particles are retained while the small-sized solutes and the solvent move across the membrane by hydrostatic pressure forces.
■ RRT can be implemented to perform diffusion or convection or both. There are three forms of RRT: dialysis (diffusion), hemofiltration (convection), and hemodiafiltration (diffusion and convection). UF is combined with dialysis or filtration as needed to remove fluid.

> **CASE STUDY 19.1** A 61-year-old male with a past medical history of uncontrolled diabetes mellitus, blindness due to diabetic retinopathy, and progressive proteinuric stage 4 chronic kidney disease (CKD) (elevated glomerular filtration rate [eGFR] 18 mL/min/1.73 m^2) is referred to the renal clinic. Medications include insulin, atorvastatin, aspirin, losartan, and furosemide. Review of the medical record indicates that his eGFR has been declining at a rate of ~8 mL/min/1.73 m^2/y for the past 5 years.
>
> **Physical examination:**
>
> Vitals: pulse, 90 beats/min; respiratory rate: 20 breaths/min; BP: 130/60 mm Hg; temperature: 98°F
> Chest: clear
> Heart: regular rate and rhythm
> Abdomen: soft with normoactive bowel sounds
> Extremities: trace edema
> Neurologic: no focal findings

Question 19.1.1: What is the etiology of CKD?

CASE STUDY 19.1 CONTINUED

The combination of diabetes mellitus, proteinuria, and diabetic retinopathy establishes the diagnosis of diabetic kidney disease as the etiology of CKD.

In view of progressive severe CKD and the prediction that he would need chronic dialysis within a year, he is referred for predialysis education. In most patients, either hemodialysis (HD) (in-center HD, self-administered home HD, or staff-assisted home HD) or peritoneal dialysis (PD) is an appropriate mode of RRT depending on patient preference. One of the purposes of predialysis education is planning for creation of appropriate access, that is, an arteriovenous fistula (AVF), arteriovenous graft (AVG), or PD catheter.

The patient chooses in-center HD and is referred to a vascular surgeon, who successfully places an AVF. The patient is followed in the renal clinic. After 1 year, he develops uremic symptoms and is started on HD.

Question 19.1.2: What are the indications for RRT in CKD?

- Symptoms and/or signs of uremia (early symptoms are anorexia, nausea, dysgeusia, myoclonus—one should not wait for late manifestations such as pericarditis or encephalopathy) (Ifudu et al., 1996; Roubicek et al., 2000)
- Persistent volume overload or electrolyte abnormalities (e.g., hyperkalemia, metabolic acidosis)
- eGFR <10 mL/min/1.73 m^2 generally in the presence of early symptoms attributable to uremia because early initiation of dialysis prior to the onset of symptoms has not been shown to improve outcome (Cooper et al., 2010).

DIALYSIS

The process of dialysis involves the removal of solutes (including toxins) from the blood and into the dialysate through diffusion across a semipermeable membrane. Dialysis is best for removal of molecules <500 Da, molecules with a decreased volume of distribution, molecules that are less protein bound, and molecules that are water soluble.

- Hemodialysis:
  - Blood is passed through a dialysis membrane at a rapid rate (300–400 mL/min). Through the process of diffusion, substances to be removed ("toxins") move from the blood into the dialysate. The purified blood is returned into the patient's bloodstream, and the dialysate is discarded (Brescia et al., 1966).
  - HD requires a vascular access, preferably a surgically created AVF. If HD needs to be started on an emergent basis in a patient without a vascular access, a double-lumen catheter may be inserted into a large vein (usually femoral or internal jugular [IJ]). A cuffed catheter may be tunneled into a vein, which decreases

the risk of infection and allows patients to be discharged home with the catheter. However, even cuffed (so-called "permanent") catheters are associated with a high rate of infection and require diligent antiseptic care.

- If a patient will need dialysis for more than a few months (as is expected with end-stage kidney disease [ESKD]), a fistula should be created as soon as feasible. HD is usually performed thrice weekly for 4 hours.
- Adequacy of HD is monitored by monthly measurements of urea clearance or Kt/V, where Kt = clearance and V = volume of distribution of urea. The goal of HD is to achieve a Kt/V of 1.2. The HEMO study demonstrated that a Kt/V of 1.6 is not superior to a Kt/V of 1.2 (Eknoyan et al., 2002).

- Types of vascular access
  - An arteriovenous fistula (native fistula or AVF) is created by connecting an artery and a vein, thereby bypassing the capillaries. The vein is now subject to the high pressures of the artery and the walls of the vein thicken or "arterialize." An arterialized vein is necessary because it is intended to undergo repeated needle puncture. It usually takes several months for the fistula to mature and be ready to use, so planning ahead is essential. Two needles are inserted into the fistula: one carries blood to the dialysis machine and the other brings it back to the fistula. After dialysis, the needles are removed, gauze is applied, and a clot seals the hole in the fistula. A native fistula can sometimes last the lifetime of the patient.
  - If the veins are too small to allow for the formation of a native fistula, an arteriovenous graft (graft fistula or AVG) is created. In the creation of a graft fistula, an artificial tube (generally made of polytetrafluoroethylene, PTFE) is used to connect an artery and a vein. A graft fistula can generally be used after a few days but is more likely to become infected and/or thrombose than is a native fistula. The longevity of a graft is thus usually only for up to 3 years.

CASE STUDY 19.1 CONTINUED

The patient does well on HD for 2 years. However, he then develops swelling of the arm housing the AVF and has increased bleeding from the needlestick sites after HD. He is referred back to the vascular surgeon.

Question 19.1.3: What are common vascular access complications?

- Failure of native fistula maturation: Angioplasty with or without stent placement may accelerate maturation and allow earlier use.
- Steal syndrome: Sometimes the fistula shunts excessive amounts of blood away from the hand, leading to an ischemic hand. Surgery may be needed to reduce or stop flow through the fistula (Hurwich, 1970).
- Aneurysm formation: An aneurysm may form in the fistula. Aneurysms in fistulae may be true or false (pseudoaneurysms). The former are due to repeated use of the fistula with weakening of the

vascular wall, occur only in native fistulae, and seldom rupture, whereas the latter are due to leakage of blood through a hole in the wall of the access. Pseudoaneurysms can occur with either native or graft fistulae though are more common with graft fistulae. They require close monitoring so that intervention can be instituted if at high risk of rupture. Risk of rupture is high in the presence of skin ulceration, an overlying scab, or the presence of infection and may require emergency ligation. The management of both true and false aneurysms requires close collaboration with an experienced vascular surgeon. Enlarging true aneurysms may require surgical removal with or without bypass or stent placement. Pseudoaneurysms can sometimes be treated with thrombin injection or ultrasound compression but often require surgical excision.

- Thrombosis: In the event of a clot in the fistula, thrombectomy with or without angioplasty is indicated (Beathard, 1995).
- Venous intimal hyperplasia may also occur, resulting in venous outflow stenosis (Roy-Chaudhury et al., 2002).
- Catheters are notorious for sepsis and thrombosis: Long-term use should be avoided if at all possible.

Question 19.1.4: How should an HD access be evaluated?

- Physical examination (Salman & Beathard, 2013)
  - Check for pulse
  - Check for bruit and thrill
  - Normally, the access is easily compressible with very little pulse
  - A pulsatile access may be indicative of outflow stenosis
  - An unusually weak pulse which does not augment with compression of the access suggests inflow stenosis
  - Discontinuity in bruit or thrill (systolic only) suggests localized stenosis
  - Upon arm elevation, AVF should collapse; lack of collapse suggests outflow stenosis (does not work for AVG)
- Indications for angiography
  - Arm swelling
  - Prolonged bleeding after needle withdrawal (suggests outflow stenosis or may be a sign of enlarging aneurysm, skin thinning, or layered thrombus).
  - Collateral veins
  - Altered pulse or thrill
  - Unexplained decrease in urea clearance (Kt/V)
  - Access flow <400 to 500 mL/min or progressive decrease in access flow
  - Bleeding on nondialysis days (may indicate loss of skin integrity, elevated pressures, or anticoagulation).
  - Dark blood in circuit (may indicate inflow or outflow stenosis).
  - High arterial pressures (indicate inflow stenosis).
  - High venous pressures (indicate outflow stenosis).
  - Clotting of dialysis filter during dialysis (may be a sign of recirculation, inflow stenosis, or outflow stenosis).
  - Positive arterial pressures (indicate high inflow or severe outflow stenosis).

- Recirculation
  - Dialyzed blood returning through the venous needle reenters through the arterial needle instead of returning to the systemic circulation. This markedly reduces the efficiency of dialysis and leads to a decrease in Kt/V. This occurs when total access flow is lower than blood flow in the dialysis circuit and suggests the presence of either inflow or outflow stenosis.

CASE STUDY 19.1 CONTINUED

The patient undergoes a fistulogram, revealing venous outflow stenosis that is treated with angioplasty and stenting.

Question 19.1.5: What are nonaccess problems that may arise in HD patients?

- Dialysis disequilibrium: HD removes solutes from the plasma and extracellular fluid but is not able to remove solutes from the brain cells as effectively. Owing to the resulting osmotic gradient between cells and extracellular fluid, brain edema may ensue. Severe dialysis disequilibrium, including syncope and seizure, is rare. Mild dialysis disequilibrium characterized by headache, fatigue, and nausea usually resolves within a few hours of dialysis cessation (Rosen et al., 1964). It is due to excessively rapid solute and water removal during dialysis.
- Hypotension: This is common on HD and is generally due to rapid fluid removal (UF). Rapid fluid removal during dialysis is associated with increased cardiovascular morbidity and mortality (Flythe et al., 2011). Other more serious causes (myocardial infarction, arrhythmia, pericardial effusion, sepsis) must be considered (Dheenan & Henrich, 2001).
- Hypokalemia post-HD: This is common if too low a dialysate potassium concentration is used and can be a cause of increased mortality (Jadoul et al., 2012). It should be kept in mind, however, that there will be a substantial rebound increase in plasma potassium once dialysis has ended because of shift of potassium from cells, so it is generally advised not to measure blood potassium levels immediately following dialysis (Blumberg et al., 1997).
- Hypophosphatemia: Because dialysate does not normally contain phosphorus, addition of phosphorus to dialysate may be necessary to avoid and treat hypophosphatemia, especially in patients undergoing daily dialysis, undergoing dialysis for intoxications in the presence of normal or near-normal kidney function, and with malnutrition.
- Anemia (see Chapter 12)
- Bone disease (see Chapter 12)
- Hypertension (see Chapter 12)
- Fatigue: Dialysis patients frequently complain of fatigue. Although inadequate dialysis is a possible cause and should be excluded, many other possibilities should also be explored. Fatigue can be due to medications, in particular, antihypertensives, analgesics, antihistamines, and psychiatric medications. The patient should be evaluated for coronary artery disease, diabetes status, chronic

viral syndromes (including hepatitis), anemia, and thyroid disorders. Dialysis patients are often very deconditioned, and exercise should be recommended to ameliorate fatigue.

■ Appetite: Patients on dialysis frequently have decreased appetite, which can lead to malnutrition. Recommendations include physical activity, nutritional consultation, and, in some cases, appetite stimulants and/or antidepressants.

■ Depression: As with any chronic disease, depression is common. Treatment includes medication reconciliation (sleeping pills, antihypertensives, antihistamines), restriction of alcohol intake, exercise, antidepressants, and referral to a psychiatrist.

■ Sexual dysfunction: Impotence in males is common and may occur because of atherosclerosis, neuropathy, smoking, diabetes, alcohol, vitamin deficiencies (B_{12} and thiamine), and thyroid disorders. Some medications may be implicated, including psychiatric medications. Women on dialysis typically have aberrant menstruation and/or anovulation. However, pregnancy can occur, and outcomes are improved by increasing frequency of dialysis.

■ Nutrition: Patients without kidney function must restrict intake of sodium, potassium, and phosphorus in order to prevent volume overload, hyperkalemia, and hyperphosphatemia, respectively. Protein restriction may result in malnutrition and is not generally recommended, though a high-biologic value low-protein diet will decrease uremic symptoms if present. Because PD is continuous, there is more freedom with dietary intake than with typical thrice weekly HD. A typical renal diet is given in Table 19.1. HD removes water-soluble vitamins, including B vitamins, vitamin C, and folate, which must be supplemented.

■ Common infections in HD patients:
  ■ HIV/hepatitis: All dialysis patients are tested for hepatitis B and C. They are also tested for tuberculosis. Pneumococcal, influenza, and hepatitis B vaccinations are indicated. Patients with hepatitis B are dialyzed in isolation. Universal precautions are used in all HD patients to prevent transmission of blood-borne infection. The risk of transmission of HIV via HD is negligible, and isolation of such patients is not required.
  ■ Bacteremia: HD patients are predisposed to bacteremia from the vascular access. The risk is as follows: catheter $>>$ graft fistula $>$ native fistula. Infections are usually due to skin organisms (Gram-positive), but up to 20% of patients can have Gram-negative bacteremia. Thus, broad-spectrum antibiotics should be used until culture and sensitivity results are available.

T A B L E 19.1	Renal Diet (Daily Amounts)

Sodium, 2 g (87 mmol)
Potassium, 2 g (51 mmol)
Phosphorus, 0.7–0.9 g (23–29 mmol)
Protein, 1.2 g/kg
Water, 1.5 L or less

CASE STUDY 19.1 CONTINUED

After 4 years on HD, the patient decides to move to a rural area where the nearest HD center is 50 miles from his home. After discussion with his dialysis team, he decides to switch to PD.

- Peritoneal dialysis:
  - Dialysate is placed into the peritoneal cavity, and toxins from the splanchnic circulation are allowed to diffuse across the peritoneum (that acts as a natural semipermeable membrane) into the dialysate, which is discarded (Miller & Tassistro, 1969). There are four types of dialysate solutions: 1.5% dextrose, 2.5% dextrose, 4.25% dextrose, and icodextrin.
  - PD requires a peritoneal catheter. A cuffed PD catheter is inserted into the peritoneal cavity either percutaneously or surgically, using a subcutaneous tunnel to the exit site. It generally takes about 2 weeks for the catheter to heal properly. Once healed, the catheter is ready to be used for an exchange. To initiate the exchange, tubing is connected to the PD catheter and to a bag full of dialysate. The dialysate bag is hung above the abdomen, and dialysate allowed to enter the abdomen. Several hours later (to allow time for toxin removal), the PD catheter is connected to an empty bag, and spent dialysate is drained from the abdomen by gravity and discarded. Most patients will perform four exchanges per day. This is referred to as continuous ambulatory peritoneal dialysis (CAPD). Cyclers are available, which automatically perform PD overnight; this is referred to as continuous cyclic peritoneal dialysis (CCPD) if dialysate is allowed to dwell in the peritoneal cavity during the day or nocturnal peritoneal dialysis (NPD) if the peritoneal cavity is dry during the day.
  - After a period of in-center training, PD is done at home on a daily basis. Patients do not have to go to a dialysis unit; PD is generally done at night when the patient is sleeping. In addition, PD allows a patient less restriction in dietary and lifestyle habits because PD preserves residual urine output and is performed daily. It is of interest that PD is usually associated with hypokalemia rather than hyperkalemia as in HD.

Question 19.1.6: **How does one determine the PD prescription? What properties of the peritoneal membrane contribute to the efficacy of diffusion? How is adequacy of the PD prescription established?**

A peritoneal equilibration test (PET) is performed to determine the peritoneal membrane transport characteristics. The ratio of creatinine concentration in dialysate and plasma (D/P) ratio at specific times (t) during the dwell is used to classify the peritoneal membrane as a high transporter, low transporter, or average transporter. The ratio of dialysate glucose at time t to the dialysate glucose at time zero (D_t/D_0) is also used to characterize the peritoneal membrane.

High transporters equilibrate rapidly and are treated with short, frequent dwells. Low transporters equilibrate slowly and are treated with longer dwells. CAPD is most appropriate for low transporters.

The peritoneal membrane has three types of pores:

- Large pores are 100 to 200 Å.
- Small pores are 40 to 60 Å.
- Aquapores are 4 to 6 Å (also called aquaporin-1).
- Most of the diffusion occurs across small pores and aquapores.
- With hypertonic dialysate, initial selective water diffusion through aquapores precedes solute transport. Therefore, with short dwells, sodium sieving can result in hypernatremia.
- Use of icodextrin prevents water loss via aquapores. Hence, sodium sieving does not happen.

A Kt/V for PD of 1.7 is recommended. Kt/V for PD is calculated as the sum of peritoneal Kt/V (dialysate urea clearance) and renal Kt/V (residual urine output).

CASE STUDY 19.1 CONTINUED

The patient is found to be a high transporter and CCPD with five 2 L exchanges over 10 hours is prescribed. Subsequently, the patient develops hypernatremia. The PD prescription is altered to increase the dwell time of each exchange to 2.4 hours (five 2 L exchanges over 12 hours) and hypernatremia resolves.

Question 19.1.7: What are common complications of PD?

- Catheter dysfunction: Catheters may become blocked, infected, or displaced.
- Peritonitis: Peritonitis due to infection results in abdominal pain, fever, chills, and cloudy dialysate. Although usually due to contamination during the procedure (intraluminal infection), an infected catheter/subcutaneous tunnel (periluminal infection) or intra-abdominal processes such as appendicitis, diverticulitis, or bowel rupture (transluminal infection) must be considered. Occasionally, noninfectious peritonitis as a result of air entry into the peritoneal space will occur. This is characterized by elevated eosinophils and monocytes in the peritoneal fluid. This typically occurs soon after surgical catheter placement. Associated bacteremia is very rare, and thus intraperitoneal antibiotics are recommended to treat peritonitis. Again, broad-spectrum antibiotics should be used until culture and sensitivity results are available. Details of treatment of peritonitis are beyond the scope of this chapter. Usually, the catheter can be salvaged unless there is (1) severe exit site or tunnel infection and (2) fungal infection. Pseudomonal infections require two antipseudomonal antibiotics; catheter removal may be necessary. Bacteremia can cause peritoneal seeding; PD peritonitis itself rarely causes bacteremia.
- Catheter obstruction
  - A two-way obstruction indicates a fibrin plug or kink.

- A one-way obstruction can signify constipation, omental wrap, or latching of the fallopian tubes onto catheter. Do catheter dye studies to clarify the cause of the one-way obstruction.
- Pain with inflow or outflow should be treated with low dwell volumes (known as tidal PD).
- Exit site infection: An infected exit site may just need change of ointment, although antibiotics can also be used. Any change in appearance should prompt suspicion of exit site infection. Antibacterial antibiotics can cause fungal infection of the exit site, treat with nystatin, remove the catheter if necessary; one-third of the patients can return to PD after a short period of HD.
- Hydrothorax can result if there is an opening in the diaphragm. A thoracentesis and pleural effusion analysis indicating high glucose concentration is diagnostic. It is possible to repair using minimally invasive surgery.
- Hydrocele can result in patients who have an open processus vaginalis (20% of patients); this is best treated with low-pressure APD or temporary HD.
- Antibiotic prophylaxis for dental procedures, endoscopy, or colposcopy is advised, though there are few data to support this practice.
- Hemoperitoneum may indicate menses, ischemic bowel, or pancreatitis.
- Chyloperitoneum may indicate lymphoma.
- Hernia repair: In the past, patients were usually switched to HD, although this is not always necessary. However, PD should be held for a few days and then restarted with low fill volumes.

CASE STUDY 19.1 CONTINUED

After 2 years of PD, the patient receives a deceased donor kidney transplant. He does well on a standard immunosuppressive regimen of mycophenolate, tacrolimus, and prednisone, maintaining good allograft function without evidence of allograft rejection. Unfortunately, he is subsequently admitted for sepsis and develops respiratory failure due to invasive aspergillosis. He is treated with liposomal amphotericin B, after which he develops acute kidney injury (AKI). He becomes oliguric and has persistent metabolic acidosis and hyperkalemia.

Blood chemistry:

Sodium: 135 mmol/L
Potassium: 6.0 mmol/L
Chloride: 100 mmol/L
Total CO_2: 10 mmol/L
Urea nitrogen: 60 mg/dL (urea: 21 mmol/L)
Creatinine: 3.5 mg/dL (309 mcmol/L)

Glucose: 255 mg/dL (14 mmol/L)
Albumin: 2.5 g/dL (25 g/L)

Arterial blood gas:

pH: 7.08
PCO_2: 40 mm Hg
Bicarbonate: 10 mEq/L
PO_2: 70 mm Hg (on 4 L NC)

Question 19.1.8: What is the etiology of AKI?

The superimposed AKI is most likely due to amphotericin B nephrotoxicity. Amphotericin B causes tubular injury and renal vasoconstriction. Reduction in GFR may be because of increased membrane permeability of the cells in the macula densa in the distal tubule, resulting in marked tubuloglomerular feedback (TGF) and excessive afferent arteriolar vasoconstriction.

CASE STUDY 19.1 CONTINUED

Laboratory findings indicate combined high–anion gap metabolic acidosis and respiratory acidosis (see Acid–Base chapter). The patient is intubated, hyperventilated, and treated with intravenous sodium bicarbonate (150 mEq bicarbonate in each liter of D5W), an insulin drip, and 30 g of sodium polystyrene sulfonate (Kayexalate). However, he remains very acidemic (pH < 7.1) and hyperkalemic. He develops hypotension unresponsive to intravenous fluids and requires pressors. On examination, there is generalized anasarca. The chest X-ray shows diffuse infiltrates.

Question 19.1.9: What are the indications for RRT in AKI?

- Hyperkalemia refractory to medical management
- Severe metabolic acidosis that cannot be corrected with sodium bicarbonate (or when sodium bicarbonate administration is contraindicated because of fluid overload) or severe metabolic alkalosis
- Fluid overload unresponsive to diuretics
- Symptoms and/or signs of uremia (anorexia, nausea, dysgeusia, myoclonus, pericarditis, encephalopathy, bleeding diathesis)
- Other severe electrolyte/metabolic abnormalities (severe hypercalcemia, hyperphosphatemia, hypermagnesemia, hyperuricemia)
- Poisoning with selected dialyzable drugs or toxins

Question 19.1.10: What type of RRT is appropriate in this patient?

Because the patient is hypotensive and requires fluid removal as well as correction of acute metabolic disturbances, continuous renal replacement therapy (CRRT) is the best option.
- Definition of CRRT
  - CRRT, as the name implies, is performed at a slow, steady rate 24 h/d.
  - CRRT can perform dialysis via diffusion or convection or both. In addition, UF is usually performed unless the patient is so hemodynamically unstable that UF is not tolerated.
  - CRRT can be venovenous or arteriovenous. Only venovenous CRRT is commonly utilized; arteriovenous circuits are no longer used because a blood flow pump is used to pull blood through the dialysis filter.
  - The major difference between intermittent RRT and CRRT is the speed at which water and solutes are removed. Rapid removal of

water and wastes during intermittent HD may be poorly tolerated in critically ill patients.
- For safety reasons, it is best not to perform CRRT with an AVF or
AVG. A central venous catheter with secure connections should
be used; IJ catheters are most commonly used, followed by femoral and, least commonly, subclavian catheters.

Question 19.1.11: What types of CRRT are available?

- There are three types of CRRT
  - Continuous venovenous hemofiltration (CVVH). CVVH uses
  convection or solvent drag to remove solutes from the blood.
  To achieve solvent drag, replacement fluid is added prefilter or
  postfilter or both; this replacement fluid plus additional fluid
  as required is removed in the effluent. Dialysate is not added;
  hence, diffusion is not utilized.
  - Continuous venovenous hemodialysis (CVVHD). CVVHD uses
  diffusion to remove solutes from the blood. Dialysate is employed
  similarly to intermittent dialysis. Replacement fluid is not added.
  - Continuous venovenous hemodiafiltration (CVVHDF). CV-
  VHDF utilized both replacement fluid and dialysate to achieve
  dialysis solute clearance through both diffusion and convection.
  - In addition, there is continuous venovenous ultrafiltration
  (CVVU), also called slow continuous ultrafiltration (SCUF).
  CVVU/SCUF functions solely to remove extra fluid from edema-
  tous patients; it is not actually RRT because solute concentra-
  tions in the blood remain unchanged.
- The extracorporeal circuits for CVVH, CVVHD, and CVVU/SCUF
are shown in Figure 19.1. Note that the CVVHD circuit is identical to that for intermittent HD of sustained low efficiency dialysis
(SLED).

Question 19.1.12: What type of RRT offers the best survival?

There is no survival difference between any of the modalities of CRRT
versus intermittent HD.

Question 19.1.13: What is the typical dose of CRRT?

An effluent (replacement fluid $+/-$ dialysate) flow rate of 20 mL/
kg/h (2 L/h in a 100-kg patient) is sufficient based on the VA/NIH
trial (Palevsky et al., 2008). KDIGO recommends an effluent volume
of 20 to 25 mL/kg/h. However, because critically ill patients typically
have interruptions of CRRT as a result of radiologic imaging and
other extenuating circumstances, a dose of 25 to 30 mL/kg/h is recommended. No benefits from more intense CRRT have been shown.

Question 19.1.14: When performing CVVH, what are benefits
and detriments of prefilter versus postfilter
replacement fluid?

Using prefilter mode will lead to some reduction in solute clearance,
but may decrease risk of filter clotting and thus obviate the need for
anticoagulation.

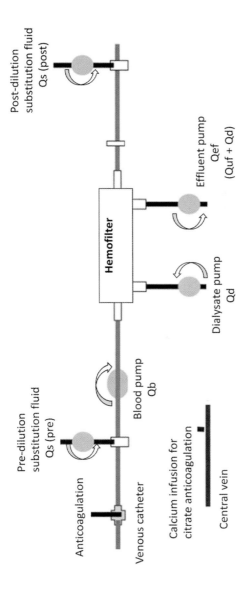

FIGURE 19.1. The continuous renal replacement therapy (CRRT) circuit consists of a blood pump that pulls blood from the patient and pumps it into the filter. Replacement fluid can be added before (prefilter) and after the filter (postfilter) for convective removal of middle molecules. Dialysate can be added into the filter for diffusion of molecules down a concentration gradient. An effluent pump exerts negative pressure on the CRRT circuit to collect the replacement fluid and dialysate in the effluent bag. CRRT can be performed with replacement fluid only (CVVH or continuous venovenous hemofiltration) or dialysate only (CVVHD or continuous venovenous hemodialysis) or with both replacement fluid and dialysate (CVVHDF or continuous venovenous hemodiafiltration). All CRRT modes can perform ultrafiltration; alternatively, pure ultrafiltration (known as SCUF or slow continuous ultrafiltration) can be performed. Anticoagulation may be necessary to keep the filter from clotting prematurely. (From Macedo E, Mehta RL. Continuous dialysis therapies: core curriculum 2016. *Am J Kidney Dis.* 2016;68(4):645–657.)

CASE STUDY 19.1 CONTINUED

The patient is begun on CVVH with postfilter replacement fluid administered at 25 mL/kg/h. However, after 12 hours, the patient remains acidotic and hyperkalemic.

Question 19.1.15: **How can you increase clearance?**

The simplest way is to increase the blood flow and replacement fluid rates. Another option with some machines is to change to CVVHDF. Filter characteristics are also important; newer filters have a larger surface area and increased filter permeability.

CASE STUDY 19.1 CONTINUED

Without heparin, the filter clots every 8 hours. Heparin is administered into the extracorporeal circuit and filter life increases to 48 hours, but the patient develops thrombocytopenia and antiheparin antibodies are positive. Heparin is discontinued. The blood flow is increased, and prefilter replacement fluid is added. However, the filter continues to clot every 12 hours.

Question 19.1.16: **What else can you do to increase filter life?**

Citrate anticoagulation can be utilized. Calcium is necessary for blood clotting. The addition of citrate to the prefilter circuit chelates calcium. The citrate–calcium complex is lost in the effluent. The calcium is added back to the postfilter circuit via a calcium infusion. This effectively prevents filter clotting, but one needs to monitor laboratory values closely to prevent hypocalcemia.

CASE STUDY 19.1 CONTINUED

Citrate anticoagulation is begun. Excessive filter clotting is prevented. Two days later, the complete metabolic panel is as follows:

Sodium: 135 mmol/L
Potassium: 4.8 mmol/L
Chloride: 100 mmol/L
Total CO_2: 18 mmol/L
Urea nitrogen: 20 mg/dL (urea: 7.1 mmol/L)
Creatinine: 1.5 mg/dL (133 mcmol/L)
Glucose: 155 mg/dL (8.6 mmol/L)
Total calcium: 12 mg/dL (3 mmol/L)
Albumin: 2.5 g/dL (25 g/L)
Systemic-ionized calcium: 0.9 mmol/L
Circuit-ionized calcium: 0.2 mmol/L
Aspartate aminotransferase (AST): 90 U/L
Alanine aminotransaminase (ALT): 120 U/L
Alkaline phosphatase: 200 U/L

Question 19.1.17: What is the cause of the metabolic acidosis, high–anion gap, elevated total calcium, reduced systemic-ionized calcium, and elevated liver function tests (LFTs)?

The patient develops citrate toxicity. Because of liver injury, there is likely impairment of citrate metabolism. Hence, citrate accumulates and metabolic acidosis results. The total calcium (including the citrate–calcium complexes as well as calcium complexed to other proteins) is high, and the systemic-ionized calcium is low. Note that the circuit-ionized calcium is at target (0.2–0.3 mmol/L), and therefore, the filter is not clotting.

One should monitor for citrate toxicity by doing labs every 6 hours. A total calcium (mg/dL) to ionized calcium (mmol/L) ratio of >10 is suggestive of citrate toxicity. Alternatively, a total calcium (mg/dL) to ionized calcium (mg/dL) ratio >2.5 is indicative of citrate toxicity.

Question 19.1.18: What alternative anticoagulant can be utilized?

An alternate anticoagulant such as argatroban (30 mcg/kg/h) can be utilized.

CASE STUDY 19.1 CONCLUDED

Citrate anticoagulation is discontinued. Argatroban is infused into the extracorporeal circuit that prevents further excessive filter clotting. A reduced dose of 15 mcg/kg/h of argatroban is used due to existing liver injury.

CVVH is necessary for about 10 days after which renal function improves. The patient fortunately eventually recovers and is discharged from the hospital.

VIGNETTE **1**

19

A 55-year-old woman with ESKD and hypertension presents for evaluation of left upper extremity swelling. She had AVG placement in the left forearm a week ago. Vital signs are normal. There is mild erythema in the path of the graft, but no warmth, purulent drainage, or bleeding.

Q: What is the cause of the left upper extremity swelling?

1. Trauma due to surgery
2. Central venous occlusion
3. Deep venous thrombosis
4. Cellulitis

A: Upper extremity swelling is commonly seen after AVG placement. This is most likely due to trauma from the AVG placement and usually resolves over 3 to 4 weeks. Elevation of the arm (especially at night) may be helpful. However, edema of an extremity following AVG insertion may also be an indication of an occult central venous stenosis or occlusion or, possibly, venous thrombosis, especially if the edema is severe and/or does not resolve over time with arm elevation. In this case, a Duplex ultrasound or venography should be performed. Erythema of a new dialysis AVG is not indicative of infection, providing the redness is limited to the path of the graft.

Q: How do you determine the direction of blood flow in the AVG?

1. Palpate the vibration throughout the graft.
2. Compress the graft and determine where the graft is pulsatile and where it is nonpulsatile.
3. It is not necessary to know the direction of blood flow.

A: It is important to know the direction of blood flow in a graft because that will indicate the correct way to insert the needles for HD. The arterial needle should be placed in the more proximal part of the AVG and the venous needle should be placed more distally in order to prevent recirculation. To determine the direction of blood flow, one must compress the middle of the graft and determine where the graft is pulsatile (i.e., arterial side) and where the blood is nonpulsatile (i.e., venous side).

VIGNETTE 2

19

A 71-year-old white man with diabetic kidney disease and coronary artery disease presents for evaluation of chest pain. A stress test is positive for coronary ischemia, and cardiac catheterization confirms a 90% right coronary artery stenosis and 90% left main disease. The patient subsequently has a coronary artery bypass graft. In recovery in the intensive care unit, he develops worsening of his kidney function.

Before surgery:
Pulse: 80 beats/min; BP: 120/84 mm Hg; respiratory rate: 20 breaths/min; temperature: 37°C; weight: 70 kg

Blood chemistry:
Sodium: 138 mmol/L
Potassium: 4.0 mmol/L
Chloride: 100 mmol/L

Total CO_2: 28 mmol/L
Urea nitrogen: 50 mg/dL (urea: 17.8 mmol/L)
Creatinine: 3.0 mg/dL (265 mcmol/L)
Glucose: 200 mg/dL (11.1 mmol/L)
eGFR: 22 mL/min/1.73 m^2
Urinary albumin to creatinine ratio: 500 mg/g (57 mg/mmol)
Urine output: 40 mL/h

One day after surgery:
Pulse: 110 beats/min; BP: 90/58 mm Hg; respiratory rate: 24 breaths/min; temperature: 37.5°C; weight: 73 kg

Blood chemistry:
Sodium: 136 mmol/L
Potassium: 5.2 mmol/L
Chloride: 100 mmol/L
Total CO_2: 22 mmol/L
Urea nitrogen: 60 mg/dL (urea: 21.4 mmol/L)
Creatinine: 3.0 mg/dL (265 mcmol/L)
Glucose: 160 mg/dL (8.9 mmol/L)
Urine output: 10 mL/h

Physical examination reveals 2+ lower extremity edema, worse from 1+ edema prior to surgery. The patient is still intubated but is oxygenating well. The cardiac index is 1.5 L/min/1.73 m^2, and the pulmonary capillary wedge pressure is 20 mm Hg.

Q: What is the next best step?

1. Catheter insertion for future HD
2. Catheter insertion for immediate HD
3. Intravenous dobutamine
4. Intravenous furosemide
5. Measurement of urinary indices
6. Both 3 and 5

A: Postoperatively, the patient appears to be in cardiogenic shock, characterized by edema and hypotension associated with low cardiac output. Worsening of renal function may be due to decreased renal perfusion and/or ischemic tubular injury. Measurement of urinary indices (fractional excretion of sodium and urea) is indicated to distinguish between prerenal failure and tubular injury.

Treatment should be geared toward hemodynamic stabilization with inotropes. Furosemide could worsen hypotension and is not necessary in view of adequate oxygenation. If oliguria and edema persist despite improvement in cardiovascular status/hypotension, dialysis may be necessary in the near future, but there is no need for HD catheter placement at this time.

References

Beathard GA. Thrombolysis versus surgery for the treatment of thrombosed dialysis access grafts. *J Am Soc Nephrol*. 1995;6:1619–1624.
Blumberg A, Roser HW, Zehnder C, et al. Plasma potassium in patients with terminal renal failure during and after haemodialysis; relationship with dialytic potassium removal and total body potassium. *Nephrol Dial Transplant*. 1997;12(8):1629–1634.

Brescia MJ, Cimino JE, Appel K, et al. Chronic hemodialysis using venipuncture and a surgically created arteriovenous fistula. *N Engl J Med.* 1966;275(20):1089–1092.

Cooper BA, Branley P, Bulfone L, et al; IDEAL Study. A randomized, controlled trial of early versus late initiation of dialysis. *N Engl J Med.* 2010;363(7):609–619.

Dheenan S, Henrich WL. Preventing dialysis hypotension: a comparison of usual protective maneuvers. *Kidney Int.* 2001;59(3):1175–1181.

Eknoyan G, Beck GJ, Cheung AK, et al. Effect of dialysis dose and membrane flux in maintenance hemodialysis. *N Engl J Med.* 2002;347(25):2010–2019.

Flythe JE, Kimmel SE, Brunelli SM. Rapid fluid removal during dialysis is associated with increased cardiovascular morbidity and mortality. *Kidney Int.* 2011;79:250–257.

Hurwich BJ. Fistula steal. *N Engl J Med.* 1970;282(10):570.

Ifudu O, Dawood M, Homel P, et al. Excess morbidity in patients starting uremia therapy without prior care by a nephrologist. *Am J Kidney Dis.* 1996;28:841–845.

Ing TS, Chebrolu SB, Cheng YL, et al. Phosphorus-enriched hemodialysates: formulations and clinical use. *Hemodial Int.* 2003;7(2):148–155.

Jadoul M, Thumma J, Fuller DS, et al. Modifiable practices associated with sudden death among hemodialysis patients in the dialysis outcomes and practice patterns study. *Clin J Am Soc Nephrol.* 2012;7(5):765–774.

Miller RB, Tassistro CR. Peritoneal dialysis. *N Engl J Med.* 1969;281(17):945–949.

Palevsky PM, Zhang JH, O'Connor TZ, et al., VA/NIH Acute Renal Failure Trial Network. Intensity of renal support in critically ill patients with acute kidney injury. *N Engl J Med.* 2008;359(1):7–20.

Rosen SM, O'Connor K, Shaldon S. Haemodialysis dysequilibrium. *Br Med J.* 1964;2(5410):672–675.

Roubicek C, Brunet P, Huiart L, et al. Timing of nephrology referral: influence on mortality and morbidity. *Am J Kidney Dis.* 2000;36(1):35–41.

Roy-Chaudhury P, Kelly BS, Miller MA, et al. Venous intimal hyperplasia in polytetrafluoroethylene dialysis grafts. *Kidney Int.* 2002;59:2325–2334.

Salman L, Beathard, G. Interventional nephrology: physical examination as a tool for surveillance for the hemodialysis arteriovenous access. *Clin J Am Soc Nephol.* 2013;8:1220–1227.

20

The Kidney During Pregnancy

THE PHYSIOLOGY OF PREGNANCY

- There is decreased systemic vascular resistance and increased arterial compliance in early pregnancy. Hence, by the second trimester, blood pressure (BP) normally decreases by 10 mm Hg.
- There is increased sympathetic tone, which increases the heart rate. Increased heart rate in conjunction with decreased afterload results in an increase in cardiac output.
- There is activation of the renin–angiotensin–aldosterone system (RAAS) and subsequent salt and water retention. Activation of the RAAS, combined with increased interstitial compliance, results in plasma volume and interstitial volume expansion, leading to edema and dilutional anemia.
- Human chorionic gonadotropin resets the osmostat so that antidiuretic hormone (ADH) is released at a lower osmotic threshold, resulting in mild hyponatremia (Davison et al., 1988).
- Glomerular filtration rate increases by ~50% by the second and third trimesters. A normal plasma creatinine thus may reflect renal impairment. Plasma urea nitrogen and uric acid concentrations also decrease.
- Protein excretion increases up to ~300 mg/d, which can result in dipstick proteinuria.
- Kidney length increases by 1.5 cm, and kidney volume increases by 30%.
- Compression of the ureters by an enlarging uterus causes hydronephrosis in most pregnant women. This rarely may cause some abdominal pain and urinary obstruction.
- Progesterone causes an increase in ventilation through its action on the respiratory center. This results in respiratory alkalosis and increased renal bicarbonate excretion, leading to a decrease in blood bicarbonate concentration.
- Most vasodilatory conditions, such as sepsis and cirrhosis, are characterized by renal vasoconstriction. However, in pregnancy, relaxin causes release of nitric oxide, which results in renal vasodilation (Conrad et al., 2005).

PREECLAMPSIA AND ECLAMPSIA

- Preeclampsia: Definition—Hypertension (BP > 140/90 mm Hg) after 20 weeks of gestation in a woman with previously normal BP *and* proteinuria >300 mg in a 24-hour urine collection (a spot urine protein to creatinine ratio of >300 mg/g [34 mg/mmol] is also suggestive). Eclampsia is preeclampsia plus seizures.

- Risk factors
  - Nulliparity
  - Positive family history of preeclampsia
  - Chronic hypertension
  - Diabetes mellitus
  - Chronic kidney disease (CKD)
  - Hypercoagulability
  - Prior history of preeclampsia
  - Multiple gestation
  - Teen pregnancy or advanced age
- Pathophysiology
  - There is placental hypoperfusion and ischemia as well as lack of transformation of cytotrophoblasts from an epithelial cell phenotype to an endothelial cell-surface adhesion phenotype (Ferris, 1991). Hence, cytotrophoblasts are unable to fully invade the uterine spiral arteries (De Wolf et al., 1980; Meekins et al., 1994). This invasion is necessary for the uterine arteries to transform from high-resistance vessels to highly compliant blood vessels, which can sustain the fetus.
  - There is an increase in hypoxia-inducible factor 1, which subsequently causes increase in transforming growth factor beta 3 (TGF-β_3) (Caniggia et al., 2000). TGF-β_3 has been shown to block cytotrophoblast invasion of the uterine spiral arteries.
  - Elevated plasma uric acid resulting from tubular reabsorption may cause endothelial dysfunction and promote preeclampsia (Khosla et al., 2005). However, an elevated uric acid level, although suggestive of the diagnosis, has not been useful in predicting outcomes.
  - Endothelial dysfunction leads to impairment of the normal decrease in peripheral vascular resistance in pregnancy. Angiogenic factors, such as soluble fms-like tyrosine kinase-1 (sFlt1), are increased and antagonize vascular endothelial growth factor (VEGF) (Levine et al., 2004; Zhou et al., 2002). VEGF is important in the stabilization of endothelial cells. sFlt1 prevents VEGF from interaction with endothelial receptors and causes endothelial dysfunction. Incubation of normal endothelial cells with serum from preeclamptic patients results in endothelial dysfunction.
- Pathology
  - Light microscopy
    - Glomerular endotheliosis (Spargo et al., 1959)
    - Cellular swelling and vacuolization
    - Loss of the capillary space
    - Thrombi are rare (unlike thrombotic microangiopathy)
  - Electron microscopy
    - Loss of glomerular endothelial fenestrae
    - Podocytes are generally intact

- Prevention
  - Aspirin has modest benefit in high-risk patients (Sibai et al., 1993).
  - Calcium and antioxidants probably of no benefit
- Treatment
  - Prompt delivery is best option.
  - Aggressive lowering of BP can cause fetal distress. Treat only if the BP is >150/100 mm Hg.
  - Magnesium infusion decreases the risk of seizures by 50% and is indicated in severe preeclampsia.

HEMOLYTIC ANEMIA, ELEVATED LIVER ENZYMES, LOW PLATELETS

- Definition: A severe variant of preeclampsia characterized by hemolytic anemia, elevated liver enzymes, and thrombocytopenia. It is associated with adverse outcomes such as placental abruption, acute kidney injury (AKI), disseminated intravascular coagulation (DIC), pulmonary edema, and hepatic hemorrhage.
- Prognosis
  - The outcome is generally good, with complete recovery postpartum, but there may be substantial acute morbidity. Chronic hypertension, microalbuminuria, cardiovascular disease, and cerebrovascular disease develop in 20% of patients over the long term.
  - Offspring may have low nephron number and be more likely to develop hypertension, diabetes mellitus, CKD, and cardiovascular disease.
  - There is a risk of recurrence with subsequent pregnancies.
- Hemolytic anemia, elevated liver enzymes, low platelets (HELLP) is difficult to distinguish from hemolytic uremic syndrome/thrombotic thrombocytopenic purpura (HUS/TTP) (see Chapter 16). A subtle distinction is that HELLP is characterized by proteinuria and hypertension prior to the development of hemolysis, thrombocytopenia, and liver injury, whereas HUS/TTP is characterized by renal failure, hemolytic anemia, and thrombocytopenia but not liver injury or coagulopathy (which can be seen with severe HELLP). HUS/TTP, but not HELLP, will benefit from plasma exchange.

CHRONIC HYPERTENSION AND GESTATIONAL HYPERTENSION

- Definition: Chronic hypertension is elevated BP that is detected before 20 weeks of gestation. Gestational hypertension is hypertension that is detected after 20 weeks of gestation but not associated with proteinuria (as opposed to preeclampsia).
- Secondary causes: Renal artery stenosis, primary hyperaldosteronism, and pheochromocytoma should be considered.
- Treatment

- Treatment of mild or moderate hypertension may impair fetal growth.
- Treatment indicated only if patient has evidence of end-organ damage or if the BP is >150/100 mm Hg.
  - Methyldopa is safe and often used.
  - Beta-blockers are usable with the exception of atenolol, which has been shown to cause intrauterine growth retardation.
  - Calcium channel blockers have also been used without adverse effects.
  - Diuretics are generally not recommended owing to concerns about decreasing placental perfusion. They may be used if the patient develops pulmonary edema.
  - Angiotensin-converting enzyme inhibitors (ACE-Is) and angiotensin-receptor blockers (ARBs) are teratogenic and are contraindicated in pregnancy.
- Intravenous drugs
  - Labetalol is effective and safe unless contraindicated.
  - Hydralazine should be used with caution owing to risk of hypotension, oliguria, placental abruption, and low APGAR scores.
  - Nitroprusside can cause fetal cyanide poisoning.
- Breastfeeding
  - Methyldopa is safe.
  - Labetalol is preferred to atenolol and metoprolol.
  - Diuretics decrease breast milk production.
  - ACE-Is are not secreted in breast milk and may be used.

ACUTE TUBULAR INJURY AND BILATERAL CORTICAL NECROSIS

- Definition: Acute tubular injury in pregnancy is generally caused by volume depletion as a result of hyperemesis gravidarum or uterine hemorrhage. Bilateral cortical necrosis is a rare and irreversible form of kidney injury associated with septic abortion or placental abruption.
- Symptoms: There may be oliguria, anuria, hematuria, and flank pain.
- Extrarenal findings such as adult respiratory distress syndrome and DIC may be present.
- Diagnosis: Acute tubular injury is diagnosed using standard criteria (see Chapter 9). Cortical necrosis is suggested by computed tomography (CT) demonstration of hypodensities in the renal cortex, which may be patchy or may involve the entire renal cortex.
- Treatment: Dialysis is often needed.

ACUTE FATTY LIVER OF PREGNANCY

Acute fatty liver of pregnancy (AFLP) is an often fatal condition characterized by liver failure characterized by elevated transaminases and hyperbilirubinemia. There may also be hyperammonemia and hypoglycemia. Preeclampsia is present in 50% of patients. Renal failure is usually mild. Treatment is supportive, and prompt delivery is prudent.

NEPHROLITHIASIS

- Pathophysiology: Pregnancy is characterized by increased vitamin D production, which results in intestinal calcium absorption and hypercalciuria (Gertner et al., 1986). Stones in pregnancy are primarily calcium oxalate and calcium phosphate.
- Diagnosis:
  - Ultrasound is the best method to diagnose stones in pregnancy.
  - 24-Hour urine studies must be done after delivery.
- Treatment:
  - Hydration, analgesia, antiemetic, antibiotics for urinary tract infection (UTI) (see below)
  - Do not use thiazides or allopurinol
  - Urinary stent is an option. Lithotripsy is contraindicated.

URINARY TRACT INFECTION

Asymptomatic bacteriuria can lead to pyelonephritis, shock, DIC, renal failure, and premature delivery and should be treated with antibiotics; avoid trimethoprim/sulfamethoxazole (TMP/SMX) (due to trimethoprim's potential effect on folic acid metabolism), tetracyclines, or quinolones. Screening for UTI is recommended only if the patient has a history of recurrent UTIs (Smaill, 2001).

DIABETES INSIPIDUS

Pregnant patients make vasopressinase, which degrades ADH. If the diabetes insipidus needs to be treated, desmopressin, which is a form of vasopressin that is not destroyed by vasopressinase, may be used.

CHRONIC KIDNEY DISEASE

- Risks: CKD is associated with preterm labor, intrauterine growth retardation, preeclampsia, and increased fetal and maternal mortality.
- Prognosis:
  - Prognosis for the pregnancy is good if the kidney injury is mild, BP is controlled, and there is no proteinuria.
  - If plasma creatinine is >2.5 mg/dL (221 mcmol/L), 70% of pregnancies will be preterm and 40% will be associated with preeclampsia (Jones & Hayslett, 1996).

DIABETIC KIDNEY DISEASE

- Patients with gestational diabetes have double the risk of albuminuria and preeclampsia (Ekbom, 1999).
- There is no clear evidence that pregnancy hastens progression of diabetic kidney disease.
- Therapy is limited because ACE-I/ARB cannot be used.

SYSTEMIC LUPUS ERYTHEMATOSUS

- Lupus nephritis is associated with higher risk of preterm delivery, intrauterine growth retardation, abortions, and preeclampsia.
- Lupus flare versus preeclampsia may be hard to distinguish. Hypocomplementemia and hematuria suggest active lupus nephritis (Buyon et al., 1992).
- Treatment:
  - Control the lupus before pregnancy.
  - Steroids and azathioprine may extend the pregnancy.

END-STAGE KIDNEY DISEASE

- Uremia impairs fertility by altering the hypothalamic–pituitary–gonadal axis (Lim et al., 1978).
- Prognosis: The majority of the fetuses are born premature, and there is significant fetal morbidity and mortality (Chao et al., 2002).
- Treatment:
  - Dialysis 20 hours or more weekly improves neonatal outcomes and increases gestation (Hou, 2002).
  - No ACE-I/ARB
  - Adjust erythropoietin to achieve a hemoglobin of 10 to 11 g/L. High hematocrit is associated with adverse fetal outcomes.

KIDNEY TRANSPLANTATION

- Kidney transplantation causes a return to fertility ~6 months after the kidney transplant.
- Prognosis:
  - One-fifth of pregnancies in transplanted patients end in the first trimester either because of miscarriage or elective termination. The remainder of the pregnancies usually produces preterm infants with low birth weight (Rizzoni et al., 1992). However, there is no increased risk of birth defects.
  - One-third of pregnant patients with kidney transplants will develop preeclampsia.
  - If allograft function is normal and BP is controlled, the rate of rejection is the same as in renal transplant patients who are not pregnant.
  - If CKD is present, there is a risk of low birth weight fetus and preeclampsia, but no clear evidence of increased progression of CKD.
- Prevention—Women are advised to wait at least 1 year (ideally 2 years) after the transplant before getting pregnant.
- Treatment
  - Immunosuppression
    - Low-dose cyclosporine or low-dose tacrolimus is acceptable.
    - Steroids can be continued with stress doses peripartum.
    - Avoid mycophenolate and sirolimus owing to teratogenicity.

A 25-year-old woman with diabetic kidney disease presents for follow-up because she is pregnant. She is in her first trimester at 8 weeks of gestation. Her BP is 145/90 mm Hg. She denies fever or dysuria, but her primary care physician tells her that her urine shows bacteria. Physical examination is negative. Urinalysis is leukocyte esterase and nitrite positive, the WBC count is 10/hpf, and there is moderate bacteriuria. The plasma creatinine is 0.5 mg/dL (44.2 mcmol/L). Urinary albumin to creatinine ratio is 100 mg/g (11.3 mg/mmol).

Q: Which of the following treatments is appropriate?

1. Methyldopa
2. Labetalol
3. Cephalexin
4. TMP/SMX
5. Ciprofloxacin

A: This patient has chronic hypertension (as defined by elevated BP prior to the 20th week of pregnancy). Decreasing the BP below 150/100 mm Hg is associated with fetal harm. Therefore, treatment for BP is undertaken only if BP is >150/100 mm Hg or if there is end-organ damage. Asymptomatic bacteriuria is associated with a risk of pyelonephritis, shock, DIC, AKI, and premature delivery and, therefore, should be treated in pregnancy. Cephalosporins are used in pregnancy to treat infections and are safe; TMP/SMX and quinolones should be avoided.

A 26-year-old woman gravida 1 para 0 with no medical history presents at 32 weeks of pregnancy for evaluation of proteinuria and hypertension. She states that her BP was previously normal but, for the past 2 weeks, has been running around 160/105 mm Hg. She denies chest pain, headaches, visual changes, hematuria, dysuria, or abdominal pain. She has had no seizures. Physical examination is significant for a BP of 155/95 mm Hg, a gravid abdomen, and 1+ bilateral leg edema. Urinalysis shows 2+ protein but is otherwise unremarkable, with no hematuria or casts seen. Urinary albumin to creatinine ratio is 600 mg/g (68 mg/mmol). Hemoglobin and hematocrit are 10 g/dL (100 g/L) and 30%, respectively, and the platelet count is 300,000/mm^3. Liver function tests are normal. The plasma creatinine is 0.5 mg/dL (44.2 mcmol/L).

Q: Which of the following is the correct diagnosis?

1. Chronic hypertension
2. Acute glomerulonephritis
3. Preeclampsia
4. Eclampsia

A: The history and physical and laboratory findings are consistent with preeclampsia, which is diagnosed as hypertension (BP > 140/90 mm Hg) after 20 weeks of gestation in a woman with previously normal BP coupled with proteinuria of >300 mg in 24 hours. Eclampsia is preeclampsia plus seizures. This patient does not have seizures. Chronic hypertension is unlikely by the history of normal BP earlier in the pregnancy and would not cause proteinuria. Acute glomerulonephritis could cause proteinuria and hypertension but is excluded by normal renal function and the absence of hematuria or cellular casts in the urine.

References

Buyon JP, Tamerius J, Ordorica S, et al. Activation of the alternative complement pathway accompanies disease flares in systemic lupus erythematosus during pregnancy. *Arthritis Rheum.* 1992;35(1):55–61.

Caniggia I, Mostachfi H, Winter J, et al. Hypoxia-inducible factor-1 mediates the biological effects of oxygen on human trophoblast differentiation through TGFβ$_3$. *J Clin Invest.* 2000;105(5):577–587.

Chao AS, Huang JY, Lien R, et al. Pregnancy in women who undergo long-term hemodialysis. *Am J Obstet Gynecol.* 2002;187(1):152–156.

Conrad KP, Jeyabalan A, Danielson LA, et al. Role of relaxin in maternal renal vasodilation of pregnancy. *Ann N Y Acad Sci.* 2005;1041:147–154.

Davison JM, Shiells EA, Philips PR, et al. Serial evaluation of vasopressin release and thirst in human pregnancy. Role of human chorionic gonadotrophin in the osmoregulatory changes of gestation. *J Clin Invest.* 1988;81(3):798–806.

De Wolf F, De Wolf-Peeters C, Brosens I, et al. The human placental bed: electron microscopic study of trophoblastic invasion of spiral arteries. *Am J Obstet Gynecol.* 1980;137(1):58–70.

Ekbom P. Pre-pregnancy microalbuminuria predicts pre-eclampsia in insulin-dependent diabetes mellitus. Copenhagen Pre-eclampsia in Diabetic Pregnancy Study Group. *Lancet.* 1999;353(9150):377.

Ferris TF. Pregnancy, preeclampsia, and the endothelial cell. *N Engl J Med.* 1991; 325(20):1439–1440.

Gertner JM, Coustan DR, Kliger AS, et al. Pregnancy as a state of physiologic absorptive hypercalciuria. *Am J Med.* 1986;81(3):451–456.

Hou S. Modification of dialysis regimens for pregnancy. *Int J Artif Organs.* 2002; 25(9):823–826.

Jones DC, Hayslett JP. Outcome of pregnancy in women with moderate or severe renal insufficiency. *N Engl J Med.* 1996;335(4):226–232.

Khosla UM, Zharikov S, Finch JL, et al. Hyperuricemia induces endothelial dysfunction. *Kidney Int.* 2005;67(5):1739–1742.

Levine RJ, Maynard SE, Qian C, et al. Circulating angiogenic factors and the risk of preeclampsia. *N Engl J Med*. 2004;350(7):672–683.

Lim VS, Kathpalia SC, Henriquez C. Endocrine abnormalities associated with chronic renal failure. *Med Clin North Am*. 1978;62(6):1341–1361.

Meekins JW, Pijnenborg R, Hanssens M, et al. A study of placental bed spiral arteries and trophoblast invasion in normal and severe pre-eclamptic pregnancies. *Br J Obstet Gynaecol*. 1994;101(8):669–674.

Rizzoni G, Ehrich JH, Broyer M, et al. Successful pregnancies in women on renal replacement therapy: report from the EDTA Registry. *Nephrol Dial Transplant*. 1992;7(4):279–287.

Sibai BM, Caritis SN, Thom E, et al. Prevention of preeclampsia with low-dose aspirin in healthy, nulliparous pregnant women. The National Institute of Child Health and Human Development Network of Maternal-Fetal Medicine Units. *N Engl J Med*. 1993;329(17):1213–1218.

Smaill F. Antibiotics for asymptomatic bacteriuria in pregnancy. *Cochrane Database Syst Rev*. 2001;(2):CD000490.

Spargo BH, McCartney C, Winemiller R. Glomerular capillary endotheliosis in toxemia of pregnancy. *Arch Pathol*. 1959;13:593–599.

Zhou Y, McMaster M, Woo K, et al. Vascular endothelial growth factor ligands and preeclampsia and hemolysis, elevated liver enzymes, and low platelets syndrome. *Am J Pathol*. 2002;160(4):1405–1423.

INDEX

Note: Page numbers followed by *f* indicate figures; those followed by *t* indicate tables.